Surgical Foundations: Essentials of Thoracic Surgery

Surgical Foundations: Essentials of Thoracic Surgery

Larry R. Kaiser, M.D.
The John Rhea Barton Professor and Chairman
Department of Surgery
University of Pennsylvania School of Medicine
Philadelphia, Pennsylvania

Sunil Singhal, M.D.
Chief Resident
Department of Surgery
The Johns Hopkins University School of Medicine
Baltimore, Maryland

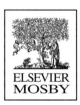

ELSEVIER
MOSBY

ELSEVIER
MOSBY

The Curtis Center
170 S Independence Mall W 300 E
Philadelphia, Pennsylvania 19106

SURGICAL FOUNDATIONS: ESSENTIALS OF THORACIC SURGERY ISBN 0-8151-2613-1

NOTICE

Surgery is an ever-changing field. Standard safety precautions must be followed, but as new research and clinical experience broaden our knowledge, changes in treatment and drug therapy may become necessary or appropriate. Readers are advised to check the most current product information provided by the manufacturer of each drug to be administered to verify the recommended dose, the method and duration of administration, and contraindications. It is the responsibility of the treating physician, relying on experience and knowledge of the patient, to determine dosages and the best treatment for the patient. Neither the publisher nor the editors assume any liability for any injury and/or damage to persons or property arising from this publication.

Library of Congress Cataloging-in-Publication Data

Kaiser, Larry R.
  Surgical foundations: essentials of thoracic surgery/Larry R. Kaiser, Sunil Singhal.—1st ed.
    p.   ; cm.
  ISBN 0-8151-2613-1
    1. Chest—Surgery.   I. Title: Essentials of thoracic surgery.   II. Singhal, Sunil.   III. Title.
    [DNLM: 1. Thoracic Survery—methods.   WF 980 K13s 2004]

RD536.K373 2004
617.5′4059—dc22   2003066602

Acquisitions Editor: Joe Rusko
Developmental Editor: Arlene Chappelle
Publishing Services Manager: Joan Sinclair
Project Manager: Mary Stermel

Printed in the United States of America

Last digit is the print number: 9 8 7 6 5 4 3 2 1

Dedication

To my wife Sanchita for her tremendous love. To my parents for
their constant support, and to my mentor Dr. Larry Kaiser
for his unending guidance.

– S.S

To Lindy, who makes it all worthwhile

– L.R.K

Preface

General thoracic surgery has evolved rapidly over the last 50 years. Only 100 years ago von Mikulicz, Brauer, and Sauerbruch among others developed methods of controlling ventilation during chest surgery when the open chest causes loss of the negative intrathoracic pressure. Another sixty years would pass, however, before thoracic surgery became a true specialty and encompassed more than simply the management of tuberculosis and bronchiectasis. Today, chest diseases affect over 2 million people in the United States alone. Thoracic surgery has become an independent entity with a wide range of procedures and topics.

Several major textbooks of thoracic surgery are now available, many on their fifth and sixth editions, and most with at least two volumes. *Surgical Foundations: Essentials of Thoracic Surgery* is one of the first textbooks that attempts to capture the true "essentials" of general thoracic surgery in an easy to read, abridged format. The fact that it is written by two authors and not by numerous contributors allows for a single very readable and approachable style. It is possible to sit and read this book cover to cover. This is not a reference text and we avoid delving into esoteric topics that can be found in the larger, more comprehensive sources. The content and presentation were designed to appeal to a diverse audience. This book should be particularly useful to medical students, surgical residents, and general surgeons who wish to acquire additional knowledge in thoracic surgery.

This book is separated into three convenient sections. The first section reviews the basic knowledge necessary for any student of thoracic surgery. The first few chapters review chest anatomy and physiology, the perioperative care of patients with chest disorders, and diagnostic and surgical procedures that relate to the chest. The second section covers the two most common chest problems encountered by the thoracic surgeon – lung cancer and emphysematous lung disease. The final section surveys the non-parenchymal thoracic diseases such as chest wall disorders, tracheal and diaphragmatic injuries, pleural diseases, and mediastinal masses.

We have proposed at the beginning of each chapter a list of key topics that should focus the reader to the most important topics in each category. At the end of each chapter, carefully selected references are provided to guide further investigation, should that be desired. Within each chapter, we have utilized carefully designed tables and figures that can be reviewed to reinforce the chapter topics.

We thank our editor at Elsevier Science, Joe Rusko, for his unflagging effort and patience during the process of writing this book. His steady support and prompt assistance has made writing this textbook a pleasure.

Contents

Non-Pulmonary Thoracic Diseases

Color Insert

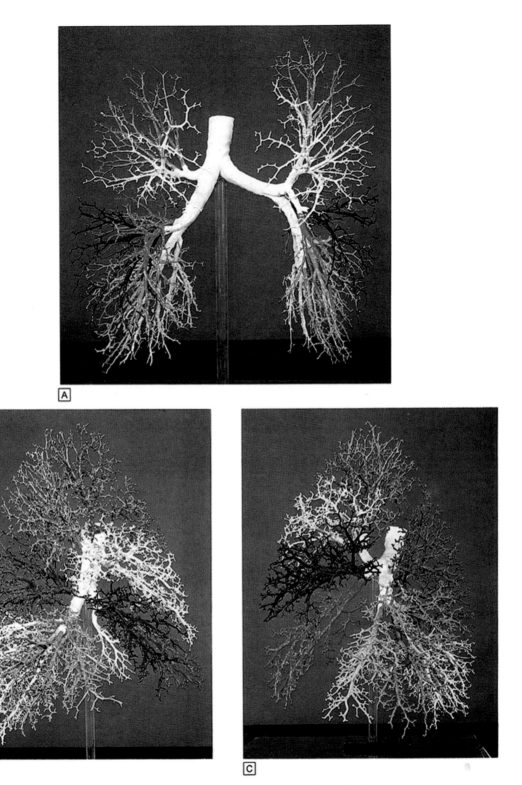

Plate 1. A, A resin corrosion cast of the adult human lower trachea and bronchial tree photographed from the anterior aspect. The segmental bronchi and their main branches have been colored: brown = apical; gray/blue = posterior; pink = anterior; dark blue = lateral (middle lobe) and superior lingular; red = medial (middle lobe) and inferior lingular; dark green = superior (apical) of inferior lobe; yellow = medial basal; orange = anterior basal; blue = lateral basal; light green = posterior basal. **B**, Corrosion cast of the bronchial tree of the right lung, color coded as in **A** to indicate the territories supplied by different segmental bronchi. **C**, Corrosion cast of the bronchial tree of the left lung, color coded as in **A**. Note that in this and other preparations shown in this figure many of the finer bronchial branches have been trimmed away to reveal the larger bronchi. (From Williams PL, *et al. Gray's anatomy*, 38th ed. New York: Churchill Livingstone, 1995:1660.)

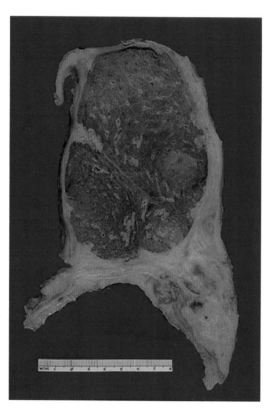

Plate 2. Gross picture of malignant mesothelioma encasing a lung.

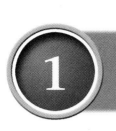

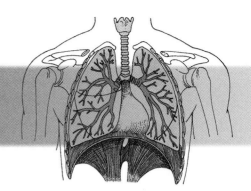

Anatomy

Anatomy: Key Points

- Know the structural components of the thoracic chest wall
- Understand the role of the diaphragm and accessory muscles in respiration
- Describe the basic anatomical units of the left and right lungs and their hilar relationships to the mediastinal structures
- Trace the passage of air from the upper airways to the alveoli and describe the structural changes that take place along this path
- Name the chief organs and structures in the mediastinum

The thorax is the area of the body between the neck and abdomen. The limits of the thorax are defined by the thoracic wall and the diaphragm. Superiorly, the thorax communicates with the neck through the thoracic inlet. The opening is bounded posteriorly by the first thoracic (T1) vertebra, laterally by the medial borders of the first rib and anteriorly by the manubrium. The opening is elliptical and broader in the direction along the shoulder girdle. It slopes downward and forward, so that the anterior part of the opening is lower than the poste-rior. The anteroposterior diameter is approximately 5 cm and transverse diameter 10 cm (Figure 1–1).

Inferiorly, the thorax is separated from the abdomen by the diaphragm. The opening is bounded posteriorly by the 12th thoracic (T12) vertebra, laterally by the curving costal margin, and anteriorly by the xiphoid process. The anterior chest is limited by the sternum and costal cartilages, which are flattened to slightly convex and angle forward.

The thorax itself can be divided between the lungs and the mediastinum. The mediastinum

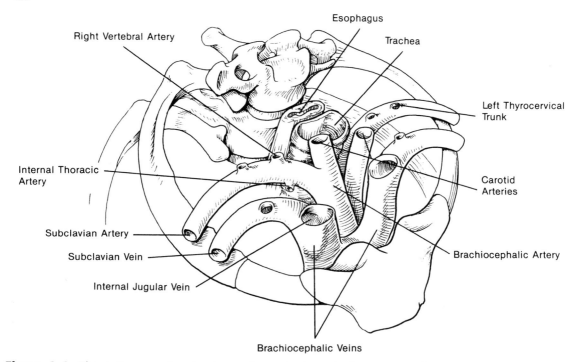

Figure 1–1. The major vascular structures that exit through the superior thoracic aperture are shown in relation to the bony skeleton, the trachea, and the esophagus. Note that the great veins are anterior to the arteries, the arteries are between the great veins and the trachea, and the esophagus lies between the trachea and the spinal column. The clavicles have been removed from this picture for clarity. (From Pearson FG, Cooper JD, Deslauriers J, *et al. Thoracic surgery*, 2nd ed. New York: Churchill Livingstone, 2002:1333.)

can be subdivided into the superior, anterior, middle, and posterior mediastinum. The lungs are separated from the mediastinum by the pleural reflections. The mediastinum lies between the right and left pleura in and near the medial sagittal plane of the chest. It extends from the sternum anteriorly to the vertebral column posteriorly and contains all the major thoracic organs except the lungs.

Surface Anatomy

Anterior and midline sits the firm, palpable surface of the sternum. The most superior aspect of the sternum is the sternal notch. The sternocleidomastoid muscle attaches to the lateral aspects of the superior border of the sternum. Slightly inferior along the sternum is the angle of Louis or sternal angle at the junction of the manubrium and the body. The sternum ends in the xiphoid process, which can be felt as a soft point at the inferior end of the sternum (Figure 1–2).

Lateral to the sternum the costal margins can be palpated, yet the majority of this space is occupied by the pectoralis muscles. The intercostal spaces can be palpated, the second and third ribs spaces are the widest, the next two are somewhat narrower, and the remainder, with the exception of the last two, are relatively narrow. The inferior boundary of the anterior thorax is formed by the xiphoid process, the cartilages of the seventh, eighth, ninth, and tenth ribs, and the ends of the cartilages of the eleventh and twelfth ribs. On either side of the thorax from the axilla downward, the flattened external surfaces of the ribs can be located (Figure 1–3). Although covered by muscles, all the ribs except the first can be palpated along the ventral and lateral aspects of the thorax. The first rib is almost completely covered by the clavicle. In the back, the angles of the ribs lie on an oblique line on either side of the spinous processes of the vertebrae.

There is a clinically important area bounded superiorly by the inferior border of trapezius, inferiorly by the superior border of latissimus dorsi, and laterally by the vertebral border of the scapula. When the scapula is drawn laterally by folding the arms across the chest and

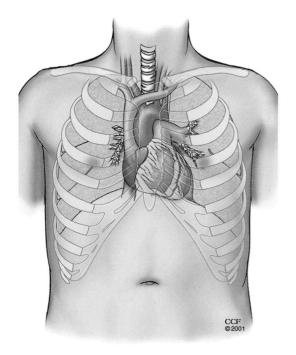

Figure 1–2. Anterior projection of major mediastinal structures through the chest wall. (© Cleveland Clinic Foundation, 2001.)

Thoracic Wall

The skeleton of the thorax is an osseocartilaginous cage, conical in shape, narrow cranially and broader caudally, longer posteriorly than anteriorly. The thoracic wall is formed by the vertebral column posteriorly, the ribs and intercostals muscles laterally, and the sternum and costal cartilages anteriorly. The thoracic portion of the vertebral column is concave forward, composed of 12 vertebrae.

The sternum is a long, flat bone, on average 17 cm long, forming the medial aspect of the anterior wall of the thorax. The sternum has three parts – the manubrium, the body, and the xiphoid process. The manubrium lies at the level of the T3–4 vertebrae and articulates with the clavicles, the first rib, and the superior portion of the second costal cartilages. The sternal body articulates with the third through seventh costal cartilages. The sternal angle or angle of Louis is formed by the articulation of the manubrium to the sternum. This is used as a reference point for the articulation with the second costal cartilage and is at the level of T4–5. Finally, the xiphoid process is the most caudal portion of the sternum.

There are 12 pairs of ribs. They are elastic arches of bone that form a large part of the thoracic skeleton. The first seven originate from the vertebral column and attach to the sternum

the trunk is bent forward, parts of the sixth and seventh ribs and the interspace between them become subcutaneous and available for auscultation. The space is known as the auscultation triangle.

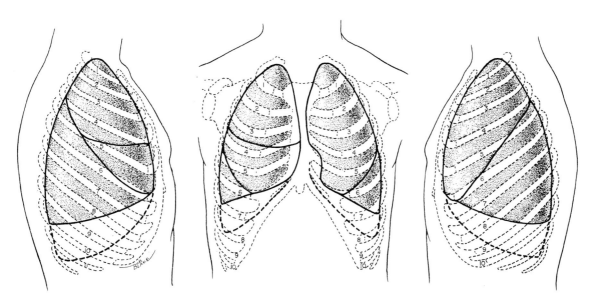

Figure 1–3. The relationships of the pleural reflections and the lobes of the lung to the ribs. The topographic anatomy and the relationships of the fissures of the lobes to ribs in inspiration and expiration are important in evaluation of the routine posteroanterior and lateral chest film. (From Townsend CM Jr. *Sabiston Textbook of surgery: The biological basis of modern surgical practice*, 16th ed. Philadelphia: WB Saunders, 2001:1206.)

via the costal cartilages. The remaining five are false ribs: the first three have their cartilages attached to the cartilage of the superior rib (vertebrochondral). The last two ribs are free anteriorly and are named floating ribs. The ribs vary in their direction: the upper ones are less oblique than the lower; the obliquity reaches its maximum at the ninth rib and gradually decreases to the 12th (Figure 1–4).

Each rib has two ends, a vertebral and a sternal articulation, and an intervening portion called the body (Figure 1–5). Its anterior surface is flat and smooth. The posterior surface is rough for the attachment of the ligament of the neck and perforated by numerous foramina. On the superior border there is a rough crest for the attachment of the anterior costotransverse ligament while the inferior border is rounded and smooth. On the posterior surface at the junction of the neck and body and closer to the inferior border is the tubercle.

The tubercle has an articular and a nonarticular aspect. The articular portion, the inferior

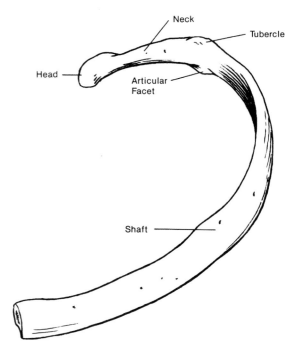

Figure 1–5. The anatomy of a rib. The head abuts on the vertebral body. The articular facet in the region of the tubercle articulates with the transverse process on the vertebral body below. The neck, after it extends to the region of the tubercle and the facet, blends with the elongated shaft. The anterior surface abuts on the corresponding costal cartilage. (From Pearson FG, Cooper JD, Deslauriers J, *et al. Thoracic surgery*, 2nd ed. New York: Churchill Livingstone, 2002:1326.)

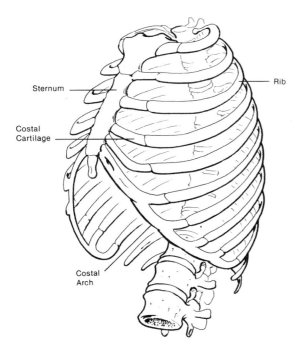

Figure 1–4. The entire bony and cartilaginous thorax is depicted in this left anterior oblique projection. The costal cartilages articulate with the sternum and the individual ribs. In the lower aspects of the costal margin, individual costal cartilages blend. Note that the 11th and 12th ribs are completely free of attachment in any way to the sternum. The spine forms the posterior articular aspects for each of the ribs. (From Pearson FG, Cooper JD, Deslauriers J, *et al. Thoracic surgery*, 2nd ed. New York: Churchill Livingstone, 2002:1327.)

and more medial of the two, has a small, oval surface for articulation with the end of the transverse process of the lower of the two vertebrae to which the head is connected (Figure 1–6). The nonarticular portion has prominences for attachments to the ligaments to the tubercle. The tubercle is much more pronounced in the superior than in the inferior ribs.

The body is thin and flat, with two surfaces (external and internal) and two borders (superior and inferior). The external surface is convex and smooth. Anterior to the tubercle, directed downward and laterally, is the angle for the iliocostal tendon attachment. The internal surface is concave, smooth, and directed superiorly. Between the inferior border is the costal groove for the intercostal vessels and nerve. The superior edge of the groove is rounded and acts as the attachment for the internal intercostal muscle. The inferior edge corresponds to the inferior margin of the rib and is the attachment for the external intercostal muscle. Within the groove are small foramina for nutrient vessels that transverse the shaft obliquely.

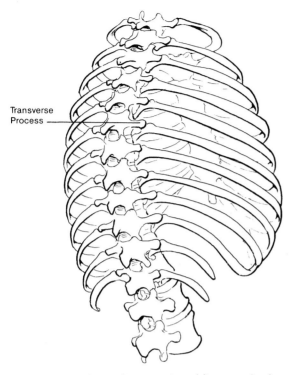

Transverse
Process

Figure 1–6. This right posterior oblique projection shows the relationship of each individual rib to the vertebral bodies and their transverse processes. Note that the head of each rib articulates with the vertebral bodies, whereas the articular processes of each rib articulate with the transverse processes. (From Pearson FG, Cooper JD, Deslauriers J, *et al. Thoracic surgery*, 2nd ed. New York: Churchill Livingstone, 2002:1327.)

The first rib is important because of its complex relationship with the lower nerves of the brachial plexus, subclavian artery, and subclavian vein. The scalenus anterior muscle attaches to the anterior inner border of the first rib. Broad and flat, the first rib is the most curved and usually the shortest of all the ribs. The head is small, rounded, and possesses only a single articular facet for articulation with the body of T1. The neck is narrow and rounded. The tubercle, thick and prominent, is on the outer border. There is no angle, but at the tubercle the rib is slightly bent upward so that the head of the bone angles inferiorly. The superior surface of the body is marked by two shallow grooves separated from each other by a slight ridge called the scalene tubercle for the attachment of the anterior scalene muscle. The anterior groove transmits the subclavian vein. The posterior groove holds the subclavian artery and the lowest trunk of the brachial plexus. Behind the posterior groove is a rough area for the attachment of the middle scalene muscle. The outer border is convex, thick, and rounded, and on its posterior aspect there is an attachment for part of the serratus anterior muscle.

The second rib is much longer than the first but has a very similar curvature. The angle is slight and situated close to the tubercle. The body is not flattened horizontally like the first rib. Its external surface is convex and slants superiorly. Near the middle of it is the origin for the serratus anterior. Behind and above this is the attachment for the scalenus posterior. The internal surface, smooth and concave, is angled inferiorly and inward; on its posterior part there is a short costal groove.

The costal cartilages are pieces of hyaline cartilage that connect ribs one through seven to the lateral edge of the sternum and are responsible for the elasticity of the thoracic cage. The first seven pairs are connected with the sternum. The next three each articulate with the inferior border of the cartilage of the preceding rib. The last two ribs have pointed extremities which terminate in the abdominal wall. Like the ribs, the costal cartilages vary in their length, breadth, and direction. They increase in length from the first to the seventh then gradually decrease to the 12th. Their width, as well as that of the intervals between them, decreases from the first to the last. They are broad at their rib attachments and taper toward their sternal insertion. They also vary in direction: the first descends a little, the second is horizontal, the third ascends slightly, while the others are angular, following the course of the ribs for a short distance and then ascending to the sternum or preceding cartilage. Each costal cartilage has two surfaces, two borders, and two extremities. The 10th rib has only a single articular facet on its head. Ribs 11 and 12 terminate in the abdominal musculature without anterior attachments. The 11th and 12th ribs each have a single large articular facet on the head. They have no necks or tubercles and are pointed at their anterior ends. The 11th rib has a slight angle and a shallow costal groove. The 12th rib is much shorter than the 11th and its head is angled inferiorly. Sometimes the 12th rib is shorter than the first.

Several muscles define the chest wall (Figure 1–7). The pectoralis major muscle extends bilaterally from the clavicle, sternum, and costal origins towards the axilla and attaches to the lateral aspect of the intertubercular sulcus of the humerus. The pectoralis major

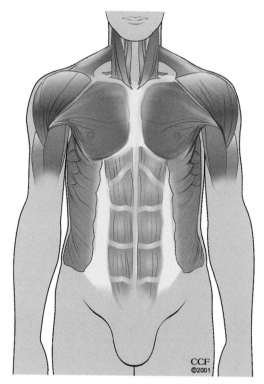

Figure 1–7. Musculoskeletal structures encountered with anterior approaches. Important muscle groups include sternocleidomastoid, pectoralis major, serratus anterior, and rectus abdominis. (© Cleveland Clinic Foundation, 2001.)

muscle is innervated by the medial and lateral pectoral nerves from the brachial plexus. These muscles are responsible for adducting and rotating the arm medially and raising and depressing the upper extremity.

The pectoralis muscle lies deep to the pectoralis minor muscle (Figure 1–8). Originating from the second to the fifth ribs, they converge upward bilaterally and attach to the coracoid process of the scapula. They are similarly supplied by the medial and lateral pectoral nerves. These muscles are active in lowering and rotating the shoulder downward.

There are three groups of intercostal muscles – the external intercostals, internal intercostals, and the transversus thoracis muscle. The intercostals are two thin planes of muscular and tendinous fibers occupying each of the intercostal spaces. In each intercostal space thin layers of fascia cover the outer surface of the external intercostal muscles and the inner intercostal muscle. There are 11 external intercostal muscles on each side. Each arises from the inferior border of a rib and inserts into the

superior border of the inferior rib. In the two lower spaces they extend to the ends of the cartilage and in the upper two or three spaces they do not reach the ends of the ribs. They are thicker than the internal intercostal muscles and their fibers are directed obliquely downward and laterally on the posterior thorax, and downward, forward, and medially on the front.

There are 11 internal intercostal muscles on each side (Figure 1–9). They originate anteriorly at the sternum, in the interspaces between the cartilages of the true ribs and at the anterior extremities of the cartilages of the false ribs. The internal intercostal muscles extend backward as far as the angles of the ribs, where they continue on to the vertebral column by a thin aponeurosis, the posterior intercostal membranes. Each arises from the ridge on the inner surface of a rib, as well as from the corresponding costal cartilage, and inserts into the superior border of the inferior rib. Their fibers are directed obliquely but pass in a direction opposite to those of the external intercostal muscles. The subcostal muscles consist of muscle fibers and an aponeurosis, which is well developed in the lower thorax. Their fibers run in the same direction as the internal intercostal muscles.

The transversus thoracis muscle is a thin plane of muscular and tendinous fibers situated along the inner surface of the anterior wall of the chest (Figure 1–10). It arises on either side from the inferior third of the posterior surface of the body of the sternum, from the posterior surface of the xiphoid process, and from the sternal ends of the costal cartilages of the inferior three or four true ribs. Its fibers diverge upward and laterally to be inserted by slips into the inferior borders and inner surfaces of the costal cartilages of the second through sixth ribs. The lowest fibers run horizontally and are continuous with the transverse abdominal muscles. The intermediate muscle fibers are oblique, while the highest are vertical. This muscle varies in its attachments, not only in different people but on opposite sides of the same individual.

The serratus anterior muscle can be visualized along the anterolateral aspects of the thoracic cage. Originating from the upper eight ribs, it attaches to the anterior surface along the medial border of the scapula. These muscles are supplied by the long thoracic nerve and are responsible for adduction and elevation of the arms above the horizontal position.

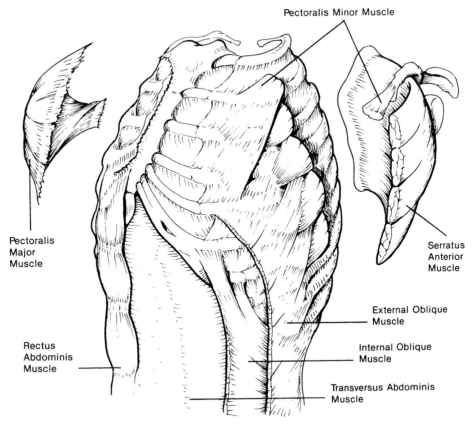

Pectoralis Minor Muscle

Pectoralis
Major
Muscle

Serratus
Anterior
Muscle

External Oblique
Muscle

Rectus
Abdominis
Muscle

Internal Oblique
Muscle

Transversus Abdominis
Muscle

Figure 1–8. The relationship of the major anterior muscles of the pectoral girdle is shown in this left anterior oblique projection. On the right side the pectoralis major muscle is shown elevated away from the chest wall. Its cut origins along the medial aspect of the sternum and costal cartilage on the right side are apparent. The pectoralis major and serratus anterior have been transected on the left side and are placed away from the chest wall for clarity. (From Pearson FG, Cooper JD, Deslauriers J, *et al. Thoracic surgery*, 2nd ed. New York: Churchill Livingstone, 2002:1331.)

The serratus posterior superior muscle is flat and thin and arises from the inferior cervical and upper thoracic spines. Its fibers pass downward and laterally and are inserted into the upper ribs. It elevates the ribs and acts as an inspiratory muscle. The serratus posterior inferior muscle is a thin flat muscle that comes from the superior lumbar and lower thoracic spines. It passes superiorly and laterally and inserts into the inferior ribs. It helps depress the ribs and acts as an expiratory muscle. The thin aponeurosis of origin is blended with the lumbodorsal fascia and aponeurosis of the latissimus dorsi.

There are 12 levator costarum muscle pairs, triangular in shape, that arise from the tip of the transverse process of the vertebrae and help raise the inferior ribs during inspiration. Each of the four inferior muscles divides into two fasciculi, one of which inserts as described above. The other passes down to the second rib below its origin.

The inferior and lateral aspects of the posterior thorax are covered by the latissimus dorsi muscle. These muscles originate from a broad aponeurosis extending from the inferior thoracic vertebrae, the lumbodorsal fascia, and the iliac crests. The muscle attaches to the intertubercular groove of the humerus. The muscle is innervated by the thoracodorsal nerve and is responsible for arm adduction, extension, and medial rotation.

The inferior border of the trapezius muscle interfaces with the superior border of the latissimus dorsi. The trapezius originates from the superior nuchal line of the occipital lobe, the ligamentum nuchae of the neck, the C7 vertebra, and supraspinous ligaments of the thoracic vertebrae. The muscle inserts on the spine and acromion of the scapula and lateral one-third of the clavicle. The trapezius muscles are supplied by the spinal accessory nerve. They act as stabilizers to the scapula and shoulders and can elevate, lower, or adduct the scapula.

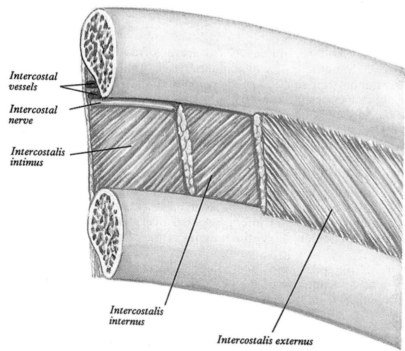

Intercostal vessels

Intercostal nerve

Intercostalis intimus

Intercostalis internus

Intercostalis externus

Figure 1–9. Dissection of a part of the thoracic wall, showing the position of the intercostal vessels and nerve relative to the intercostal muscles. (From Williams PL. *Gray's anatomy*, 38th ed. New York: Churchill Livingstone, 1995:814.)

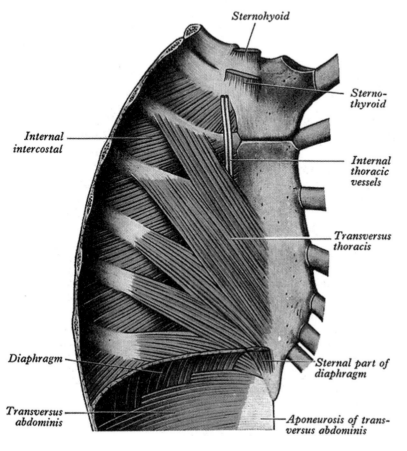

Sternohyoid

Sterno-thyroid

Internal intercostal

Internal thoracic vessels

Transversus thoracis

Diaphragm

Sternal part of diaphragm

Transversus abdominis

Aponeurosis of trans-versus abdominis

Figure 1–10. The left transversus thoracis, exposed and viewed from its posterior aspect. Note that, in the interval between the sternal and costal origins of the diaphragm, the lower border of transversus thoracis is in contact with the upper border of transversus abdominis. (From Williams PL. *Gray's anatomy*, 38th ed. New York: Churchill Livingstone, 1995:814.)

The intercostal neurovascular bundle runs between the intermediate and deepest layer of the transversus thoracis muscle. The bundle is arranged as vein, artery, and nerve from the lowest to the highest along the inferior aspect of each rib (Figure 1–11). Posteriorly, there is a single large intercostal artery. The first two spaces derive their artery from branches of the superior intercostal artery, a branch of the costocervical trunk of the subclavian artery. The posterior intercostal arteries for the lower nine spaces come off the descending thoracic aorta (Figure 1–12). The corresponding posterior intercostal veins drain back into the azygous or hemiazygous veins. Anteriorly, there are two small anterior intercostal arteries in each intercostal space. The first six spaces are branches of the internal thoracic artery. The lower spaces are branches of the musculophrenic artery, which is a continuation of the internal thoracic artery. The veins in this region drain to the internal thoracic veins and musculophrenic veins.

The intercostal nerves are the anterior rami of the first 11 thoracic spinal nerves. The first intercostal nerve is joined to the brachial plexus by a large branch that is equivalent to the lateral cutaneous branch of typical intercostal nerves. The remainder of the intercostal nerves are small and there is no anterior cutaneous branch. The second intercostal nerve is joined to the medial cutaneous nerve of the arm by an important branch called the intercostobrachial nerve. This nerve supplies the skin of the axilla and the superior medial side of the arm. In coronary artery disease, pain is referred along this nerve to the medial side of the arm. The anterior ramus of the 12th thoracic nerve lies in the abdomen and is referred to as the subcostal nerve. The first six intercostal nerves supply the skin, the parietal pleura, the intercostal muscles and the serratus posterior muscles. The next five nerves supply the skin, the parietal peritoneum, and the anterior abdominal muscles.

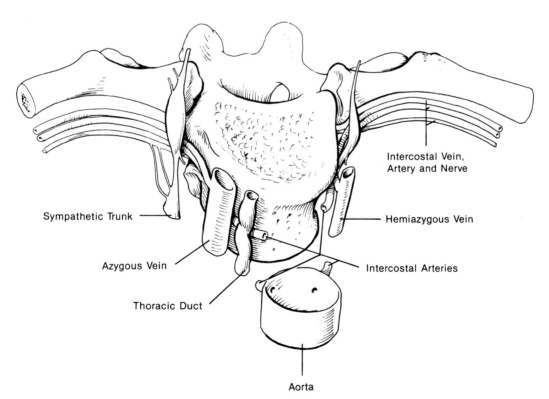

Intercostal Vein, Artery and Nerve

Sympathetic Trunk

Hemiazygous Vein

Azygous Vein

Intercostal Arteries

Thoracic Duct

Aorta

Figure 1–11. The relationship of the intercostal arteries, veins, and nerves is shown. Note that the intercostal arteries are directly caudad to each rib. Sequentially below these are the intercostal artery and nerve. The veins drain into the azygos system on the right and into the hemiazygos system on the left. The intercostal nerves arise from the spinal cord, exit the spinal canal, and are joined by communicating branches from the sympathetic trunks. (From Pearson FG, Cooper JD, Deslauriers J, *et al. Thoracic surgery*, 2nd ed. New York: Churchill Livingstone, 2002:1330.)

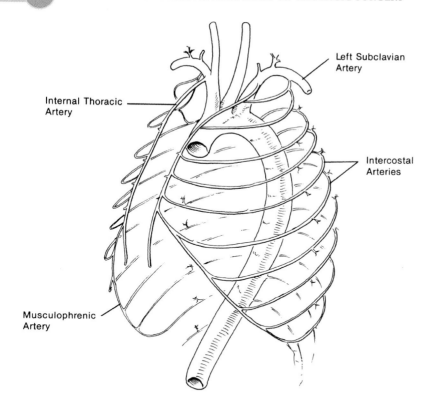

Internal Thoracic Artery

Left Subclavian Artery

Intercostal Arteries

Musculophrenic Artery

Figure 1–12. The arterial supply of the chest wall is shown in this left anterior oblique projection. Note that the intercostal arteries arise from the aorta posteriorly for the lower 10 intercostal spaces. The highest intercostal arteries branch off from the subclavian. The paired internal thoracic arteries arise from the subclavian and course down along the posterolateral aspect of the sternum. They give rise to a major branch, the musculophrenic artery, which goes along the costal cartilages to anastomose with the intercostal arteries. The continuation of the internal thoracic artery becomes the superior epigastric artery. (From Pearson FG, Cooper JD, Deslauriers J, *et al. Thoracic surgery*, 2nd ed. New York: Churchill Livingstone, 2002: 1329.)

The internal thoracic artery supplies the anterior wall of the thorax and abdomen (Figure 1–13). It is a branch of the first part of the subclavian artery in the neck. It descends vertically on the pleura posterior to the costal cartilages, lateral to the sternum, and terminates in the sixth intercostal space by dividing into the superior epigastric and musculophrenic arteries. The following branches come off this vessel:

- Two anterior intercostals arteries from the superior six intercostal spaces
- Perforating arteries, which accompany the terminal branches of the corresponding intercostal nerves
- The pericardiophrenic artery, which accompanies the phrenic nerve and supplies the pericardium
- Mediastinal arteries to the anterior mediastinum
- The superior epigastric artery, which enters the rectus sheath and supplies the rectus muscle as far as the umbilicus
- The musculophrenic artery, which runs around the costal margin of the diaphragm and supplies the inferior intercostal spaces and diaphragm.

Diaphragm and Accessory Muscles of Respiration

The diaphragm is a dome-shaped muscle with right and left domes (Figure 1–14). The right dome reaches as high as the superior border of the fifth rib and the left dome can reach the inferior border of the fifth rib. The central tendon lies at the level of the xiphisternal joint. The domes support the right and left lungs, whereas the central tendon supports the heart. The diaphragm varies significantly at various stages of breathing, standing or sitting, and after a large meal.

The muscular fibers may be grouped according to their origin into three parts—sternal, costal, and lumbar. The sternal part arises from two fleshy slips from the posterior xiphoid process. The costal part comes off the inner surfaces of the cartilages and adjacent parts of the inferior six ribs on each side, interdigitating with the transversus abdominis muscle. The lumbar part originates from the lumbocostal aponeurotic arches and from the lumbar vertebrae. There are two lumbocostal arches, a medial and a lateral, on either side. The internal arcuate

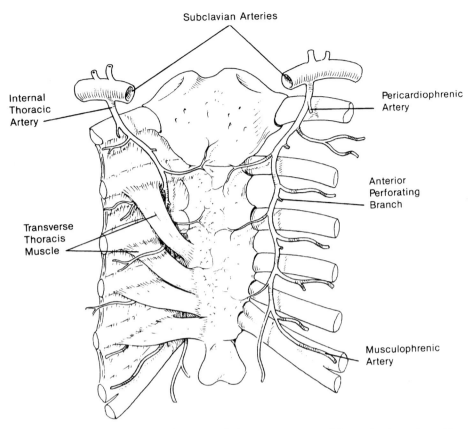

Subclavian Arteries

Internal
Thoracic
Artery

Pericardiophrenic
Artery

Anterior
Perforating
Branch

Transverse
Thoracis
Muscle

Musculophrenic
Artery

Figure 1–13. Illustrated is the detail of the internal thoracic artery and its major branches. The pericardio-phrenic arteries arise from the proximal portion of the internal thoracic arteries. They join with the pericardio-phrenic veins, which are usually paired, and progress to the diaphragm with the phrenic nerve. The perforators arising from each internal thoracic are shown, as are the communications with the intercostal vessels. The internal thoracic arteries provide the major blood supply to the sternum. The distal arteries arising from the internal thoracic include the musculophrenic, which goes laterally into the costophrenic sinus at the edge of the diaphragm, and the superior epigastric, which penetrates the diaphragm between the costal and sternal portions of the musculature. (From Pearson FG, Cooper JD, Deslauriers J, *et al. Thoracic surgery*, 2nd ed. New York: Churchill Livingstone, 2002:1330.)

ligament is a tendinous arch in the fascia covering the superior part of the psoas major. Medially, it is continuous with the lateral tendinous margin of the corresponding crus and is attached to the side of the vertebral bodies of L1 and L2. Laterally, it is fixed to the anterior of the transverse process of L1. The external arcuate ligament arches across the superior part of the quadratus lumborum. It attaches medially to the anterior of the transverse process of the L1 vertebra and laterally to the tip and inferior margin of the 12th rib.

The central tendon of the diaphragm is a thin but strong aponeurosis located near the center of the muscle, though slightly more anterior than posterior, therefore the posterior muscular fibers are longer. It has three divisions separated from each other by slight indentations. The right muscle fibers are the largest, the middle muscle fibers are directed toward the xiphoid process, and the left muscle fibers are the smallest. The tendon is composed of several planes of fibers which intersect each other at different angles and come together into straight or curved bundles in order to give it additional strength.

The thoracic outlet has three main openings:

• The caval opening at the level of the T8 vertebra. Elliptical in shape and the highest of the three openings, the opening is at the junction of the right and middle leaflets of the central tendon so that its margins are tendinous. The inferior vena cava and the terminal branches of the right phrenic nerve pass through this opening.

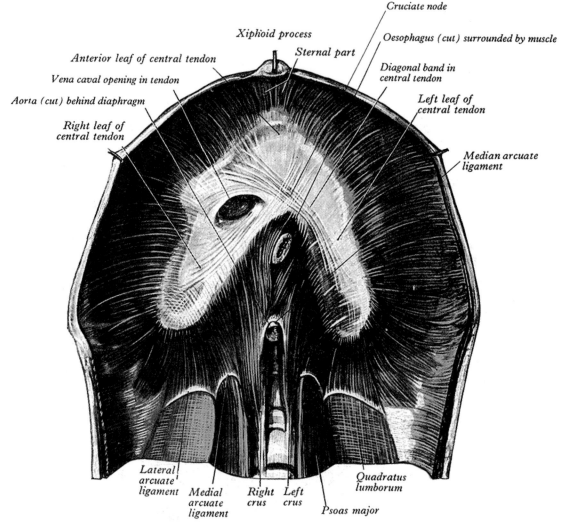

Figure 1-14. Abdominal aspect of the diaphragm. Note that the fibers descend from their relatively 'high' anterior sternocostal attachments steeply and obliquely to their complex 'low' posterior attachments. (From Williams PL, *et al. Gray's anatomy*, 38th ed. New York: Churchill Livingstone, 1995:814.)

- The esophageal opening at the level of the T10 vertebra. The opening is formed by a sling of muscle fibers from the right crus. It transmits the esophagus, the right and left vagus nerves, the esophageal branches of the left gastric vessels, and the lymphatics from the inferior one-third of the esophagus.
- The aortic opening at the level of T12 vertebra. This hiatus is situated slightly to the left of the midline and is bounded by the crura anteriorly and posteriorly by L1. The aorta, thoracic duct, and the azygous vein pass through this foramen.

Other structures that pass through the diaphragm include the greater, lesser, and low-est splanchnic nerves, which pierce the crura. The sympathetic trunks pass posterior to the median arcuate ligament on both sides and the superior epigastric vessels pass between the sternal and costal origins of the diaphragm on each side.

The phrenic nerves provide both the sensory and the motor function of the diaphragm. The right phrenic nerve penetrates the diaphragm just lateral to the caval foramen and the left just lateral to the left heart border. Each nerve divides into roughly four trunks: an antero-lateral trunk, a posterolateral trunk, a sternal trunk, and a crural trunk. After giving off the sternal trunks, the nerves penetrate the diaphragm and therefore cannot be seen from the thoracic cavity.

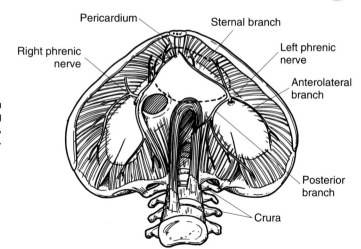

Figure 1–15. Anatomy of the diaphragm from the abdominal perspective, showing innervation. (Redrawn from Sabiston DC, Spencer FC. *Surgery of the chest*, 6th ed. Philadelphia: WB Saunders, 1995:1082.)

The arterial supply to the diaphragm comes from the left and right phrenic arteries, which originate from the abdominal aorta at the level of the aortic hiatus (Figure 1–15). They bifurcate posteriorly near the dome and travel along the margin of the central tendon. A large anterior branch runs anteriorly and superiorly and anastomoses with the pericardiophrenic vessels, and a smaller posterior branch courses laterally and posteriorly along the dorsal, lumbar, and costal origins of the diaphragm and anastomoses with the intercostal vessels. Venous drainage is from the right and left inferior phrenic veins, which drain into the inferior vena cava.

The diaphragm has several functions.

- *Abdominal straining.* The diaphragm aids in contracting the anterior abdominal wall and raising intra-abdominal pressure. This mechanism has multiple effects. It can be used to evacuate the pelvic contents (micturition, defecation, parturition). This increased pressure also supports the vertebral column and prevents flexion in lifting heavy weights.
- *Venous pump.* The descent of the diaphragm decreases the intrathoracic pressure and at the same time increases the intra-abdominal pressure. This pressure change compresses the blood in the inferior vena cava and forces it up into the right atrium to increase cardiac preload. The pressure is also important for regulating lymph return through the thoracic duct.
- *Inspiration.* The diaphragm is the principal muscle of inspiration (Figure 1–16). The dome is concave down towards the abdomen. During inspiration the lowest

ribs remain fixed in space, and the peripheral muscular fibers contract, drawing the central tendon down and anteriorly with the attached pericardium. In this movement the curvature of the diaphragm does not change. The dome moves downward parallel to its original position and pushes down on the abdominal viscera. The descent of the abdominal viscera is permitted by the elasticity of the abdominal wall.

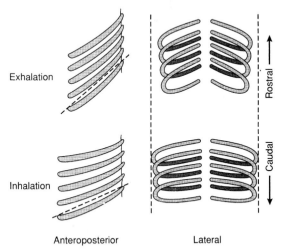

Figure 1–16. Chest wall dimensions. Contraction of the diaphragm causes the basal floor of the thoracic cavity to move downward, displacing the abdominal contents downward and increasing the rostral–caudal dimensions of the thoracic cavity. Contractions of the external intercostal muscles, the scalenus muscles, and the sternocleidomastoid muscles lift the rib cage superiorly and laterally, increasing the anteroposterior and lateral dimensions of the chest wall. (From Leff AR, Schumacker PT. *Respiratory physiology: basics and applications.* Philadelphia: WB Saunders, 1993:48.)

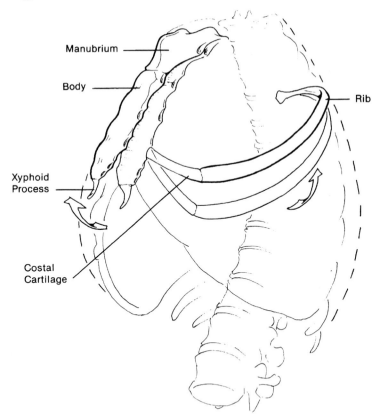

Manubrium

Body

Xyphoid
Process

Costal
Cartilage

Rib

Figure 1–17. The expansion and contraction of the chest wall are governed by the motion of the individual ribs, costal cartilages, and sternum. The sternum works as a handle on a water pump. As it is moved upward, the xiphoid process and body go more anteriorly and cephalad, whereas the manubrium articulates with the first rib and clavicle and rotates anteriorly and cephalad. The bucket handle motion of the ribs and costal cartilages is facilitated by articulations both posteriorly and anteriorly. The posterior articulations of the rib, with the head, the vertebral body, and the articular facet, move against the transverse process of the vertebral body below. The costal cartilage articulates with the sternum and moves upward on forced inspiration and downward on forced expiration. (From Pearson FG, Cooper JD, Deslauriers J, *et al. Thoracic surgery*, 2nd ed. New York: Churchill Livingstone, 2002:1326.)

Once the maximum diaphragmatic tension against the abdominal viscera is reached, the inferior ribs elevate and push the body of the sternum and the upper ribs forward. The right aspect of the diaphragm which lies over the liver has a greater resistance to overcome than the left side of the diaphragm, which lies over the stomach. To compensate for this the right crus and the fibers of the right side are generally stronger than those of the left. Before sneezing, coughing, laughing, crying, vomiting, or expelling urine or feces, a deep inspiration takes place.

The height of the diaphragm constantly changes during respiration. It also varies with the degree of distention of the stomach and intestines and with the size of the liver. The position of the diaphragm in the thorax depends upon three main factors:

- The elastic recoil of the lung tissue, tending to pull it upward
- The pressure exerted on its inferior surface by the viscera; this tends to be a negative pressure, or downward suction, when the patient sits or stands. Alternatively it is an upward pressure when a person lies down
- The intra-abdominal tension due to the abdominal muscles. These are in a state of contraction in the standing position. Therefore, the diaphragm is pushed up higher when a patients stands than when he sits.

During quiet respiration, the ribs are elevated by contraction of the intercostal muscles. The thoracic cage increases in dimensions upward and laterally along the midaxillary line. The greatest excursion occurs at the level of the longest ribs – ribs five through seven. The bucket-handle motion swings the ribs upward and laterally (Figure 1–17). Additional help in elevating the ribs comes from the costal muscle fibers of the diaphragm.

Additional muscles of respiration include (Figure 1–18, Table 1–1):

- *Scalene muscles*: assist in elevation of the rib cage during inspiration
- *Serratus posterior inferior muscles*: stabilize the thoracic cage by resisting the upward and medial pull of the diaphragm

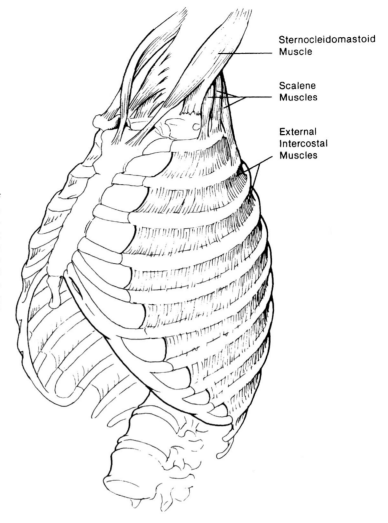

Sternocleidomastoid Muscle

Scalene Muscles

External Intercostal Muscles

Figure 1–18. Accessory muscles of inspiration. Note that all this musculature is directed at raising the fibromuscular skeleton and extending it anteriorly. This coordinated motion increases the intrathoracic diameters and allows further expansion of the lungs. (From Pearson FG, Cooper JD, Deslauriers J, *et al. Thoracic surgery*, 2nd ed. New York: Churchill Livingstone, 2002: 1328.)

TABLE 1–1 • *Thoracic muscles*

Muscle Function	Origin	Insertion	Respiratory
External intercostal muscle	Inferior rib border	Superior border of rib below	Inspiratory/expiratory
Internal intercostal muscle	Inferior rib border	Superior border of rib below	Inspiratory/expiratory
Transversus thoracis	Adjacent ribs	Adjacent ribs	Inspiratory/expiratory
Diaphragm	Xiphoid process; lower six costal cartilages; L1–3	Central tendon	Inspiratory
Levatores costarum	Tips of transverse process of C7, T1–T11	Rib below	Inspiratory
Serratus posterior superior	Lower cervical and upper thoracic spines	Upper ribs	Inspiratory
Serratus posterior inferior	Upper lumbar and lower thoracic spines	Lower ribs	Inspiratory

- *Quadratus lumborum*: stabilizes the 12th rib, but its effect on respiration is minimal
- *Sternocleidomastoid*: acts in elevating the first rib in respiration
- *Serratus posterior superior*: acts in elevation of the ribs. Serratus posterior inferior draws the inferior ribs down and posteriorly, elongating the thorax and assisting with inspiration
- *Levatoris costarum*: active in elevating the ribs.

Expiration is a passive process that occurs when intrapulmonic pressures exceeds atmospheric pressure. Elastic resistance of the lung causes recoil and rise in intrapulmonic pressure. Additional recoil of the rib cage hastens the process. During forced expiration, abdominal straining can cause rapid diaphragmatic elevation and rigid air transit.

Lungs

The lungs are respiratory organs on either side of the thorax, separated from each other by the heart and structures in the mediastinum. The lung has a light, porous, spongy texture and is highly elastic. The surface is smooth, shining, and divided into numerous polyhedral areas.

The lungs are pinkish white at birth and develop a dark gray color with age as carbonaceous substances deposit in the areolar tissue near the pleural surface. The posterior border of the lung is darker than the anterior. The right lung weighs on average 625 g, the left 575 g.

Each lung is pyramidal, with a rounded apex that extends 3–4 cm into the neck above the level of the sternal end of the first rib. The base is broad, concave, and rests on the convex surface of the diaphragm, which separates the right lung from the right lobe of the liver, and the left lung from the left lobe of the liver, the stomach, and the spleen. Since the diaphragm extends higher on the right than on the left side, the base of the right lung is deeper than the left. The base of the lung descends during inspiration and ascends during expiration.

The costal surface of the lungs is smooth and matches the chest cavity (Figure 1–19). It is in contact with the costal pleura and has slight grooves corresponding with the overlying ribs. The mediastinal surface of the lungs interfaces with the mediastinal pleura. It has a

cardiac impression that is deeper on the left than on the right. Superior and posterior to the cardiac impression is the hilum, where the structures enter that form the root of the lung. These structures are covered by pleura, which, inferior to the hilum and posterior to the pericardial impression, forms the pulmonary ligament. On the right lung, immediately superior to the hilum, is an arched groove for the azygos vein, while running upward, and then angling laterally some distance inferior to the apex, is a wide groove for the superior vena cava and right innominate vein. Behind this, and closer to the apex, is a groove for the innominate artery. Behind the hilum and the attachment of the pulmonary ligament is a vertical groove for the esophagus; this groove becomes less distinct caudally because of the shift of the inferior part of the esophagus to the left of the midline. Anterior and to the right of the inferior part of the esophageal groove is a deep concavity for the thoracic part of the inferior vena cava. On the left lung, immediately above the hilum, is a well-marked curved impression produced by the aortic arch, and running upward from this towards the apex is a groove for the left subclavian artery. There is an impression anterior to the groove and close to the margin of the lung where the left innominate vein runs. Behind the hilum and pulmonary ligament is a vertical groove produced by the descending aorta. Anteriorly, near the base of the lung, the inferior part of the esophagus causes a shallow impression.

The inferior border is thin and sharp where it separates the base from the costal surface and extends into the costophrenic sinus. The posterior border is broad and rounded, and drops into the deep concavity on either side of the vertebral column. It is much longer than the anterior border and projects into the costophrenic sinus. The anterior border is thin and sharp and overlaps the anterior of the pericardium. The anterior border of the right lung is almost vertical and projects into the costomediastinal sinus. On the anterior border of the left lung the pericardium is exposed at the cardiac notch. Opposite this notch the anterior margin of the left lung is situated laterally to the line of reflection of the corresponding part of the pleura.

The left lung is divided into two lobes, superior and inferior, by an interlobar fissure, which extends from the costal to the mediastinal surface of the lung both superior and inferior to

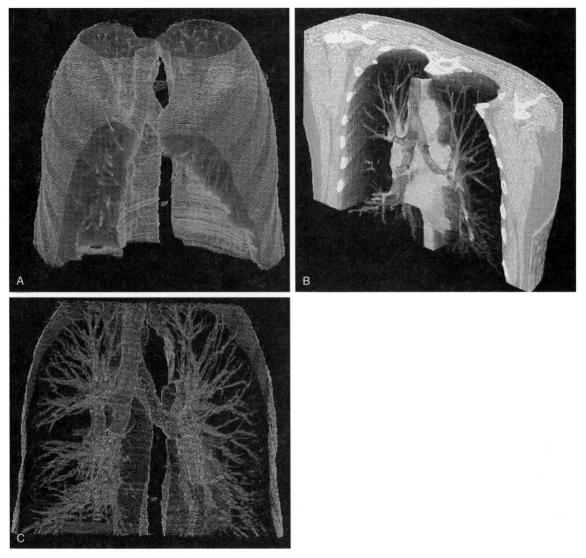

Figure 1-19. Helical computed tomographic data. **A, B,** Anterior views of the thorax demonstrating the spatial interrelationship between lung parenchyma and the chest wall. **C,** Anterior view of the thorax demonstrating normal bronchial anatomy. (Courtesy of GA Johnson, PhD, Department of Radiology, Duke University Medical Center, Durham, North Carolina.)

the hilum (Figure 1–20). As seen on the surface, this fissure starts on the mediastinal surface of the lung at the superior and posterior part of the hilum and extends to the third and fifth posteriorly. It extends inferiorly and anteriorly over the costal surface and reaches the inferior border a little behind its anterior surface around the sixth to seventh costochondral junction. The superior lobe lies superior and anterior to this fissure and includes the apex, the anterior border, and a considerable part of the costal surface and the greater part of the mediastinal surface of the lung. The lower lobe, the larger of the two, is situated inferior and

posterior to the fissure. It comprises the base, a large portion of the costal surface, and most of the posterior border of the left lung.

The right lung is divided into three lobes (superior, middle, inferior) by two interlobar fissures. One of these separates the inferior from the middle and superior lobes and corresponds closely with the fissure in the left lung (Figure 1–21). The other fissure separates the superior from the middle lobe (see Figure 1–20). It starts in the previous fissure near the posterior border of the lung. This fissure runs anteriorly and separates the anterior lung border on a plane with the sternal end of the fourth costal

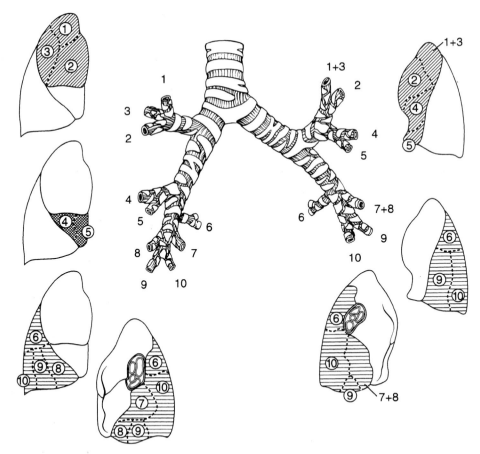

Figure 1–20. The lobes and segments of the lung. Right upper lobe segments: 1, apical; 2, anterior; 3, posterior. Right middle lobe segments: 4, lateral; 5, medial. Right lower lobe segments: 6, superior; 7, medial basal; 8, anterior basal; 9, lateral basal; 10, posterior basal. Left upper lobe segments: 1 and 3, apical posterior; 2, anterior; 4, superior (lingular); 5, inferior (lingular). Left lower lobe segments: 6, superior; 7 and 8, anteromedial basal; 9, lateral basal; 10, posterior basal. (From Pearson FG, Cooper JD, Deslauriers J, *et al. Thoracic surgery*, 2nd ed. New York: Churchill Livingstone, 2002:428.)

cartilage. Variations in fissure do occur. There is incomplete fusion of the middle and anterior portion of the superior lobe in over 50% of the lung examined. The middle lobe, the smallest lobe of the right lung, is wedge-shaped and includes the inferior part of the anterior border and the anterior part of the base of the lung. The right lung is 2.5 cm shorter than the left because the diaphragm rises higher on the right side to accommodate the liver. It is also broader because of the tilt of the heart to the left side. Overall, its total capacity is greater and it weighs more than the left lung.

A little above the middle of the mediastinal surface of each lung and nearer its posterior border is the lung root. The root is formed by the bronchus, the pulmonary artery, the pulmonary veins, the bronchial arteries and veins, the pulmonary plexuses of nerves, lymphatic vessels, and bronchial lymph glands,

all of which are enclosed by a reflection of the pleura. The root of the right lung lies posterior to the superior vena cava and part of the right atrium and inferior to the azygos vein. The left lung root passes beneath the aortic arch and anterior to the descending aorta. The phrenic nerve, the pericardiacophrenic artery and vein, and the anterior pulmonary plexus, lie anterior to the lung root on each side. The vagus and posterior pulmonary plexus are posterior to the root. Below each is the pulmonary ligament. The chief structures composing the root of each lung are arranged with the two pulmonary veins anteriorly, the pulmonary artery in the middle, and the bronchus and bronchial vessels posteriorly.

The lungs are composed of the visceral pleura, a subserous areolar tissue, and the pulmonary parenchyma. The subserous areolar tissue contains a large proportion of elastic fibers. It covers

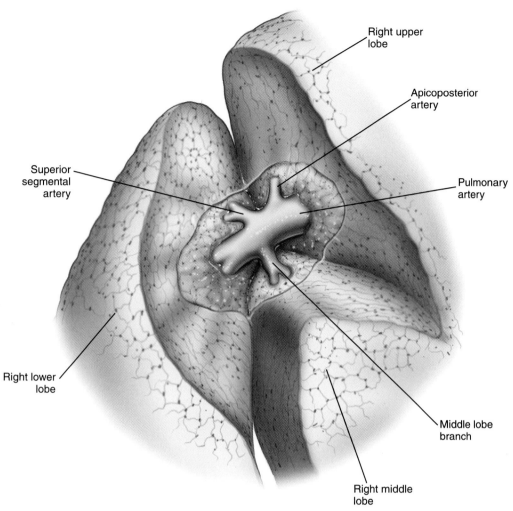

Figure 1–21. View into the right major fissure from the front. The fissure has been opened widely to expose and identify the segmental arteries to the upper, middle, and lower lobes. Anomalies of these vessels are common. The location of the posterior segmental artery to the right upper lobe is most variable; this artery may be a branch of the superior segmental artery. Occasionally, this segmental arterial branch is absent. (From Pearson FG, Cooper JD, Deslauriers J, *et al. Thoracic surgery*, 2nd ed. New York: Churchill Livingstone, 2002:986.)

the entire surface of the lung and extends inward between the lobules. The parenchyma is composed of secondary lobules connected together by interlobular areolar tissue. Each secondary lobule is composed of several primary lobules, the anatomical units of the lung. The primary lobule consists of an alveolar duct, the air spaces connected with it and their blood vessels, lymphatics, and nerves (Figure 1–22).

The pulmonary artery carries the venous blood to the lungs; it divides into branches, which accompany the bronchial airways, and ends in a dense capillary network in the alveolar walls (Figure 1–23). In the lung the branches of the pulmonary artery are usually superior

and anterior to the bronchial airway. The pulmonary capillaries form plexuses that lie immediately beneath the lining epithelium, in the walls and septa of the alveoli. The pulmonary veins start in the pulmonary capillaries and coalesce into larger branches that run through the lung, independent of the pulmonary arteries and bronchi. After freely communicating with other branches they form large vessels, which ultimately come into relation with the arteries and bronchial tubes and accompany them to the hilum. Finally they open into the left atrium.

The bronchial arteries supply blood for the nutrition of the lung; they are derived from the

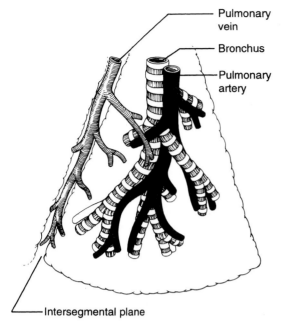

Figure 1–22. The bronchopulmonary segment. (From Pearson FG, Cooper JD, Deslauriers J, *et al. Thoracic surgery*, 2nd ed. New York: Churchill Livingstone, 2002:428.)

thoracic aorta or from the upper aortic intercostal arteries and accompany the bronchial airways. They perfuse the bronchial glands and the walls of the larger bronchial airways and pulmonary vessels. Those supplying the bronchi form a capillary plexus in the muscular coat that gives off a second plexus in the mucous coat. This plexus communicates with small venous trunks that empty into the pulmonary veins. Others are distributed in the interlobular areolar tissue and terminate partly in the deep and partly in the superficial bronchial veins. Lastly, some terminate on the surface of the lung, beneath the pleura, where they form a capillary network (Figure 1–24). The bronchial vein is formed at the root of the lung, receiving superficial and deep veins corresponding to branches of the bronchial artery. It does not receive all the blood supplied by the artery, as some of it passes into the pulmonary veins. It ends in the azygos vein on the right and in the highest intercostal or in the accessory hemiazygos vein on the left.

Pleura

Each lung is covered by a thin serous membrane in the form of a closed invaginated sac. A portion of the serous membrane called the

visceral pleura covers the surface of the lung and extends into the fissures between its lobes. The rest of the membrane, called the parietal pleura, lines the inner surface of the chest wall, covers the diaphragm, and reflects over the structures occupying the middle of the thorax (Figure 1–25). The two layers are continuous with one another around and inferior to the lung root. The potential space between them is known as the pleural cavity. When the lung collapses or when air or fluid collects between the two layers, the cavity becomes apparent. The right and left pleural sacs do not communicate (Figure 1–26).

Like other serous membranes, the pleura is covered by a single layer of flattened, nucleated cells, sealed at their edges by cement substance. These cells are modified connective-tissue corpuscles and rest on a basement membrane. Beneath the basement membrane there are networks of yellow elastic and white fibers, imbedded in ground substance that contains connective-tissue cells. Blood vessels, lymphatics, and nerves are distributed in the substance of the pleura. The arteries of the pleura are derived from the intercostal, internal mammary, musculophrenic, thymic, pericardiac, and bronchial vessels.

Trachea and Bronchi

The trachea is a cartilaginous and membranous airway in the anterior mediastinum that extends from the inferior part of the larynx to the level of the T5 vertebra, where it divides into the two bronchi, one for each lung. The trachea is somewhat elliptical but flattens posteriorly (Figure 1–27). It is approximately 11 cm in length and 2 cm in diameter.

The anterior surface of the trachea is convex and is covered in the neck by the thyroid isthmus, the sternothyroid and sternohyoid muscles, the cervical fascia, and branches of the anterior jugular veins (Figure 1–28). Laterally, in the neck, it borders the common carotid arteries, the right and left lobes of the thyroid gland, the inferior thyroid arteries, and the recurrent nerves. In the thorax, the trachea is bordered by the manubrium, thymus remnants, the left innominate vein, the aortic arch, the innominate and left common carotid arteries, and the deep cardiac plexus (Figure 1–29). Posteriorly it is in contact with the esophagus and the right and left paratracheal lymph node chains (Figure 1–30). At the tracheal bifurcation, there is a

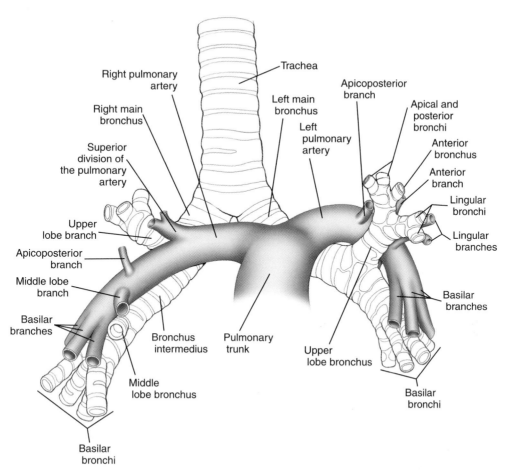

Figure 1-23. Anteroposterior view of the pulmonary artery branching and its relationship to the bronchial tree. (From Pearson FG, Cooper JD, Deslauriers J, *et al. Thoracic surgery*, 2nd ed. New York: Churchill Livingstone, 2002:1015.)

sharp carina, which measures approximately 1.5 cm in diameter, dividing into the left and right bronchus. The septum separating the trachea into the two bronchi is left of the midline and the right bronchus appears to be a more direct continuation of the trachea than the left. Any solid object entering the trachea is directed toward the right bronchus. This tendency is aided by the larger diameter of the right bronchus.

Each lobe of the right and left lungs is divided into bronchopulmonary segments (see Figure 1–20). There are 10 segments in the right lung and eight in the left (Figure 1–31). Subdivisions in the bronchial tree correspond to the anatomic segments and are named accordingly. These tertiary bronchi were regarded by Jackson and Huber as the final branches but the advent of the fiberoptic bronchoscope has led to introduction of additional nomenclature for the fourth, fifth, and sixth

divisions, since these can now be visualized. A convenient numerical system is used in which segmental bronchi are numbered from 1 to 10 on each side and are identified by the capital letter B for bronchus. This may be prefixed by a capital letter R or L for the appropriate side, so that RB3 identifies the bronchus to the anterior segment of the right upper lobe. The apical posterior segment of the left upper lobe is LB1 + 2, and anteromedial basal segment of the same side becomes LB8, since each of these paired segments is supplied by a single tertiary bronchus (Figure 1–32).

Segmental or fourth-order bronchi are indicated by the lower case letter a for posterior and b for anterior. The letter c may also be used when necessary for additional bronchi. Fifth-order bronchi are designated by the Roman numerals i (posterior) and ii (anterior). Finally, those at the level of the sixth order are characterized by α and β.

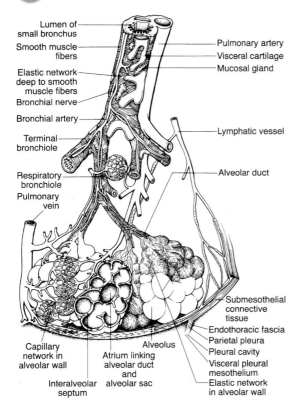

Figure 1–24. The interrelationships of the anatomic structures involved in lung anatomy. (From Williams PL, Warwick R, Dyson M, Bannister LH, eds. *Gray's anatomy*, 37th ed. Edinburgh: Churchill Livingstone, 1989:1279.)

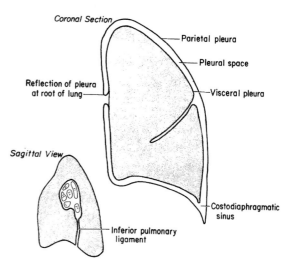

Figure 1–25. Schematic coronal section of a hemithorax and sagittal view of the root of the lung showing the pleural coverings. Note the location of the costodiaphragmatic sinus. (From Sabiston DC, Spencer FC. *Surgery of the chest*, 6th ed. Philadelphia: WB Saunders, 1995:524.)

The right bronchus is wider and shorter and more vertical in direction than the left. It is about 2.5 cm long and enters the right lung opposite T5. The azygos vein arches over it from behind; and the right pulmonary artery runs inferiorly to anteriorly. About 2 cm from its take off it gives off a branch to the upper lobe of the right lung. The bronchus passes inferior to the right pulmonary artery. It divides into two branches for the middle and lower lobes (Figure 1–33). The right bronchus gives off a branch for the superior lobe approximately 2.5 cm from the bifurcation of the trachea. All the other main stem divisions come off inferior the pulmonary artery. The first of these is distributed to the middle lobe, and the main tube then passes downward and backward into the lower lobe, giving off in its course a series of large ventral and small dorsal branches. There are four ventral and four dorsal branches, which arise alternately. The branch to the middle lobe is regarded as the first of the ventral series.

The left bronchus is smaller in caliber but longer than the right, being nearly 5 cm long.

It enters the root of the left lung opposite T6. It passes beneath the aortic arch and crosses anterior to the esophagus, the thoracic duct, and the descending aorta. The left pulmonary artery runs superiorly and then anteriorly. The left bronchus passes inferior to the level of the pulmonary artery before it divides. The first branch of the left bronchus arises about 5 cm from the bifurcation of the trachea and enters the superior lobe (see Figure 1–33). The main stem then enters the lower lobe, where it divides into ventral and dorsal branches similar to those in the right lung. The branch to the superior lobe of the left lung is regarded as the first of the ventral series.

The trachea and extrapulmonary bronchi are composed of incomplete rings of hyaline cartilage, fibrous tissue, muscular fibers, mucous membrane, and glands. There are 16–20 tracheal cartilages, which form rings around the anterior two-thirds of the circumference of the trachea. The ring does not extend posteriorly. Instead the trachea is supported by fibrous tissue and unstriped muscular fibers. The cartilages are placed horizontally above each other, separated by narrow intervals. They measure about 4 mm in depth and 1 mm in thickness. Their outer surfaces are flattened in a vertical direction but the internal surfaces are convex. The cartilages are thicker in the middle than at the margins. Two or more of the cartilages often unite and they are sometimes bifurcated at their ends. They are highly elastic but may become calcified with advanced age. In the right

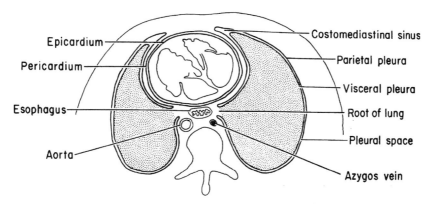

Figure 1–26. Schematic cross-section of the thorax. The shape of the pleural space is shown by the invagination of the lung buds, and the pleura is divided into its parietal and visceral parts. Note the location of the costomediastinal sinus anteriorly. (From Sabiston DC, Spencer FC. *Surgery of the chest*, 6th ed. Philadelphia: WB Saunders, 1995:523.)

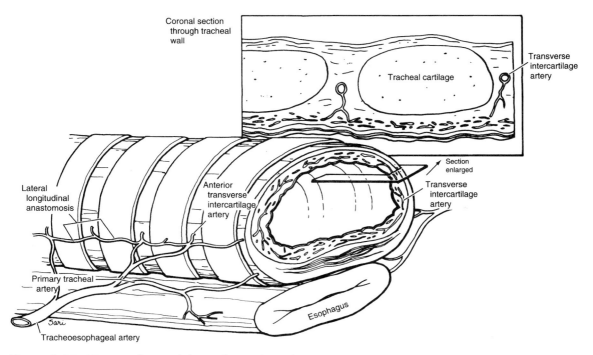

Figure 1–27. Microcirculation of the trachea and esophagus. There is a rich submucosal plexus but no similar plexus of vessels on the external surface. Tracheal cartilage is nourished entirely from the submucosal circulation. (From Salassa JR, Pearson BW, Payne WS. Gross and microscopical blood supply of the trachea. *Ann Thorac Surg* 1977;24:100.)

bronchus the cartilages vary in number from six to eight; in the left, from nine to 12. They are shorter and narrower than those of the trachea but have the same shape and arrangement.

The first cartilage is broader than the rest and is connected to the inferior border of the cricoid cartilage by the cricotracheal ligament. The last cartilage is thick and broad in the middle and curves inferiorly and posteriorly between the two bronchi. It ends on each side in an imperfect ring that encloses the beginning of the bronchus. The cartilage above the last is somewhat broader than the others at its center.

The muscular tissue consists of two layers of nonstriated muscle, longitudinal and transverse. The longitudinal fibers are external and consist of a few scattered bundles. The transverse fibers are internal and form a thin layer that extends transversely between the ends of the cartilages.

The mucous membrane is continuous from the larynx to the bronchi. It consists of

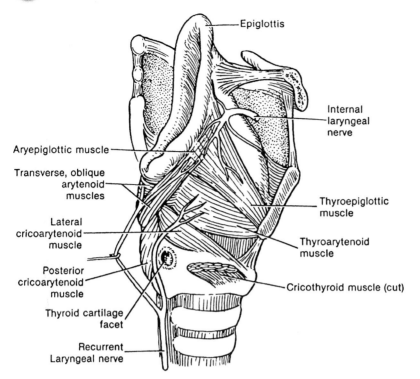

Figure 1–28. Lateral view of laryngeal muscles and nerves. (From Cummings C, *et al.*, eds. *Otolaryngology, head and neck surgery.* St Louis: CV Mosby, 1986.)

areolar and lymphoid tissue and presents a well-marked basement membrane supporting a stratified epithelium. The surface layer is columnar and ciliated, while the deeper layers are composed of oval or rounded cells. Beneath the basement membrane there is a distinct layer of longitudinal elastic fibers with a small amount of intervening areolar tissue. The submucous layer is composed of a loose meshwork of connective tissue, containing large blood vessels, nerves, and mucous glands.

The intrapulmonary bronchi divide and subdivide throughout the entire organ, the smallest subdivisions constituting the lobular bronchioles. The larger divisions consist of:

- An outer coat of fibrous tissue that is supported at intervals by irregular plates of hyaline cartilage, usually at the points of bifurcation
- A middle layer of circular smooth muscle fibers
- An internal mucous membrane lined by columnar ciliated epithelium resting on a basement membrane.

The lobular bronchioles differ from the larger airways in containing no cartilage, and the ciliated epithelial cells are cubical in shape. The lobular bronchioles are about 0.2 mm in diameter. Each bronchiole divides into two or more respiratory bronchioles with scattered

alveoli. Each of these divides into several alveolar ducts with a greater number of alveoli connected to them. Each alveolar duct is connected to a variable number of irregularly spherical spaces called acini. Within each acinus is a variable number (two to five) of interconnected alveolar sacs. The alveoli are lined by a delicate layer of simple squamous epithelium, the cells of which are united at their edges by a cement substance.

The right main bronchus gives rise to three lobar bronchi: upper, middle, and lower. Any two of these may occasionally have a common stem. The apical segment of the right upper lobe forms the apex of the right lung. It extends into the root of the neck as high as the vertebral end of the first rib. Toward the lateral aspect of the lung, the apical segment dips downward slightly between the posterior and anterior segments. This boundary line is roughly at the level of the first rib anteriorly and almost down to the second rib posteriorly. The anterior segment extends from the apical segment above down to the horizontal fissure at about the level of the fourth rib.

The middle lobe bronchus branches into two segmental bronchi, the complete branchings of which become the lateral segment and medial segment of the lobe. These segments are separated by the vertical plane extending from the hilus out to the costal surface of the

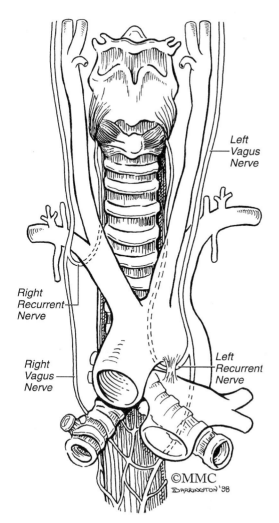

Figure 1–29. Anatomy of the right and left recurrent laryngeal nerves. Tracheal and esophageal branches are not shown. (From Pearson FG, Cooper JD, Deslauriers J, *et al. Thoracic surgery*, 2nd ed. New York: Churchill Livingstone, 2002:333.)

into four basal segmental bronchi: medial, anterior, lateral, and posterior. The basal segments of the lower lobe form the base of the lung and rest upon the diaphragm. The medial basal segment is sometimes partially separated from other basal segments by an extra fissure; in this event it has sometimes been called the cardiac lobe of the lung. The major vascular relationship on the right is the right pulmonary artery, which crosses anteriorly to the right mainstem bronchus at its origin and extends down on the anterolateral surface of the bronchus.

The upper lobe bronchus in the left lung subdivides into a superior division bronchus and an inferior or lingular division bronchus. The superior division can be thought of as corresponding to the right upper lobe, with the lingular division corresponding to the right middle lobe; there is usually no fissure separating the two and their segmental subdivisions are not the same. Unlike the situation on the right, the superior division of the left upper lobe has only two segments: the apical posterior segment – which corresponds to a combination of the right apical and posterior segments – and the anterior segment. The inferior or lingular division also has two segments, superior and inferior.

The left lower lobe segments are similar to the right lower lobe, except that the portion corresponding to the right anterior basal and medial basal segments is supplied on the left by two bronchi that have a common stem, and thus forms a single anteromedial basal segment. Other left lower lobe segments are: superior, lateral basal, and posterior basal. The left main-stem bronchus is larger than the right main-stem bronchus because it passes inferior to the aortic arch. The left pulmonary artery crosses the bronchus to lie on the posterolateral aspect of the mainstem bronchus and its divisions.

The major airways have a dual blood supply from bronchial arteries and pulmonary circulation. The bronchial arterial circulation is the main source of blood flow to the central airways. It may be divided into anterior branches, which arise from the subclavian, internal mammary, or coronary arteries, and the posterior branches, which arise from the thoracic aorta or intercostal arteries.

In the proximal airway, the bronchial arteries divide within the peribronchial connective tissue sheath surrounding the main bronchi, resulting in two or three branches that wind around the wall of the bronchus to the level of

lung and reaching its inferior border just anterior to the inferior end of the oblique fissure. These segments are related to the anterior parts of the fourth and fifth ribs and their costal cartilages.

The lower lobe bronchus gives off a posteriorly directed superior segmental bronchus just inferior to the level of the orifice of the middle lobe bronchus. The superior segment of the lower lobe occupies the entire superior part of the lower lobe and extends from the upper part of the oblique fissure at about the level of the vertebral end of the third rib to the level of the vertebral end of the fifth or six rib.

Inferior to the level at which the superior segmental bronchus arises, the lower lobe divides

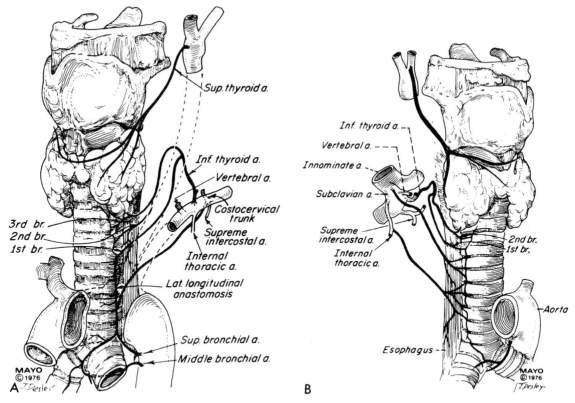

Figure 1–30. A, Left anterior view of arteries supplying the trachea. In this specimen, the lateral longitudinal anastomosis links branches of the inferior thyroid, costocervical trunk, and bronchial arteries. **B,** Right anterior view of vessels supplying the trachea. In this specimen, the lateral longitudinal anastomosis links branches from the inferior thyroid, subclavian, internal thoracic, and superior bronchial arteries. (From Salassa JR, Pearson BW, Payne WS. Gross and microscopical blood supply of the trachea. *Ann Thorac Surg* 1977;24:100. Reprinted with permission of the Society of Thoracic Surgeons.)

the terminal bronchiole. The arteries anastomose to form a peribronchial plexus and also penetrate the bronchial wall to form a submucosal plexus. In the distal airways, the bronchial and pulmonary circulations anastomose.

Mediastinum

The mediastinum is defined by the following borders: the thoracic inlet superiorly, the diaphragm inferiorly, the sternum anteriorly, the vertebral column posteriorly, and the parietal pleura laterally (Figure 1–34).

Anterior Mediastinum

The anterior mediastinum is bounded anteriorly by the sternum, laterally by the pleura, and posteriorly by the pericardium. It is narrow superiorly but widens inferiorly. Its anterior wall is formed by the left transversus thoracis muscle and the fifth, sixth, and seventh left costal cartilages. It contains the thymus, a quantity of loose areolar tissue, some lymphatic vessels that ascend from the convex surface of the liver, two or three anterior mediastinal lymph glands, and branches of the internal mammary artery.

Thymus

The thymus reaches maximum size at puberty, then it involutes and almost disappears. During most active growth, it consists of two lateral lobes placed in close contact along the midline, situated partly in the thorax, partly in the neck, and extending up from the fourth costal cartilage as high as the inferior border of the thyroid gland. It is covered by the sternum and by the origins of the sternohyoid and sternothyroid. Caudally, it sits on the pericardium, separated from the aortic arch and great vessels by a layer of fascia. The thymus is a pinkish gray color and lobulated on its surfaces. The lobes are usually fused in the

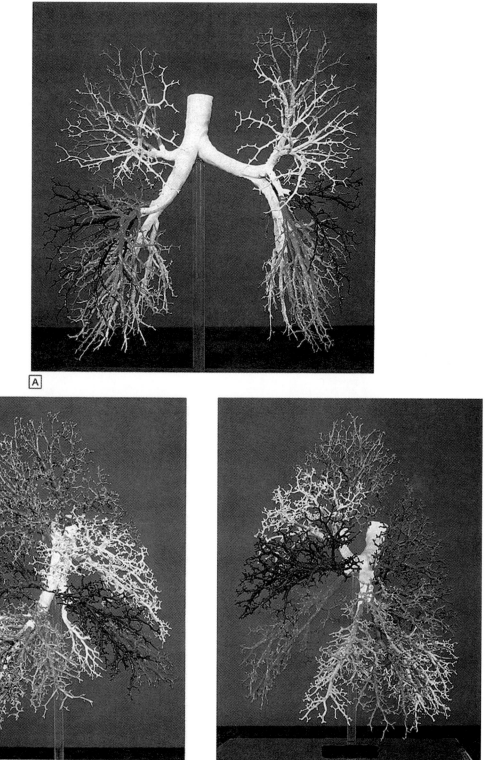

Figure 1–31. A, A resin corrosion cast of the adult human lower trachea and bronchial tree photographed from the anterior aspect. The segmental bronchi and their main branches have been colored: brown = apical; gray/blue = posterior; pink = anterior; dark blue = lateral (middle lobe) and superior lingular; red = medial (middle lobe) and inferior lingular; dark green = superior (apical) of inferior lobe; yellow = medial basal; orange = anterior basal; blue = lateral basal; light green = posterior basal. **B,** Corrosion cast of the bronchial tree of the right lung, color coded as in **A** to indicate the territories supplied by different segmental bronchi. **C,** Corrosion cast of the bronchial tree of the left lung, color coded as in **A.** Note that in this and other preparations shown in this figure many of the finer bronchial branches have been trimmed away to reveal the larger bronchi. (From Williams PL, *et al. Gray's anatomy,* 38th ed. New York: Churchill Livingstone, 1995:1660.) [See color insert, plate 1]

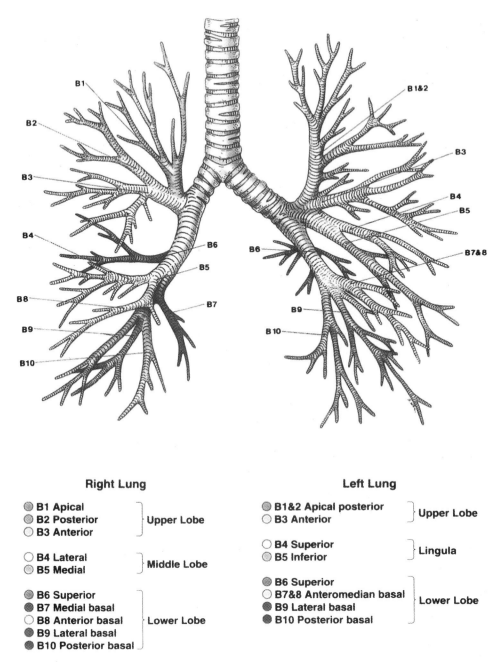

Right Lung

- ◕ B1 Apical
- ◕ B2 Posterior   } Upper Lobe
- ○ B3 Anterior

- ○ B4 Lateral
- ◕ B5 Medial   } Middle Lobe

- ● B6 Superior
- ● B7 Medial basal
- ○ B8 Anterior basal   } Lower Lobe
- ● B9 Lateral basal
- ● B10 Posterior basal

Left Lung

- ◕ B1&2 Apical posterior
- ○ B3 Anterior   } Upper Lobe

- ○ B4 Superior
- ◕ B5 Inferior   } Lingula

- ● B6 Superior
- ○ B7&8 Anteromedian basal   } Lower Lobe
- ● B9 Lateral basal
- ● B10 Posterior basal

Figure 1–32. The segmental anatomy of the bronchial tree with the universally adopted descriptive and numeric identification. (From Roth JA, Ruckdeschel JC, Weisenburger, TH. *Thoracic oncology*, 2nd ed. Philadelphia: WB Saunders, 1995:131.)

midline, giving the gland an H-shaped configuration. Averaging 5 cm by 4 cm by 6 mm in thickness, at birth it weighs about 15 g and by puberty it weighs about 35 grams; by 70 years of age it is a mere 6 g.

Each lobe is composed of lobules held together by delicate areolar tissue. The entire gland is enclosed in a capsule of denser struc-

ture. The primary lobules vary in size from that of a pinhead to that of a small pea and are composed of a number of small irregular nodules or follicles. Each follicle is 1–2 mm in diameter and has a medullary and a cortical portion. The cortical portion is composed of lymphoid cells, supported by a network of finely branched cells, which is continuous

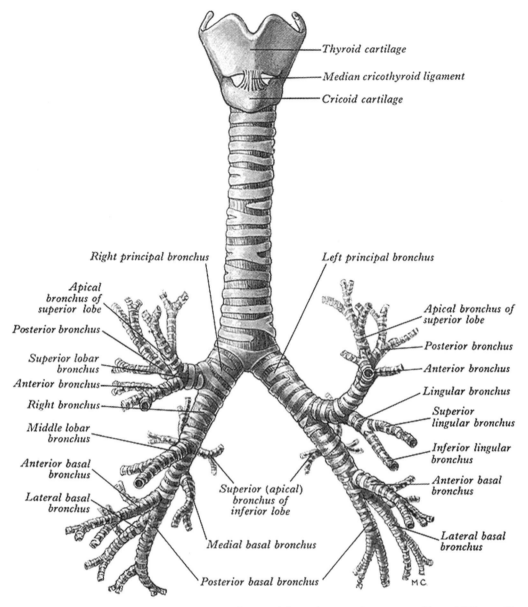

Figure 1–33. The cartilages of the larynx, trachea and bronchi: anterior aspect. (From Williams PL, *et al. Gray's anatomy*, 38th ed. New York: Churchill Livingstone, 1995:1654.)

with a similar network in the medullary portion. This network forms the adventitia for the blood vessels. In the medullary portion the reticulum is coarser than the cortex, the lymphoid cells are relatively fewer in number and there are peculiar concentric nest-like bodies called Hassall corpuscles. Each follicle is surrounded by a vascular plexus from which vessels pass into the interior and radiate from the periphery toward the center, forming a second zone just within the margin of the medullary portion.

The arterial supply of the thymus is provided laterally by the internal mammary artery, superiorly by the superior and inferior thyroid arteries, and inferiorly from the pericardiophrenic branches. The veins terminate in the left innominate vein and in the thyroid veins. The relation of the thymus to the phrenic nerve is critical because both nerves descend through the thymus gland in its middle portion, becoming intimate with the gland as they pass from the chest into the neck at the level of the thoracic inlet.

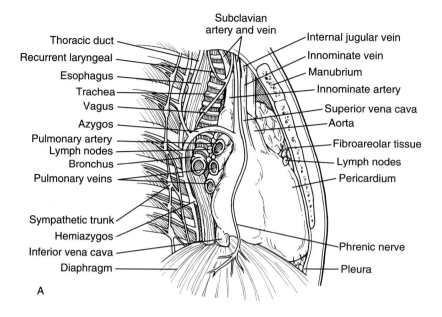

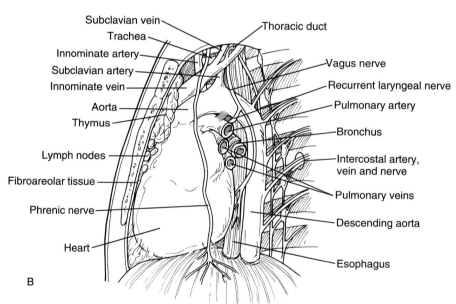

Figure 1–34. The anatomic structures of the mediastinum as seen from the right side (**A**) and from the left side (**B**).

Superior Mediastinum

The superior mediastinum lies between the manubrium anteriorly and the upper thoracic vertebrae posteriorly. It is bounded inferiorly by a slightly oblique plane passing backward from the junction of the manubrium and body of the sternum to the inferior part of T4 and laterally by the pleura. It contains the aortic arch, the innominate artery and the thoracic section of the left common carotid and the left subclavian arteries, the innominate veins and the superior half of the superior vena cava, the left highest intercostal vein, the vagus, cardiac, phrenic, and left recurrent nerves, the trachea, esophagus, and thoracic duct.

Middle Mediastinum

The middle mediastinum is the broadest part of the interpleural space. It contains the heart enclosed in the pericardium, the ascending aorta, the inferior half of the superior vena cava with the azygos vein, the bifurcation of the trachea and the two bronchi, the pulmonary artery dividing into its two branches, the right and left pulmonary veins, the phrenic nerves, and some bronchial lymph glands.

Posterior Mediastinum

The posterior mediastinum runs parallel with the vertebral column; it is bounded anteriorly by the pericardium, inferiorly by the posterior surface of the diaphragm, posteriorly by the vertebral column from the inferior border of T4 to T12, and laterally by the mediastinal pleura (Figure 1–35). It contains the thoracic part of the descending aorta, the azygos and the two hemiazygos veins, the vagus and splanchnic nerves, the esophagus, the thoracic duct, and some lymph glands

Esophagus

The esophagus is a muscular canal, approximately 23–25 cm long, extending from the pharynx to the stomach. It starts in the neck at the inferior border of the cricoid cartilage opposite C6, descends anteriorly along the vertebral column, through the superior and posterior mediastinum, passes through the diaphragm, and, enters the abdomen opposite T11. The general direction of the esophagus is vertical but it has two slight curves in its course. Near the neck it is midline but it angles to the left side and gradually passes to the midline again

at the level of the T5 and finally deviates to the left again as it passes forward to the esophageal hiatus in the diaphragm. The esophagus also has anteroposterior twists corresponding to the curvatures of the cervical and thoracic portions of the vertebral column. The narrowest part of the digestive tract is where the esophagus passes into the diaphragm (Figure 1–36).

The cervical portion of the esophagus borders the trachea and the thyroid gland posteriorly, sits on the vertebral column, and borders the common carotid artery and parts of the lobes of the thyroid gland laterally. The recurrent laryngeal nerves ascend between the esophagus and the trachea (tracheoesophageal groove). On the esophagus's left side is the thoracic duct. The thoracic portion of the esophagus is situated in the superior mediastinum between the trachea and the vertebral column slightly left of the midline. It passes posterior and to the right of the aortic arch, descends in the posterior mediastinum along the right side of the descending aorta, and then runs anterior and left of the aorta. The esophagus finally enters the abdomen through the diaphragm at the level of the T10. In the inferior part of the posterior mediastinum the thoracic duct lies to the right of the esophagus. Cranially, it lies posteriorly and crosses at the level of the T4, continuing superiorly on its left side. The abdominal portion of the esophagus lies in the esophageal groove on the posterior surface of the left lobe of the liver and only its anterior and left aspects are covered by peritoneum.

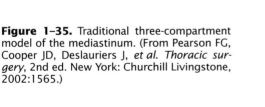

Figure 1–35. Traditional three-compartment model of the mediastinum. (From Pearson FG, Cooper JD, Deslauriers J, *et al. Thoracic surgery*, 2nd ed. New York: Churchill Livingstone, 2002:1565.)

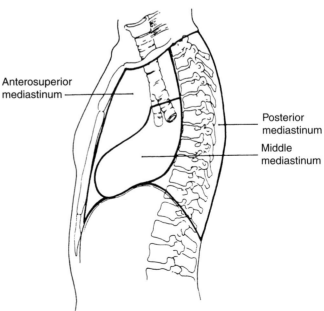

Anterosuperior mediastinum

Posterior mediastinum

Middle mediastinum

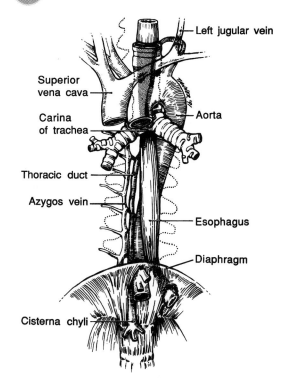

Figure 1–36. Anatomic figure demonstrating the relationship of the esophagus to other structures within the mediastinum. (From Wolfe WG, Sebastian MW. *Complications in thoracic surgery.* St Louis: CV Mosby, 1992:245.)

The esophagus has four layers: external, muscular, submucosal, and mucosal. There is no serosal layer to the esophagus. The muscular layer is composed of external longitudinal and an internal circular fibers. The longitudinal fibers are arranged in three fasciculi: one in front, which is attached to the vertical ridge on the posterior surface of the lamina of the cricoid cartilage, and one on either side, which is continuous with the muscular fibers of the pharynx. The circular fibers are continuous with the pharyngeal constrictor muscles. Their direction is transverse at the superior and inferior parts of the esophagus but oblique in the intermediate part. The submucosal layer contains blood vessels, nerves, and mucous glands. The mucous layer is studded with small papilla and is covered with a thick layer of stratified squamous epithelium. Between mucosa and submucosa is a layer of longitudinally arranged nonstriped muscular fibers called the muscularis mucosa.

The arteries supplying the esophagus are derived from the inferior thyroid branch of the thyrocervical trunk, from the descending thoracic aorta, from the left gastric branch of the celiac artery, and from the left inferior phrenic

of the abdominal aorta. The nerves come from the vagus and the sympathetic trunks. They form a plexus in which there are a groups of ganglion cells between the two muscular layers and a second plexus in the submucosal tissue.

Thoracic Duct

The thoracic duct carries most of the lymph and chyle into the blood. It is the endpoint for most of the lymphatic vessels of the body except those from the right side of the head, neck, and thorax, the right upper extremity, the right lung, the right side of the heart, and the convex surface of the liver. In the adult it varies from 38 to 45 cm in length and extends from L2 to the root of the neck.

It begins in the abdomen by a triangular dilatation, the cisterna chyli, which is situated anterior to the L2 vertebral body, to the right side and posterior to the aorta, by the side of the right crus of the diaphragm. It enters the thorax through the aortic hiatus of the diaphragm and ascends through the posterior mediastinal cavity between the aorta and azygos vein. Posteriorly lies the vertebral column, the right intercostal arteries, and the hemiazygos veins as they cross to open into the azygos vein; anteriorly is the diaphragm, esophagus, and the pericardium. Opposite T4 it angles towards the left side, enters the superior mediastinal cavity, and ascends behind the aortic arch and the thoracic part of the left subclavian artery and between the left side of the esophagus and the left pleura to the upper orifice of the thorax. Passing into the neck it forms an arch which rises about 3–4 cm above the clavicle and crosses anterior to the subclavian artery, the vertebral artery and vein, and the thyrocervical trunk. It also passes anterior to the phrenic nerve and the medial border of the anterior scalene muscle. Anterior to the thoracic duct is the left common carotid artery, vagus nerve, and internal jugular vein. It ends by opening between the left subclavian vein with the left internal jugular vein.

The thoracic duct varies in size. It is smaller in the middle of the thorax and dilates just before emptying into the circulatory system. It has a varicose appearance. Up to 50% of individuals have an anomalous pattern. Occasionally, it divides in the middle of its course into two vessels of unequal size, which reunite or subdivide into several branches that form a plexiform interlacement. It occasionally divides superiorly into two branches, right and left. The left ends in the usual manner while the right opens into the right subclavian vein, in connection with the right lymphatic duct. The thoracic duct has several valves to prevent the passage of venous blood into the duct.

The cisterna chyli receives the two lumbar lymphatic trunks and the intestinal lymphatic trunk (Figure 1–37). The lumbar trunks are formed by the union of the efferent vessels from the lateral aortic lymph glands. They receive the lymph from the lower limbs, from the walls and viscera of the pelvis, from the kidneys and suprarenal glands and the deep lymphatics of the greater part of the abdominal wall. The intestinal trunk receives the lymph from the stomach and intestine, from the pancreas and spleen, and from the lower and front part of the liver.

Opening into the thoracic duct on either side is a descending trunk from the posterior intercostal lymph glands of the lower six or seven intercostal spaces. It also receives the efferents from the posterior mediastinal lymph glands and from the posterior intercostal lymph glands of the superior six left spaces. In the neck it is joined by the left jugular and left subclavian trunks. The right lymphatic duct courses along the medial border of the anterior scalene muscle at the root of the neck and ends in the right subclavian vein, at its angle of junction with the right internal jugular vein.

The right lymphatic duct receives the lymph from the right side of the head and neck through the right jugular trunk; from the right upper extremity through the right subclavian trunk; from the right side of the thorax, right lung, right side of the heart, and part of the convex surface of the liver through the right bronchomediastinal trunk. These three collecting trunks frequently open separately in the angle of union of the two veins.

There are multiple valves throughout the length of the thoracic duct, particularly in the cephalic end, which ensures unidirectional flow. The wall of the thoracic duct contains smooth muscle cells with an intrinsic contraction interval of 10–15 seconds. Movement of the chyle through the thoracic duct is modulated primarily by the intrinsic contraction of the chest wall and the pressure gradient between the abdomen and thorax. The flow rate varies between 0.4 ml/min and 4 ml/min, depending on the rate of lymph formation in the intestines and liver.

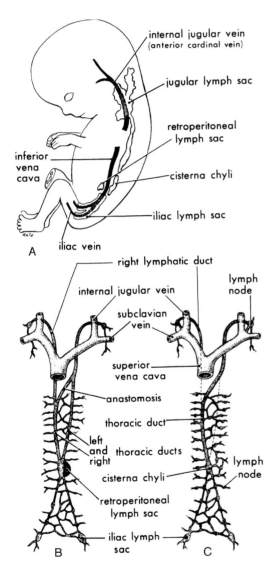

Figure 1–37. Embryonic origin of the lymphatic channels and the thoracic duct in the human embryo. **A,** Left side of a 7-week-old embryo with the six lymph sacs. **B,** Ventral view at 9 weeks showing the paired thoracic ducts. **C,** Later stage showing the formation of the adult thoracic duct and the right lymphatic duct. (From Moore KL, Persaud TVN. *The developing human,* 5th ed. Philadelphia: WB Saunders, 1993.)

Key Reading

Williams P, ed. *Gray's anatomy,* 38th ed. New York: Churchill Livingstone, 1995. *The classic textbook on thoracic anatomy.*

Selected Readings

Blevins CE. Anatomy of the thorax. In: Shields TW, ed. *General thoracic surgery.* Philadelphia: Williams & Wilkins, 1994:13–31.

Ellis H, Colborn GL, Skandalakis JE. Surgical embryology and anatomy of the breast and its related anatomic structures. *Surg Clin North Am* 1993; 73:611–632.

Kurihara Y, Yakushiji YK, Matsumoto J, *et al*. The ribs: anatomic and radiologic considerations. *Radiographics* 1999;19:105–119.

Reede DL. The thoracic inlet: normal anatomy. *Semin Ultrasound CT MR* 1996;17:509–518.

Snell R. Clinical anatomy. New York: Little, Brown & Co., 1995.

Symbas PN. Surgical anatomy of the great arteries of the thorax. *Surg Clin North Am* 1974;54: 1303–1312.

Wang NS. Anatomy of the pleura. *Clin Chest Med* 1998;19:229–240.

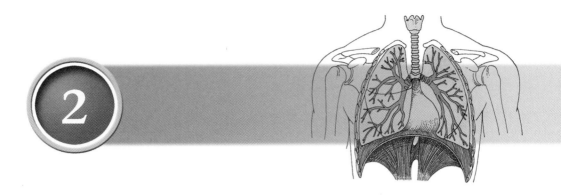

2

Pulmonary Physiology

VENTILATION

PERFUSION

PHYSIOLOGY OF BLOOD–GAS EXCHANGE

PATHOPHYSIOLOGY

Pulmonary Physiology: Key Points

- Understand the anatomic and physiological changes that occur along the airway from the trachea to the alveoli
- Describe the mechanism behind respiration
- Know the process by which oxygen passes from the alveoli into the bloodstream and finally to the target tissue
- Name the chief factors that can cause hypoxemia and hypercapnia

The lungs are responsible for oxygenating the blood that perfuses the body. They are responsible for transferring oxygen into the blood stream. The lungs occupy the greatest volume of any organ in the body, have a greater surface area and are exposed to the external environment more than any other organ except the skin. The lung is the lightest organ per volume and receives 100% of the cardiac output at the lowest perfusion of any organ.

Ventilation

Atmospheric oxygen can enter the blood stream only if it is delivered to the alveoli. Air must enter through the oropharynx or nasopharynx and then travel past the larynx into the trachea, through the conducting airways of the tracheobronchial tree, and then into the alveoli. The pressure gradient required for air movement is generated by the primary and accessory respiratory muscles. These are regulated by components of the central nervous system.

Airways

The upper airway is composed of the mouth, pharynx, and larynx. The conducting zone of the lung is composed of the trachea and the first 16 generations of the airways. This zone is the anatomical dead space because there is an absence of alveoli, and thus gas exchange is not possible while air dwells within them. The 17th to 19th generations consist of the respiratory bronchioles, from which the first alveoli emerge. This region is termed the 'transitional zone' of the lung. Generations 20–23 are lined with alveolar ducts and sacs and are known collectively as the respiratory zone (Figure 2–1).

The conducting airways distal to the pharynx have cartilaginous walls with minimal smooth muscle. They are lined with ciliated epithelium interspersed with mucus-secreting goblet cells. The cilia and mucus are involved in the clearance of inhaled or aspirated particles. The mucociliary escalator carries particles in the tracheobronchial tree to the pharynx where they are either swallowed or expectorated. The cilia beat synchronously at 1000–1500 cycles per minute and can move particles 2–10 μm in diameter at a rate of 16 nm/min. Smokers demonstrate abnormalities in both mucous production and ciliary motility that contribute to their difficulties with secretion clearance. Bronchiectasis is a condition in which the bronchi are dilated and a loss of ciliary action occurs. Secretions pool and can become chronically infected, a situation that may be associated with hemoptysis.

The transition zone is composed of membranous and terminal bronchioles. They do not contain cartilage and are innervated by the autonomic nervous system. Bronchoconstriction occurs due to cholinergic stimulation of muscarinic receptors in this zone while adrenergic receptors cause bronchodilation. Several other chemokines, including leukotrienes, thromboxane, and prostacyclins act on the bronchial lumen in this region.

The histological morphology of the respiratory zone differs markedly from the conducting and transitional zones. There are 300 million alveoli with a total surface area of around 7 mm². The only component of the alveoli that is critical to air movement is the elastin that is embedded within the basal lamina in the alveolar septal interstitium. Elastin provides elastic recoil properties that prevent hyperextension of lung tissue. There are two major types of alveolar epithelial cell. Type I cells, the major lining cells, are large, flat, squamous cells with cytoplasmic extensions and are primarily responsible for gas exchange. Type II granular pneumocytes are thicker and are responsible for producing surfactant (Figure 2–2).

Surfactant, a dipalmitoyl phosphatidylcholine, reduces alveolar surface tension, a force that decreases alveolar size and results in alveolar collapse. By Laplace's law, the distending pressure (P) required to overcome the surface tension (T) is inversely proportional to the radius (r), $P = 2T/r$. Therefore, as the alveolus gets smaller, the surfactant becomes more concentrated, and its effect on lowering the surface tension becomes more critical as a means of keeping the alveolus open. This decrease in surface tension also helps to equalize pressures within alveoli of differing sizes that would otherwise result in emptying of smaller alveoli into larger ones and subsequent collapse of smaller alveoli. Surfactant also counterbalances the hydrostatic pressure of blood. Without surfactant, unopposed surface tension would result in a hydrostatic force of 20 mm Hg pushing fluid from the blood into the alveolus. Surfactant levels are increased by thyroid hormone and glucocorticoids. They are decreased in respiratory distress syndrome, acute pancreatitis, smokers, and at high oxygen tensions. The alveoli also contain pulmonary alveolar macrophages that pass through lung capillaries into the pulmonary interstitium. These cells can phagocytose particles smaller than 2 μm.

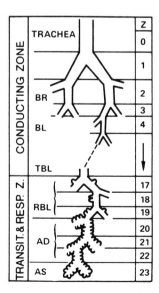

Figure 2–1. Diagram of the human bronchial tree. Gas exchange cannot take place prior to division 17, and this volume constitutes the anatomic dead space. (AD, alveolar ducts; AS, alveolar sacs; BL, bronchioli; BR, bronchi; RBL, respiratory bronchioli; TBL, terminal bronchioli; Z, number of airway generations.) (From Weibel ER. *Morphometry of the human lung.* Berlin: Springer-Verlag, 1963.)

Mechanics of Ventilation

Ventilation is achieved by air movement to and from the alveoli. Ventilation is assessed by the

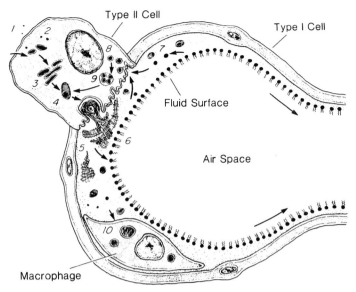

Figure 2–2. Schematic diagram of the surfactant system. A single alveolus is shown, with the location and movement of surfactant components depicted. Surfactant components are synthesized from precursors (1) in the endoplasmic reticulum (2) and transported via the Golgi apparatus (3) into lamellar bodies (4), which are the intracellular storage granules for surfactant. After secretion into the liquid that lines the alveolus, the surfactant forms tubular myelin (5), which is thought to generate the surface monolayer (6), which lowers surface tension. Subsequently, surfactant components are taken back into type II cells, possibly in the form of small vesicles (7), apparently by a specific pathway involving endosomes (8) and multivesicular bodies (9) and culminating again in storage of surfactant in lamellar bodies. Some surfactant in the liquid layer is also taken up by alveolar macrophages (10). A single transit of the phospholipid components of surfactant through the alveolar lumen normally takes a few hours. The phospholipids in the lumen are taken back into the type II cell and used approximately 10 times before being degraded. (From Hawgood S, Clements JA. Pulmonary surfactant and its apoproteins. *J Clin Invest* 1990;86:1.)

measurement of the partial pressure of arterial carbon dioxide (P_{CO_2}). Alveolar ventilation ($\dot{V}_A$) is dependent on the depth of inspiration (tidal volume, V_T), the volume of the conducting airways (dead space, V_{DS}), and the rate of respiration (R). Mathematically, alveolar ventilation can be defined as:

$$\dot{V}_A = (V_T - V_{DS}) \times R.$$

Air can move down the tracheobronchial tree when a force is generated that is sufficient to overcome the combined pressures of the elastic recoil of the lung, the frictional resistance to airflow, and the inertial resistance of the tracheobronchial air column, lungs, and chest wall (Figure 2–3). With inspiration, the increased negative pressure generated by the respiratory muscles (chiefly the diaphragm) initially overcomes the elastic recoil of the lung. Once overcome, the alveoli will enlarge. The end of inspiration is achieved when the summed forces of the elastic recoil of the lung and the chest wall equal the force generated by inspiratory muscle contraction (Figure 2–4).

The force generated by the diaphragm generates peak force at approximately 130% of its resting length. The decline in force generated with decreasing muscle length, which corresponds to an increase in resting lung volume, assumes clinical importance. For example, in chronic obstructive pulmonary disease, hyperinflation of the lung produces flattening of the diaphragm. The flattened diaphragm has a shorter length and produces less force.

The force of contraction is also a function of the frequency of muscle fiber stimulation and the velocity of fiber shortening. Up to a point, force generation increases with increasing stimulation frequency. Thereafter, force remains constant, despite further increase in stimulation frequency. Less tension is generated with higher velocities of muscle shortening. Therefore, for a given level of stimulation of the respiratory muscles, less force is generated at higher airflow rates, because higher airflow rates correlate with higher muscle shortening velocities.

During normal exhalation, the muscles of inspiration relax and the elastic recoil of the

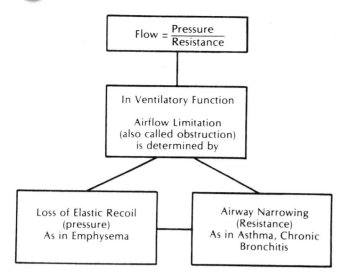

Figure 2–3. Origins of airflow. Airflow is a function of alveolar pressure and airways resistance. Expiratory pressure is caused by elastic recoil and muscular effort. Airways resistance is caused by anything that compromises the conducting air passages, such as mucus, bronchospasm, inflammation, mucosal edema, dynamic airways collapse, or combinations. (From Petty TL. Office spirometry. *Semin Respir Med* 1983;4:184.)

lung results in a passive decrease in alveolar volume, which produces a positive alveolar pressure. There is a pressure gradient for air to move out of the lungs until functional residual capacity (FRC) is reached. At this point, the alveolar and atmospheric pressures are equal; thus, there is no gradient for air movement. Additional air can be forcefully exhaled until the fixed outward recoil of the chest is equal to the force exerted by the expiratory muscles (intercostal and abdominal muscles).

The driving pressure for airflow through the entire system (from alveoli to atmosphere) is the difference between the alveolar pressure and pressure at the airway opening (atmospheric pressure; Figure 2–5). Alveolar pressure consists of two components, the elastic recoil pressure and the pleural pressure. Furthermore, elastic recoil pressure is determined by the intrinsic elastic properties of the alveoli and the degree of stretch imposed on the lung. The pleural pressure is generated by the elastic recoils of the lung and chest wall. At FRC, pleural pressure is approximately −5 cm water. It becomes more negative with deeper inspiration and more positive with forced expiration. The pressure generated within the alveoli is dissipated in overcoming the resistance to airflow, including frictional resistance.

During the respiratory cycle, alveolar forces are balanced between the elastin, which allows recoil and prevents alveolar hyperextension, and surfactant, which reduces alveolar surface tension that would cause alveolar collapse. The compliance of the lung is a measure of the resistance of the lungs to expansion (Figure 2–6). Therefore, lungs with decreased compliance require greater work to allow alveolar expansion.

Control of Ventilation

Normal ventilation is involuntary and is mediated by the respiratory center in the medulla, primarily in a dorsal nucleus and in a ventral group of nuclei (Figure 2–7). No definite pacemaker cells have yet been identified to explain the rhythmic nature of normal ventilation. Rather, one major theory suggests that within major clusters of respiratory neurons is a collection of cells whose pooled firing patterns produce inspiration and expiration – an oscillating respiratory network. Voluntary ventilation is mediated by the cerebral cortex via the corticospinal tracts. The efferent neurons from the pons and medulla are in the white matter of the spinal cord between the lateral and ventral corticospinal tracts. All of the nerves concerned with inspiration join in the ventral horns of C3–5, in the phrenic motor neurons, or in the external intercostal motor neurons, which can be found in the ventral horns throughout the thoracic spinal cord. Dysfunction of any of these neural pathways, by either local inflammation, trauma, tumor, or systemic disease, can impair the ability to create an effective negative inspiratory effort.

Inspiratory and expiratory muscles are alternately inhibited and stimulated. Inspiratory neurons are located primarily in the dorsal nuclei group of the medulla. Expiratory neurons are at either end of the ventral group of nuclei, with additional inspiratory neurons

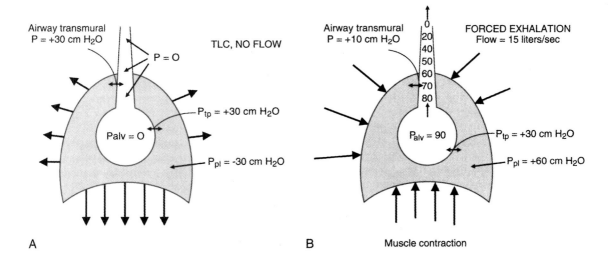

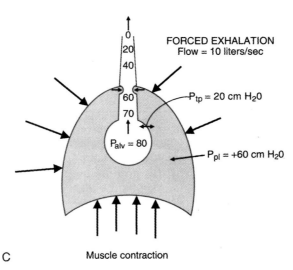

Figure 2–4. A, End inspiration, before the start of exhalation. **B**, At the start of a forced exhalation. **C**, Expiratory flow limitation later in a forced exhalation. Expiratory flow limitation occurs at locations where airway diameter is narrowed as a result of a negative transmural pressure. (From Leff AR, Schumacker PT. *Respiratory physiology: basics and applications.* Philadelphia: WB Saunders, 1993:42.)

in its midposition. Both are influenced by receptor afferents from the airways and the carotid and aortic bodies. Chemoreceptors located bilaterally in the carotid bodies and in the aortic bodies near the aortic arch are composed of type I and type II glomus cells (Figure 2–8). These cells contain several neurotransmitters, including large quantities of dopamine and other catecholamines, serotonin, acetylcholine, and several neuropeptides. Glomus cells are considered the actual chemosensing cells.

Receptors in the ventrolateral medulla are stimulated to increase ventilation by increased CO_2 or a decrease in pH. The carotid body cells are affected primarily by hypoxemia. In general, the respiratory minute volume is proportional to the metabolic rate. The effective stimuli are mediated by CO_2. Elevated CO_2 levels stimulate an increased rate and depth of inspiration, with a resultant rise in minute volume, whereas low CO_2 levels decrease the respiratory drive. In addition, there are medullary chemoreceptors that respond to

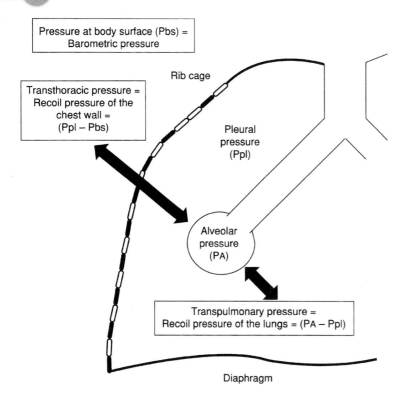

Figure 2–5. Schematic diagram illustrating the relationship between the lungs and chest wall. (From Pearson FG, Cooper JD, Deslauriers J, *et al.*, ed. *Thoracic surgery*, 2nd ed. New York: Churchill Livingstone, 2002:13.)

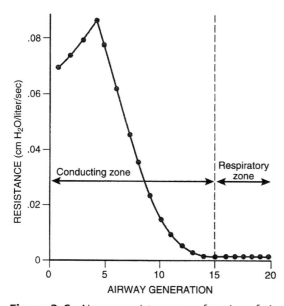

Figure 2–6. Airways resistance as a function of airway generation. In the normal lung, most of the resistance to airflow occurs in the first eight airway generations. (Redrawn from Pedley TJ, Schroter RC, Sudlow MF. The prediction of pressure drop and variation of resistance within the human bronchial airways. *Respir Physiol* 1970;9:387.)

The inherent rhythm of breathing is the result of complex interactions in the dorsal and ventral respiratory groups of the medulla that mediate the depth and the rate of breathing in response to a number of different stimuli. The pneumotaxic center in the pons is responsible for alternating between inspiration and expiration. There are stretch receptors within the lung that produce feedback signals to shut off inspiration (the Hering–Breuer reflex). These same stretch receptors indicate the degree of deflation and signal the respiratory center to initiate inspiration. Chemoreceptors also exist in the carotid and aortic bodies that respond primarily to changes in oxygen and carbon dioxide tensions. Other chemoreceptors in the ventral lateral medulla are pH-sensitive and can initiate a ventilatory effort in response to altered CO_2 levels.

Perfusion

The lung has a dual blood supply. The pulmonary circulation receives the entire cardiac output from the right ventricle under low pressure and is composed of mixed venous blood with an approximate oxygen saturation of 68–76% in normal individuals. This blood consists of the systemic venous return mixed with cardiac venous return, which enters the

cerebral spinal fluid pH, which is primarily related to the amount of dissolved CO_2 in the serum (Figure 2–9). This pH change could reflect CO_2 changes of respiratory or metabolic origin.

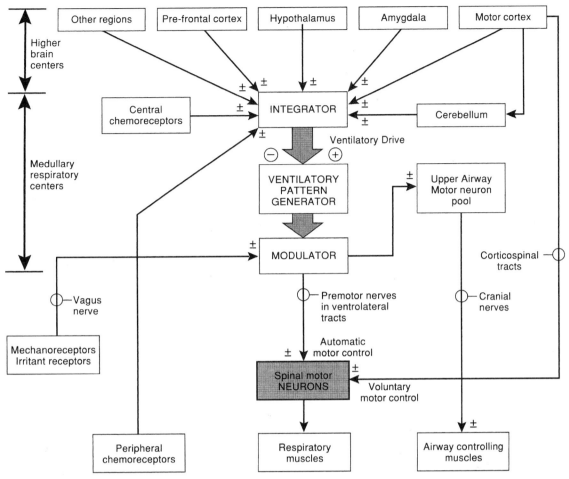

Figure 2–7. Schematic overview of the medullary respiratory control center, its inputs, and its output to the motor neurons controlling the muscles of respiration. Note that voluntary control of the respiratory muscles competes with automatic ventilatory control at the level of the respiratory muscle motor neurons. (From Leff AR, Schumacker PT. *Respiratory physiology: basics and applications.* Philadelphia: WB Saunders, 1993, p 112.)

right heart via the thesbian veins and the coronary sinus. The bronchial circulation arises from the aorta, receives only 1% of the left ventricular cardiac output and has an oxygen saturation near 100%. The pulmonary arterial vessels are thin-walled, containing much less vascular smooth muscle than the systemic vessels. This results in a vasculature that, under normal conditions, is more distensible and thus maintains relatively low pressure and low resistance within the pulmonary circulation. Normal pulmonary arterial pressure is one fifth of that of the systemic circulation.

The main pulmonary artery branches into the left and right pulmonary arteries, which subdivide into the lobar, segmental, and subsegmental branches. These are intimately related to the airways, with one or more branches of the pulmonary artery supplying each bronchopulmonary segment. These large elastic arteries give rise to the morphologically distinct arterioles that comprise the precapillary pulmonary vessels. The arterioles, capillaries, and venules comprise the microcirculation of the lung and establish the blood–air interface required for gas exchange. Other cellular components are important in the pulmonary microcirculation. Pericytes are found in the alveolar capillaries and are thought to be phagocytic and to control vascular contraction. Mast cells are found in the connective tissue of the pulmonary vessels that provide the vasoactive substances mediating pulmonary hypoxic vasoconstriction.

Blood returns to the pulmonary capillary network, pulmonary veins, and left atrium. These veins lack valves and drain into distinct superior and inferior pulmonary veins on

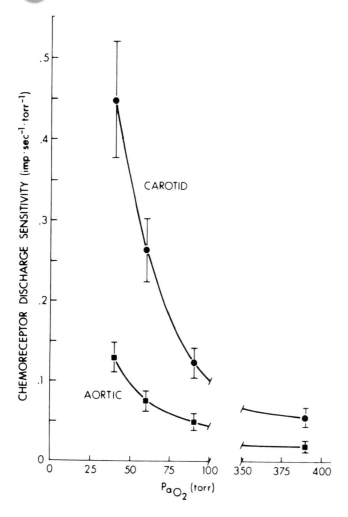

Figure 2–8. Response of aortic and carotid body receptors to hypoxia. (From Lahiri S, Mokasi A, Mulligan E, Nishino T. Comparison of aortic acid and chemoreceptor responses to hypercapnia and hypoxia. *J Appl Physiol* 1981;51:55.)

either side. They do not follow the bronchial anatomy as closely as the pulmonary distribution. Of note, some bronchial arteries drain directly into the pulmonary venous system without entering the capillary network, and contribute to physiological shunting. The lungs may contain up to 20% of the total body volume, although only 10% of that volume is in the capillaries. The velocity of flow through the capillary bed depends on cardiac output; however, a red cell passes through the alveolar–capillary gas exchange area in 0.3–0.8 seconds.

The distribution of the blood flow to the lung is not uniform. Gravity and alveolar pressures influence regional lung perfusion. Ventilation ($\dot{V}$) and perfusion ($\dot{Q}$) increase from the top to the bottom of the lung; however, $\dot{Q}$ increases more rapidly (Figure 2–10). Classic descriptions of the lung describe three zones based on the interrelationship between alveolar pressure (P_A), pulmonary arterial

pressure (P_a), and pulmonary venous pressure (P_V). Zone 1 conditions ($P_A > P_a > P_V$) are those at the apex of the lung, where pulmonary arterial pressure falls below alveolar pressure (normally close to atmospheric pressure). If this occurs, the capillaries are flattened and no flow is possible (Figure 2–11). This zone does not occur under normal conditions, because the pulmonary arterial pressure is just sufficient to raise blood to the top of the lung, but may be present if the arterial pressure is reduced (following severe hemorrhage, for example) or if alveolar pressure is raised (during positive pressure ventilation). This ventilated but unperfused lung is useless for gas exchange and is called alveolar dead space.

Further down the lung (zone 2), pulmonary arterial pressure increases because the hydrostatic effect exceeds alveolar pressure. ($P_a > P_A > P_V$) However, venous pressure is still very low and is less than alveolar pressure,

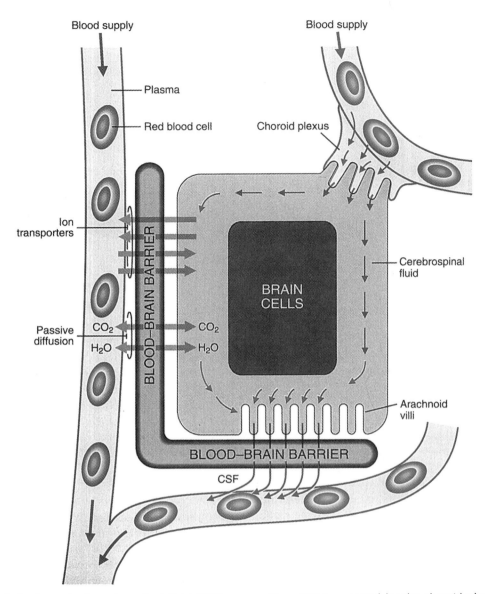

Figure 2–9. Control of cerebrospinal fluid (CSF) composition. CSF is secreted by the choroid plexus from plasma and bathes the central nervous system. Its composition reflects the extracellular environment for the brain cells. The blood–brain barrier has a low permeability to ions and separates blood from CSF. Ion transporters in the blood–brain barrier can alter the ionic composition of CSF, thereby regulating its pH. Carbon dioxide diffuses rapidly through the blood–brain barrier, so changes in arterial P_{CO_2} produce rapid parallel changes in the P_{CO_2} of the CSF. (From Leff AR, Schumacker PT. *Respiratory physiology: basics and applications.* Philadelphia: WB Saunders, 1993:118.)

and this leads to remarkable pressure–flow characteristics. Under these conditions, blood flow is determined by the difference between arterial and alveolar pressures (not the usual arterial–venous pressure difference). Indeed, venous pressure has no influence on flow unless it exceeds alveolar pressure. Since arterial pressure is increasing down the zone but alveolar pressure is the same throughout the lung, the pressure dif-

ference responsible for flow increases. In addition, increasing recruitment of capillaries occurs down this zone.

In zone 3, venous pressure exceeds alveolar pressure ($P_a > P_V > P_A$), and flow is determined in the usual way by the arterial–venous pressure difference. The increase in blood flow down this region of the lung is apparently caused by distention of the capillaries. The pressure within them (lying between arterial

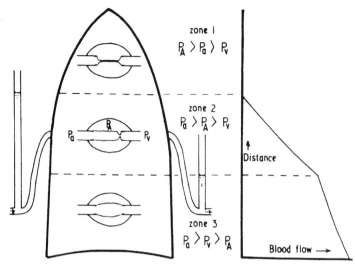

Figure 2–10. Diagram of blood flow in the isolated lung. Uneven distribution of blood flow in the lung is based on the relationship between perfusion pressure and the pressures affecting the capillaries within the lung. *Zone 1*: Alveolar pressure exceeds perfusion pressure in the apex of the lung, and theoretically, no flow occurs. This zone is unlikely to exist in healthy individuals. ($P_A > P_a > P_V$). *Zone 2*: Pulmonary arterial pressure now exceeds alveolar pressure, but alveolar pressure is greater than pulmonary venous pressure. In this zone, the capillaries behave like Starling's resistors, and flow increases down the zone owing to the increasing hydrostatic pressure that is secondary to gravitational effects; i.e. flow is determined by the arterial–alveolar pressure difference, which is the 'waterfall' area of the lung. *Zone 3*: In this area, pulmonary venous pressure exceeds alveolar pressure and flow is determined by the pulmonary arterial–venous pressure difference, which remains constant throughout the region. As the base of the lung is approached, flow can be shown to decrease despite increasing hydrostatic pressure. This area, *zone 4*, is caused by constriction of arterioles due to the increased mass of tissue that is compressed owing to the effects of gravity. This area varies and depends on the degree of expansion. With reference to previous discussion, this area decreases with increased age. (From West JB, Dollery CT, Naimark A. Distribution of blood flow in isolated lung; relation to vascular and alveolar pressures. *J Appl Physiol* 1964;19:713.)

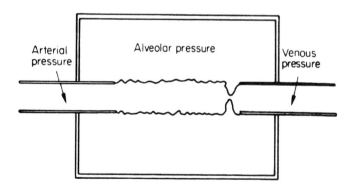

Figure 2–11. Diagram of a Starling resistor or flutter valve. The capillary network can be visualized as a collapsible tube within the alveolar pressure chamber. This model accounts for the increased blood flow down zone 2 of the lung. (From West JB. *Ventilation – blood flow and gas exchange*, 4th ed. Oxford: Blackwell, 1985.)

and venous) increases down the zone while the pressure outside (alveolar) remains constant. Thus their transmural pressure rises and, indeed, measurements show that their mean width increases. Recruitment of previously closed vessels may also play some part in the increase in blood flow down this zone.

The thin-walled arteries contain smooth muscle that dilates in response to pain, sympathetic stimulation with acetylcholine, beta-sympathetic receptor stimulation (epinephrine and norepinephrine), bradykinin, prostaglandin (PG)E$_1$, and prostacyclin. They constrict with alpha-receptor stimulation, histamine, serotonin, thromboxane A$_2$, PGF, and hypoxemia. Pulmonary arteries produce endothelial-derived relaxing factor (EDRF) or nitric oxide (NO), which have important implications towards ventilation and selective pulmonary venodilation.

Physiology of Blood–Gas Exchange

The lungs' fundamental place of gas exchange is the acinus, which composes the terminal airway and its surrounding alveoli. There are around 300 million alveoli in an adult lung; each one is 0.25 mm in diameter. The total available surface area available for gas exchange is around 100 m². The alveoli are interdigitated with a capillary network. The alveolar-capillary border is anywhere from 0.2–0.3 mm thick, permitting the rapid exchange of gaseous compounds.

Gas exchange occurs at the alveolar level at the interface of the alveolar epithelium and the capillary endothelium (Figure 2–12). The alveoli are outpouchings of the respiratory bronchioles, alveolar ducts, and alveolar sacs. The alveolar septa are made up of a continuous flattened epithelium comprising type I and type II alveolar epithelial cells covering a thin layer of interstitial tissue. Type I alveolar cells cover approximately 95% of the alveolar surface and

functionally are involved in resorbing pathological alveolar fluid or ingesting intra-alveolar particulate material. The type II epithelial cells are the source of alveolar surfactant and are also involved in the renewal of the alveolar surface by differentiation into type I cells. A continuous basal lamina underlies both type I and type II cells and is in apposition to the underlying endothelial cell. The alveolar septal interstitium is also composed of connective tissue made of a proteoglycan matrix embedded with elastin and collagen. Alveolar macrophages are important in clearance of intra-alveolar material, production of inflammatory mediators, and antigen presentation.

After delivery of oxygen to the alveoli, it diffuses through the alveolar–capillary interface. At the blood–air interface, there are approximately 500 million alveoli with a combined surface area of 100 m². Thus 120 L of air will come into contact with 25 L of blood per minute. For oxygen to be delivered to the blood, it must first dissolve into the layer of pulmonary surfactant, thus moving from the

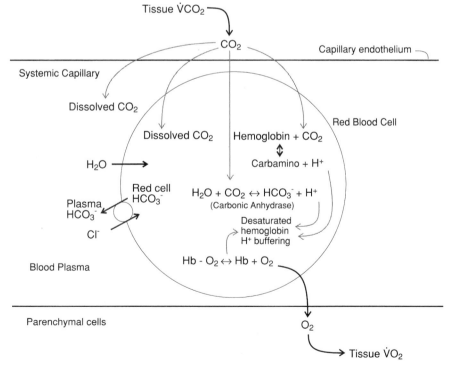

Figure 2–12. Summary of events that occur as a red blood cell passes through a systemic capillary. Oxygen unloading along the capillary is enhanced by increases in Pco_2 and decreases in pH (the Bohr effect), while CO_2 loading into blood is enhanced by the simultaneous desaturation of hemoglobin (the Haldane effect). Most of the oxygen is bound to hemoglobin in the red blood cells, whereas most of the bicarbonate produced in the red blood cells is transported to the plasma. (From Leff AR, Schumacker PT. *Respiratory physiology: basics and applications.* Philadelphia: WB Saunders, 1993:81.)

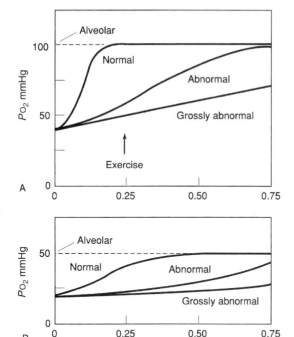

Figure 2–13. Alveolar capillary Po_2 versus the amount of time spent in the capillary by deoxygenated blood. **A,** Graph is plotted with normal alveolar Po_2 levels. **B,** Graph is plotted with an alveolar Po_2 of 50 mm Hg. Both graphs are plotted with normal and abnormal alveolar membranes. Normal capillary transit time is approximately 0.75 sec and may be reduced to as little as 0.25 sec during exercise or other states of high cardiac output. End-capillary Po_2 is a function of transit time, alveolar membrane function, and alveolar Po_2. (From West JB. *Respiratory physiology – the essentials*, 3rd ed. Baltimore: Williams & Wilkins, 1985:28.)

gas phase to the liquid phase. Oxygen then diffuses through the alveolar epithelium, interstitium, and capillary endothelium and into the plasma. Once in the plasma, some oxygen will remain dissolved. However, the majority of oxygen enters the erythrocyte, where it becomes bound to hemoglobin (Figure 2–13).

The relationship between ventilation and perfusion determines alveolar and thus arterial Po_2 and Pco_2. Ideally, alveolar ventilation and perfusion should allow for complete hemoglobin saturation and removal of sufficient carbon dioxide to result in a normal pH level. This does not occur uniformly, as described by the different zones of the lung. The extremes of these ratios are pure shunts (low $\dot{V}/\dot{Q}$) or pure dead space (high $\dot{V}/\dot{Q}$). Under normal conditions, alveolar Po_2 is 100 mm Hg and Pco_2 is 40 mm Hg. The mixed venous blood in the pulmonary arterial system has a Po_2 of

about 40 mm Hg and a Pco_2 of 45 mm Hg. The resulting gradients favor diffusion of oxygen into the blood and carbon dioxide into the alveolar space.

The amount of air inhaled does not equal the amount of gas seen by alveoli because of the inherent dead space in the conducting airways. On inspiration, the amount of gas reaching the alveoli (V_A) is less than the tidal volume (V_T) and is dependent on the volume of the dead space (V_{DS}):

$$V_A = V_T - V_{DS}.$$

In each breath, the vast majority of gas is not exchanged. Each breath increases the alveolar P_AO_2 and decreases the alveolar P_ACO_2 by only 5% to 10%. The small changes are due to the buffer effect of the gas remaining in the lungs at the end of a normal breath (the functional residual capacity, FRC). Normal V_A is 300 cc and the normal FRC is 3 liters.

The pulmonary arterial blood enters the lung with a mixed venous oxygen tension and a mixed venous carbon dioxide tension that is determined by the cardiac output and the metabolic rate of tissues. In blood, oxygen is carried both in dissolved form and on hemoglobin. Hemoglobin is composed of globin folded around heme, an iron-containing O_2 carrier. Each gram of hemoglobin can bind up to 1.39 mL O_2. The strength with which O_2 binds to the heme molecule decreases with each of four binding sites in a non-linear fashion called the oxyhemoglobin dissociation curve (Figure 2–14). The dissolved oxygen comprises only a small amount of the oxygen carried in the blood. The oxygen content of the blood can be described by:

$$O_2 \text{ content (mL/dL blood)} = \text{(Hemoglobin content in grams)} \times (1.39) \times (O_2 \text{ saturation}) + 0.003 \times Po_2.$$

Many factors influence the relation between the partial pressure of oxygen and the blood content (Table 2–1). Factors that are involved in increased O_2 use (increased Pco_2 and higher temperature and reduced pH) decrease the affinity of the hemoglobin for O_2, causing a rightward shift of the curve, and facilitate the release of O_2 to tissues. The leftward shift causes increased loading of O_2 by hemoglobin. Factors such as increased production of 2,3-diphosphoglycerate move the curve to the right. Carbon monoxide competes with O_2 for hemoglobin binding sites and shifts the curve to the left. Temperature and acidosis similarly affect curve movement. Increased adenosine

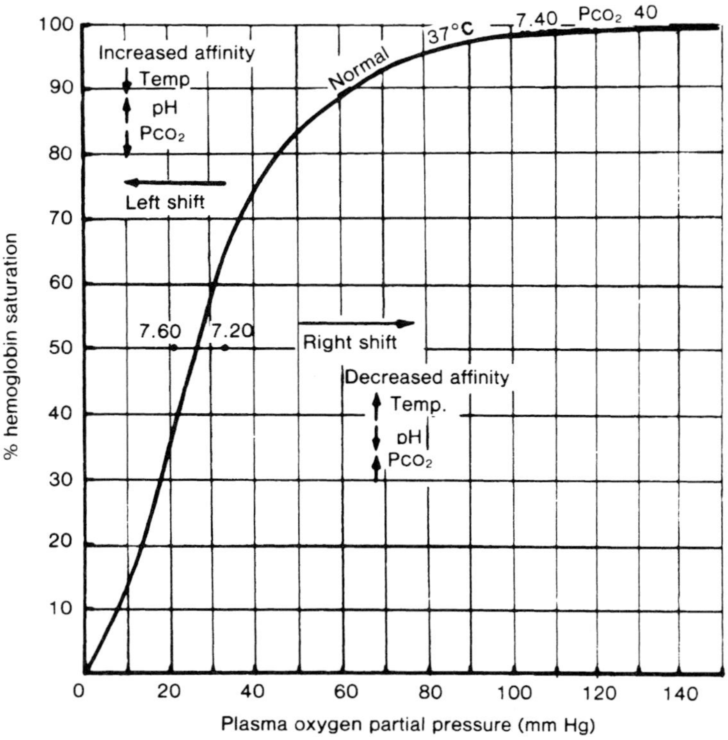

Figure 2–14. The oxygen–hemoglobin dissociation curve. This figure highlights the effects of temperature and acid-base as well as the effect of changes in the partial pressure of carbon dioxide on the curve. The points 7.6 and 7.2 represent the left and right shifts that occur secondary to pH. (From Margand PMD, Brooks CG Jr, Hunter JW. *Preoperative pulmonary preparation: a clinical guide.* Baltimore: Williams & Wilkins, 1981.)

TABLE 2–1 • *Factors that Influence the Relation Between the Partial Pressure of Oxygen and the Blood Content*	
Factors that Decrease the Affinity of the Hemoglobin for O_2 (Right-shift)	**Factors that Increase the Affinity of the Hemoglobin for O_2 (Left-shift)**
Hypercapnia	Carbon monoxide
Acidosis	Alkalosis
Increased production of 2,3-diphosphoglycerate	Hypocapnia
Increased adenosine triphosphate	Hypothermia
Increased cortisol levels	
Increased aldosterone levels	
Hyperthermia	
Exercise	
Propranolol	

triphosphate (ATP) concentrations, cortisol levels and aldosterone levels move the curve to the right.

After oxygenation within the lungs, arterial blood is distributed to the body where oxygen is released and diffuses into tissues. Oxygen delivery to peripheral tissues and oxygen consumption by organs can be calculated based on oxygen content:

O_2 delivery (mL/dL blood) = Cardiac output × O_2 content (mL/dL blood).

O_2 consumption (mL/dL blood) = Cardiac output × (arterial O_2 content − venous O_2 content).

In situations where arterial oxygen content remain constant, a fall in the mixed venous saturation indicates a fall in cardiac output. Clinically, a mixed venous specimen for oxygen saturation can be used as a 'poor man's cardiac output.'

Carbon dioxide is transported through the blood in three forms: 90% as bicarbonate,

5% carried by hemoglobin, and 5% dissolved in plasma. In contrast to the frequent problems with oxygen, problems with CO_2 gas exchange become clinically important only with advanced pulmonary disease. CO_2 is 20 times more soluble in blood than oxygen and rapidly forms carbonic acid.

The rate at which oxygen and carbon dioxide can transfer between the alveoli and pulmonary arterial blood depends on:

- the inspired gas concentration
- the mixed venous oxygen tension and mixed venous carbon dioxide tension
- the diffusion capacity of the alveoli–capillary interface
- the ratio of ventilation to perfusion ($\dot{V}/\dot{Q}$) in each acinus.

The rate of diffusion of a gas, governed by Fick's law of diffusion, is proportional to the area available for diffusion, the diffusion coefficient of a particular gas, and the partial pressure gradient across the barrier, and is inversely proportional to the thickness of the barrier. The area available for diffusion is relatively constant; however, during exercise, additional capillaries can be recruited, thus increasing diffusion. In hypovolemia, the reverse may be true. The diffusion coefficient is proportional to the solubility of a given gas and inversely proportional to its molecular weight. When comparing oxygen and carbon dioxide, although carbon dioxide is larger than oxygen, it is about 25 times more soluble in the liquid phase and thus diffuses more rapidly through the air–blood barrier. The diffusing capacity of oxygen is difficult to measure, so the diffusing capacity of carbon monoxide ($D_L CO$) is measured.

Pathophysiology

Hypoxemia

Hypoxemia can result from four distinct processes: hypoventilation, diffusion gradients, shunt, and ventilation/perfusion mismatch.

Hypoventilation

Hypoventilation can be caused by drugs (opiates, barbiturates), mechanical impairments of the chest wall (painful incisions and binders), and paralysis of the respiratory muscles (muscular dystrophy, polio virus, and neuromuscular blockade). Since the level

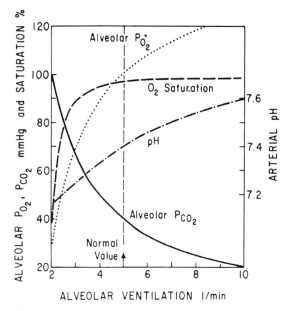

Figure 2–15. Changes in gas exchange during hypoventilation. Note the rapid rise in P_{CO_2}, compared with the so-called slow fall in arterial oxygen saturation. (From West JB. *Pulmonary pathophysiology: the essentials.* Baltimore: Williams & Wilkins, 1977.)

of alveolar P_{O_2} is a function of the balance between oxygen supply and oxygen consumed, any process that causes hypoventilation will cause the alveolar P_{O_2} to drop. As a result of hypoventilation, there is a subsequent rise in alveolar P_{CO_2} (Figure 2–15). This relationship can be described by the alveolar gas equation:

$$P_A O_2 = P_{INSP} O_2 - P_A CO_2/(0.8).$$

Hypoventilation is always accompanied by hypercarbia and is secondary to a low minute ventilation, either on the basis of low tidal volume or rate. The addition of supplemental oxygen to the inspired gas of a hypoventilating patient will readily overcome the hypoxia of hypoventilation.

Increased diffusion gradients

Increased diffusion gradients cause failure of equilibration between the hemoglobin in the red cell and the gas in the alveoli. Under normal conditions the red cell has fully equilibrated with alveolar oxygen within one third of its passage through the alveolar capillary. However, any process such as collagen vascular disease, sarcoidosis, and idiopathic interstitial fibrosis can cause arterial hypoxemia.

Shunt

Shunt, another cause of hypoxemia, is the fraction of blood that enters the systemic arterial system without passing through a ventilated portion of the lung. Shunts occur because of intracardiac communications such as occur in congenital heart disease, arteriovenous malformations of the lung, lung consolidation (i.e. pneumonia), and the use of vasodilators such as nitroprusside. Of the four causes of hypoxemia, shunt is the only one that cannot be corrected by oxygen therapy because the shunted blood is never exposed to the airway. Also unlike the other three causes, P_aco_2 is typically low to normal. An approximation of the shunt can be described by:

$$\text{Shunt flow/total flow} = \dot{Q}_S/\dot{Q}_T$$
$$= (F_iO_2/2) - (P_aO_2/10).$$

A calculated shunt of less than 10% is compatible with normal lungs, 10–20% is rarely of clinical importance, 20–30% indicates significant pulmonary disease, and greater than 30% is life-threatening.

Ventilation/perfusion mismatch

Finally, ventilation/perfusion mismatch (i.e. 'partial shunting') is the most common cause of hypoxemia. Conditions, such as oversedation, chronic obstructive pulmonary disease, and the inability to take a deep breathe, that describe perfusion exceeding ventilation (shunts) or ventilation exceeding perfusion (dead space) create a mismatch. In patients with pulmonary disease, the lung will have alveoli with varying $\dot{V}/\dot{Q}$ ratios (Figure 2–16). The hyperventilatory response to hypoxia, which results from chemoreceptors at the carotid bifurcation and below the aortic arch, is more effective in correcting hypercarbia than hypoxia. Thus the net result of $\dot{V}/\dot{Q}$ mismatch is hypoxemia and hyperventilation. Ventilation/perfusion mismatch is diagnosed primarily by exclusion of the other three causes of hypoxia.

Pulmonary blood flow can be actively redistributed to optimize the $\dot{V}/\dot{Q}$ relationship by a process called 'hypoxic pulmonary vasoconstriction.' Alveolar hypoxia (Po_2 <70 mm Hg), hypercarbia, or collapse results in local pulmonary arteriolar vasoconstriction. The exact mechanism for this response remains unclear but may involve local release of vasoactive mediators. This vasoconstriction will divert blood from areas that will undergo little gas exchange (low $\dot{V}/\dot{Q}$), thus lowering Po_2 and increasing Pco_2 to areas that are better ventilated (high $\dot{V}/\dot{Q}$).

Hypercapnia

An increase in P_aCO_2 is often due to a compensation for an underlying metabolic alkalosis. However, if this is not the case, other primary respiratory causes need to be considered. The CO_2 level in arterial blood is directly proportional to the rate of CO_2 production by oxidative metabolism ($\dot{V}CO_2$) and inversely proportional to the rate of CO_2 elimination by alveolar ventilation ($\dot{V}_A$). Alveolar ventilation is the fraction of the total expired ventilation ($\dot{V}_E$) that is not dead space ventilation ($\dot{V}_d/\dot{V}_E$). Therefore,

$$P_aco_2 \text{ is proportional to } (\dot{V}co_2/\dot{V}A)$$
$$= (\dot{V}co_2)/[(\dot{V}_E)(1-\dot{V}_d/\dot{V}_E)].$$

From this equation, it can deducted that there are three major sources of hypercapnia:

- Increased CO_2 production ($\dot{V}co_2$)
- Hypoventilation
- Increased dead space ventilation ($\dot{V}_d/\dot{V}_E$).

Increased CO_2 production ($\dot{V}CO_2$)

Increased CO_2 production (i.e. hypermetabolism) is normally accompanied by an increase in minute ventilation. The ventilatory response tends to eliminate excess CO_2 and maintain a constant arterial Pco_2. Therefore, excess CO_2 production does not normally cause hypercapnia. However, when CO_2 exertion is prevented by an increase in dead space ventilation, an increase in CO_2 production can result in an increase in the arterial Pco_2. Therefore, increased CO_2 production is relevant in causing hypercapnia in patients with underlying lung disease. The rate of CO_2 production can be measured at the bedside by metabolic carts that assess body nutritional status. They measure total CO_2 excreted per minute. The normal $\dot{V}co_2$ is 90–130 L/min/m^2, which is roughly 80% of the $\dot{V}o_2$. An increase in $\dot{V}co_2$ is evidence for one of the following abnormalities: generalized hypermetabolism, overfeeding, or organic acidoses.

Hypoventilation

Increased alveolar hypoventilation can occur due to either a primary neurological defect or a muscular process. Oversedation with narcotics, obesity, shock, myasthenia gravis or

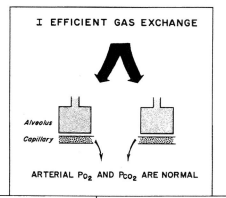

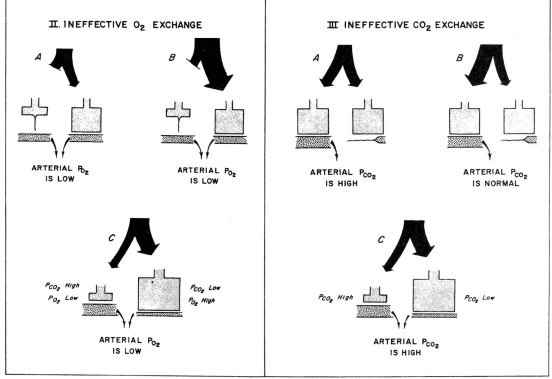

Figure 2–16. Variations in ventilation and perfusion that cause disturbances in exchange of oxygen and carbon dioxide. **I,** Adequate and well-matched ventilation and perfusion maintain normal arterial oxygenation and elimination of carbon dioxide. **IIA, IIB,** Collapse of terminal airway leads to arterial hypoxemia even if ventilation to unaffected areas increases. The reduction in P_{O_2} depends on the amount of blood that continues to flow through the collapsed pulmonary segments. Alveolar hypoxia invokes hypoxic pulmonary vasoconstriction, which tends to limit the amount of wasted perfusion or 'shunt' blood flow. **IIC,** Marked maldistribution of ventilation and perfusion can also lead to hypoxia (i.e. if most of the perfusion goes to poorly ventilated areas, inefficient gas exchange results). This condition is seen in later examples as the patient's position or cardiac output is changed. **III,** Continued ventilation of a nonperfused alveolus results in wasted or dead-space ventilation. In addition, hypotension or reduced cardiac output can result in reduced perfusion of ventilated alveoli with similar effects. In the presence of dead-space units, an increase in total minute ventilation can accommodate rising CO_2 tension and return P_{CO_2} levels to normal limits. Therefore, it is important to look not only at blood gas results when assessing the respiratory status of a patient but also at the effort required to obtain the measured values. Dead space can obviously be seen to be of two types: (1) Anatomic dead space ($V_{D\ anat}$) – areas of conducting airways in which no blood-gas exchange occurs; and (2) alveolar dead space ($V_{D\ alv}$) – areas of lung parenchyma in which blood–gas exchange is expected but is decreased as a result of, for example, pulmonary embolism or hypoperfusion. The total contribution of dead space is the sum of (1) and (2) and is called the physiologic dead space ($V_{D\ phys}$). (From Sabiston DC Jr, Spencer FC. *Surgery of the chest*, 6th ed. Philadelphia: WB Saunders, 1995:25.)

other neuromuscular diseases may result in a decreased drive to move gas. Opiates and benzodiazepines are the most common culprits causing hypoventilation. Muscular weakness can also cause alveolar hypoventilation. The standard measure for evaluating respiratory muscle strength is the maximum inspiratory pressure (MIP) and maximal voluntary ventilation (MVV). Most healthy adults have an MIP above 80 cm H_2O. Carbon dioxide retention develops when the MIP falls to less than 40% normal value.

Increased dead space ventilation ($\dot{V}_d/\dot{Q}_E$)

Dead space ventilation increases when the alveolar–capillary interface is destroyed (i.e. emphysema), when blood flow is reduced (e.g. heart failure, pulmonary embolus) or when alveoli are overdistended by positive pressure ventilation.

End-tidal carbon dioxide can often be measured off ventilators. This attempts to approximate P_aCO_2. Typically, end-tidal CO_2 is 5 mm Hg higher than arterial carbon dioxide levels. An increasing gradient between end-tidal carbon dioxide and arterial carbon dioxide suggests increased dead space ventilation. A proportionate increase in end-tidal carbon dioxide and arterial carbon dioxide indicates the patient is either hypoventilating or increasing metabolic activity.

Key Readings

West JB. *Respiratory physiology*. Baltimore: Williams & Wilkins, 1990. *Classic textbook that should be part of any thoracic surgeon's library.*

West JB. *Pulmonary pathophysiology – the essentials.* Baltimore: Williams & Wilkins, 1998. *By the same author; attempts to describe the physiology behind hypoxia and hypercapnia.*

Selected Readings

Ferguson GT, Enright PL, Buist AS, Higgins MW. Office spirometry for lung health assessment in adults: a consensus statement from the National Lung Health Education Program. *Chest* 2000;117:1146–1161.

Grippi MA. *Pulmonary pathophysiology*. Lippincott's pathophysiology series. Philadelphia: JB Lippincott, 1995.

Hlastala MR, Thomas H. *Complexity in structure and function of the lung.* Lung biology in health and disease 121. New York: Marcel Dekker, 1998.

Palecek F. Hyperinflation: control of functional residual lung capacity. *Physiol Res* 2001;50:221–230.

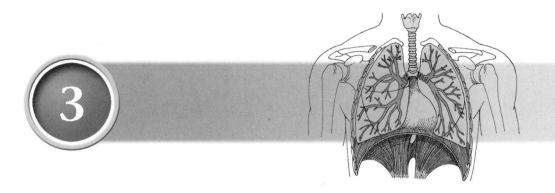

Perioperative Care

PULMONARY FUNCTION TESTS
PREOPERATIVE ASSESSMENT
POSTOPERATIVE CARE

MECHANICAL VENTILATION
ACUTE RESPIRATORY DISTRESS
SYNDROME

Perioperative Care: Key Points

- Recognize who needs a preoperative assessment
- Know the tests that should be performed prior to operative management
- Describe the spectrum of pulmonary function tests and the indications for each
- Know the options for mechanical ventilation
- Know the pathophysiology and current aspects of management of acute respiratory distress syndrome

Pulmonary Function Tests

Pulmonary function tests provide an objective measurement of lung function. An enormous amount of pulmonary function parameters can be measured (Table 3–1). The main categories of data that are helpful in assessing pulmonary function include static lung volumes, dynamic lung volumes, diffusing capacity, respiratory muscle strength, and arterial blood gas.

Static lung volumes

Static lung volumes describe several properties that exist when there is no airflow in or out of the lungs. By convention, maximally inflated lungs and airways are described by being filled with four separate volumes of gas and four capacities (Figure 3–1).

The four static lung volumes conventionally described are as follows:

- *Tidal volume (TV)* is the volume of gas inspired with each normal breath. The metabolic needs of a patient and the efficiency of gas exchange determine the minute ventilation.
- *Residual volume (RV)* is the volume of gas remaining in the lung following a maximal expiratory effort. In young individuals, RV is determined by the combined effect of the

TABLE 3–1 • *Typical Values in Pulmonary Function Tests*

These values are for a healthy, resting, recumbent young man (1.7 m² surface area) breathing air at sea level, unless other conditions are specified. They are presented to give approximate figures. These values may change with position, age, size, sex, and altitude; there is variability among members of a homogeneous group under standard conditions.

Pulmonary Volumes	
Inspiratory capacity, mL	3600
Expiratory reserve volume, mL	1200
Vital capacity, mL	4800
Residual volume (RV), mL	1200
Functional residual capacity, mL	2400
Thoracic gas volume, mL	2400
Total lung capacity (TLC), mL	6000
RV/TLC × 100, %	20
Ventilation	
Tidal volume, mL	500
Frequency, respirations/min	12
Minute volume, mL/min	6000
Respiratory dead space, mL	150
Alveolar ventilation, mL/min	4200
Distribution of Inspired Gas	
Single-breath test (% increase N_2 for 500 mL expired alveolar gas), % N_2	<1.5
Pulmonary nitrogen emptying rate (7 min test) % N_2	<2.5
Helium closed circuit (mixing efficiency related to perfect mixing), %	76
Diffusion and Gas Exchange	
O_2 consumption (STPD), mL/min	240
CO_2 output (STPD), mL/min	192
Respiratory exchange ratio, R (CO_2) output/O_2 uptake)	0.8
Diffusing capacity, O_2 (STPD) resting, mL O_2/min/mm Hg	>15
Diffusing capacity, CO (steady state) (STPD) resting, mL CO/min/mm Hg	17
Diffusing capacity, CO (single-breath) (STPD) resting, mL CO/min/mm Hg	25
Diffusing capacity, CO (rebreathing) (STPD) resting mL CO/min/mm Hg	25
Alveolar Ventilation/Pulmonary Capillary Blood Flow	
Alveolar ventilation (L/min) blood flow, L/min	0.8
Physiologic shunt/cardiac output × 100, %	<7
Physiologic dead space/tidal volume × 100, %	<30
Pulmonary Circulation	
Pulmonary capillary blood flow, mL/min	5400
Pulmonary artery pressure, mm Hg	25/8
Pulmonary capillary blood volume, mL	75–100
Pulmonary 'capillary' blood pressure (wedge), mm Hg	8
Alveolar Gas	
Oxygen partial pressure, mm Hg	104
CO_2 partial pressure, mm Hg	40
Arterial Blood	
O_2 saturation (% saturation of Hb with O_2), %	97.1
O_2 tension, mm Hg	100
CO_2 tension, mm Hg	40

TABLE 3-1 • *Typical Values in Pulmonary Function Tests (Continued)*

Alveolar–arterial PO_2 difference (100% O_2), mm Hg	33
O saturation (100% O_2), %	100
O_2 tension (100% O_2), mm Hg	640
pH	7.4
Mechanics of Breathing	
Maximal voluntary ventilation, L/min	125–170
Forced expiratory volume, % in 1 sec	83
% in 3 sec	97
Maximal expiratory flow rate (for 1 L), L/min	400
Maximal inspiratory flow rate (for 1 L), L/min	300
Compliance of lungs and thoracic cage, L/cm H_2O	0.1
Compliance of lungs, L/cm H_2O	0.2
Airway resistance, cm H_2O/L/sec	1.6
Work of quiet breathing, kg-M/min	0.5
Maximal work of breathing, kg-M/breath	10
Maximal inspiratory and expiratory pressure, mm Hg	60–100

From Comroe JH Jr. *The lung*, 2nd ed. Chicago: Year Book, 1962.

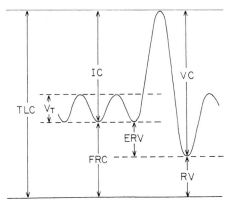

Figure 3-1. Spirometry. Subdivision of lung volumes. TLC, total lung capacity; V_T, tidal volume; IC, inspiratory capacity; FRC, functional residual capacity, i.e. lung volume at end-expiration; ERV, expiratory reserve volume; RV, residual volume, i.e. lung volume after forced expiration from FRC; VC, vital capacity, i.e. the maximal volume of gas inspired from RV. (From Sabiston DC Jr. *Textbook of surgery: the biological basis of modern surgical practice*, 15th ed. Philadelphia: WB Saunders, 1997:1787.)

expiratory muscles and the inward recoil of the lung to compress the chest wall. With obstructive lung disease, maximal expiratory flow at low lung volumes becomes small. Patients with severe airway obstruction are unable to maintain an expiratory effort long enough to reach minimum volume. In patients with chronic obstructive pulmonary disease, expiratory flow never

ceases completely. They produce a small expiratory flow until they can no longer resist the urge to inspire.

- *Expiratory reserve volume (ERV)*: Functional residual capacity (FRC) − RV.
- *Inspiratory reserve volume (IRV)*: Total lung capacity (TLC) − (FRC + TV).

Pulmonary volumes can be described by four capacities.

- *Total lung capacity (TLC)* is a sum of these four volumes and can be described by a single equation:

$$TLC = IRV + TV + ERV + RV.$$

Total lung capacity is the amount of gas contained within the lung during a maximal voluntary inspiratory effort. It is determined by the balance between the maximal inspiratory force arising from the respiratory muscles and the opposing expiratory force applied by the elastic properties of the lung and chest wall. The major muscles involved in inspiration to TLC are the diaphragm and the inspiratory intercostal muscles. Increases in TLC occur when there are reductions in the inward elastic recoil of the lung. This occurs most commonly with the destruction of the elastic alveolar walls of the lung parenchyma by emphysema. TLC may be decreased by a variety of factors unrelated to pulmonary disease. TLC can be underestimated when inspiratory effort is impaired or when pain arising from the lung, pleura, chest wall, or abdomen produces conscious or reflex inhibition of inspiration. Neuromuscular diseases or muscle weakness due to metabolic abnormalities can reduce maximal inspiratory force. Skeletal abnormalities of the spine or rib cage, increased abdominal volume due to ascites or pregnancy, and morbid obesity overloading both abdomen and rib cage also reduce TLC.

- *Vital capacity (VC)* is the volume of air that can be inspired or expired by alternating between maximal inspiratory and expiratory efforts. Mathematically it can be expressed as: VC = TLC − RV. VC is a sensitive but nonspecific test of lung function. VC is usually reduced in moderate to severe acute or chronic airway obstruction because RV is increased much more than TLC.
- *Functional residual capacity (FRC)* is the volume of gas remaining in the lungs at end-expiration. At FRC, the inward elastic recoil of the lung is balanced by the outward elastic recoil of the chest wall, producing a negative pleural pressure.
- *Inspiratory capacity (IC)*: TV + IRV.

Total gas in the lungs is commonly measured by one of three methods:

- Washout of an inert gas (N_2)
- Equilibration with an inert test gas (helium)
- Whole-body plethysmography.

Lung volume measurements initially determine FRC because that lung volume is most easily reproduced by the patient and is independent of patient compliance. Exhalation from FRC gives the ERV. RV can then be calculated by subtracting ERV from FRC. TLC can be calculated by adding the VC to RV.

Accurate measurements of lung volume done by washing out nitrogen or by equilibrating with an inert gas (helium) requires that the test gas communicate to or from all compartments of the lung. All gas-containing compartments must be freely washed out or exchanged. Poorly communicating blebs or bullae can cause lung volumes to be significantly underestimated when using N_2 washout or helium dilution techniques. Lung volumes can also be measured by body plethysmography, which involves placing the subject in a large airtight box and breathing through a mouthpiece connected to the outside. A shutter occludes the mouthpiece and, as the patient breathes rapidly over a closed shutter, the volume of gas in the chest is compressed and expanded, creating a similar change in gas volume in the box. This process allows all gas contained in the thorax to be measured.

Dynamic Lung Volumes

Dynamic measurements of lung volume can be obtained by spirometric measurements. Three variables remain the most useful though in predicting pulmonary function: FEV_1, FVC, and the ratio of FEV_1:FVC. FVC (forced vital capacity) is the maximal volume of gas that can be exhaled during a forced exhalation beginning at TLC. FEV_1 is the volume of gas that can be exhaled during the first 1 second of a forced exhalation maneuver beginning at TLC.

Non-smokers lose FEV_1 at a rate of 20–30 mL/year. In some smokers, this rate of decline can increase by two- or threefold. The magnitude of functional impairment in obstructive lung disease can be assessed using pulmonary function testing. When a predicted FEV_1 is close to 4 L, the patient should not have a history of significant exercise impairment until the FEV_1 falls below 3 L/second. If the FEV_1 is 2–3 L/second, this would be consistent with mild exercise limitation. An FEV_1 of 1–2 L/second correlates with a moderate degree of exercise impairment. Anything less would suggest severe exercise impairment. In combination with history and physical examination, these results can be quite powerful in predicting pulmonary function.

Reductions in FEV_1:FVC reflect significant airway obstruction that may be related to spasm, secretions, compression, or an intraluminal mass. Therapy may entail bronchodilators, mucolytic agents, suctioning, bronchoscopy, relief of airway compression, or removal of an endobronchial mass. A reduced FEV_1 usually reflects the presence of chronic obstructive pulmonary disease, which may have an active (reversible) component (bronchospasm) as opposed to a fixed irreversible defect. For this reason, FEV_1 measurements are usually obtained with and without bronchodilators to help identify therapeutic possibilities.

$FEF_{25\%-75\%}$ (forced mid-expiratory flow) is another useful measurement of airway obstruction. This measurement is defined by the slope (volume vs time) of the line between the points at 25% and 75% on the expiratory curve. To perform these flow measurements, the patient is asked to inspire maximally to TLC and then, with maximal forced expiratory effort, air is blown out of the lungs to RV. Using a spirometer, air volumes can be measured as a function of time, and the FEV_1, FVC, $FEF_{25\%-75\%}$, and other volumes can be determined.

Diffusing Capacity

The diffusing capacity (D_LCO) of the lung is defined as the lung's ability to take up an inhaled non-reactive test gas, such as carbon monoxide, which binds to hemoglobin with a high affinity. Thus virtually all the CO that reaches an alveolar space crosses the alveolar air–blood barrier and reaches a red cell. Measurements of lung diffusing capacity are critically influenced by three parameters:

- The ability of the test gas to reach the alveolar gas-exchanging surfaces
- The ability of the test gas to cross the alveolar septa
- The mass of the red cells in the pulmonary capillary bed available to bind the test gas.

Respiratory Muscle Strength

To evaluate problems with muscle contraction, a patient can be asked to make a maximal inspiratory or expiratory effort against a pressure gauge, and the resultant pressure, generated isometrically, is measured. The force developed by the respiratory muscles are directly related to the lung volume. Maximal inspiratory pressure (MIP) is achieved at the smallest lung volume (RV) when the length–tension relationship of the diaphragm is optimized. Conversely, maximal expiratory pressure (MEP) is achieved at total lung capacity.

A useful test of the patient's overall pulmonary function, including muscle strength, is the maximal voluntary ventilation (MVV). In this maneuver, the patient breathes as rapidly and as deeply as possible over a 12-second interval. The resultant exhaled volume is measured and extrapolated over a minute. Empirically, it has been observed that the MVV is 35–40 times the FEV_1.

Arterial Blood Gas

Acid–base analysis is a useful adjunct to pulmonary function testing. There are four primary acid–base disorders: respiratory acidosis and alkalosis, and metabolic acidosis and alkalosis.

When hypercapnia ($P_aCO_2 > 44$ mmHg) arises as a result of alveolar hypoventilation or significant ventilation–perfusion mismatching, respiratory acidosis develops. A rise in P_aCO_2 produces a fall in pH. A persistent increase in CO_2 stimulates the renal tubular cells to secrete hydrogen ions and to retain HCO_3^-. As a consequence, serum bicarbonate concentrate rises, tending to restore pH towards normal. The pH is not completely restored to normal; however, the process is referred to as a compensated respiratory acidosis. The increase in bicarbonate from renal compensation is termed the base excess.

When hypocapnia ($P_aCO_2 < 36$ mmHg) arises as a result of alveolar hyperventilation, respiratory alkalosis develops. Although bicarbonate concentration falls, pH rises. With persistent hypocapnia, renal tubular cells excrete additional bicarbonate, restoring pH towards normal. Restoration of pH may be nearly complete, and the process is referred to as compensated respiratory alkalosis.

Preoperative Assessment

Before surgery in the chest, a decision must be made regarding other studies that should be carried out (Table 3–2). The type and extent of the evaluation depend on a number of clinical factors. For patients with a lung mass, a recent chest radiograph and computed tomographic (CT) scan of the chest should be obtained. Most, but not all, should have a recent set of pulmonary function studies. The decision to search for disseminated disease with a bone scan and a CT or magnetic resonance imaging (MRI) scan of the brain is a difficult one, and precise criteria to define when they should be obtained do not exist. It is always better to obtain a complete evaluation for disease if there is any reason at all to do so. This would include any organ-specific or nonspecific signs or symptoms. Nonspecific signs include weight loss, easy fatigability, or anemia; organ-specific signs include bone pain, elevated liver enzyme levels, or localizing neurologic findings. If any of these findings is present, a complete staging evaluation is obtained, not just the study pointed to by the organ-specific complaint. Any patient with a past history of malignancy should have a complete extent of disease workup, as should the patient who is at a higher risk for operation,

TABLE 3–2 • *Evaluation of Risk of Pulmonary Resection in Patients with Pulmonary Disease*

Function	Test	Patient at Risk – Needs Preoperative Optimization or Further Evaluation	Prohibitive Risk
Mechanical ventilatory	FEV_1 postoperative predicted	<1.0 L/sec	<0.8 L/sec
	FVC preoperative	<2.0 L	<1.5 L
	MBC preoperative	<55%	<35%
Parenchymal pulmonary	Po_2 preoperative (rest)	50–60 mm Hg	<50 mm Hg
	Pco_2 preoperative (rest)	40–44 mm Hg	>45 mm Hg
	$\dot{Q}_S/\dot{Q}_T$ preoperative	10–20%	>20%
Cardiac	ECG at rest	Abnormal, especially ischemic changes	Acute MI, ventricular arrhythmias
	ETT	<85% MPHR	Early (+) ETT
	Ventricular function (rest–exercise ejection fraction by radionuclide studies)	EF < 50% or deterioration with exercise	EF < 30%
Cardiopulmonary capacity	Chronic Hb level	>17 g/100 mL	>20 g/100 mL
	Cardiac: ETT	Unable to complete Stage IV secondary to dyspnea on exertion	Unable to complete Stage I (cardiac ischemia or arrhythmias)
	Stairwalking	Unable to complete three flights of stairs	Unable to walk one flight
Cardiopulmonary exercise testing	Postexercise arterial blood gases	Fall in Po_2	Fall in Po_2 to <49 mm Hg or CO_2 retention

ECG, electrocardiogram; EF, ejection fraction; ETT, exercise tolerance test; FFV_1, forced expiratory volume at 1 sec; FVC, forced vital capacity; Hb, hemoglobin; MI, myocardial infarction; MBC, maximal breathing capacity; MPHR, maximum predicted heart rate.
From Sabiston DC Jr. *Textbook of surgery: the biological basis of modern surgical practice*, 15th ed. Philadelphia: WB Saunders, 1997;1793.

such as an individual with multiple medical problems or borderline pulmonary function. Additionally, any patient with locally advanced disease in whom the indications for operation are being extended (i.e. N2 disease) or a non-smoker with a lung mass should have disseminated disease ruled out. The aim is to avoid operating on a patient who proceeds to manifest disseminated disease within 1 year of operation, which is a finding that ideally should have been identified preoperatively.

An important aspect of the preoperative evaluation of a patient undergoing a thoracic procedure is the assessment of pulmonary function. Not all patients undergoing thoracotomy require pulmonary function testing, but the majority of patients with lung cancer also have some element of underlying lung disease as a result of the same risk factor that is associated with their cancer – cigarette smoking.

Assessment of pulmonary function serves to identify patients at a significantly increased likelihood of postoperative morbidity as well as to identify patients who stand to benefit from preoperative manipulations designed to attenuate those risks. There is no single best test to evaluate pulmonary function in a patient who is slated to undergo pulmonary resection. Also, there are no absolute values that contraindicate resection, although using a combination of studies it is at least possible to make a judgment as to which patients are at an increased risk for postoperative morbidity or mortality.

Preoperative spirometry to measure flows and volumes should be performed. Important measurements include FEV_1, MVV, diffusing capacity, FEV_1:FVC ratio, and the ratio of the RV to TLC. An FEV_1 less than 40% of predicted has been associated with increased postoperative morbidity and mortality. Reduced diffusing capacity has also been associated with postoperative problems (Figure 3–2).

Any assessment of postoperative morbidity and mortality must take into account the extent of the proposed resection. Often this is difficult to determine, and the experience of the surgeon is closely related to the likelihood of pneumonectomy. The surgeon operating on patients with compromised lung function should be experienced in the performance of segmental resections, sleeve resections, and nonanatomic resections. Techniques of video-assisted thoracic surgery may also be of use in patients with limited pulmonary reserve who require pulmonary resection. There are a number of measures that can be instituted that are designed to attenuate the postoperative risk in these patients with compromised lung function. The sobering truth, however, is that it often comes down to a judgment on the part of the surgeon based on both objective and subjective factors that may be most important. There are some patients who are just not candidates for pulmonary resection for a variety of reasons that sometimes may be difficult to articulate.

Recent experience with lung volume reduction surgery in patients with severe end-stage emphysema has changed our thinking regarding surgery for lung cancer in patients with compromised lung function. Nutritional assessment and therapy and a supervised program of pulmonary rehabilitation may further optimize borderline patients for pulmonary resection. Currently, our tendency is to be quite aggressive in considering patients with pulmonary malignancies for resection. Rarely is a patient turned down for resection solely on the basis of pulmonary function. At times, the resections have to be somewhat creative, and there are a number of intraoperative factors that may contribute to a reduction in postoperative problems.

Patients with borderline lung function must be strongly motivated toward resection. These patients are not the ones to be talked into an operation even if their other treatment options are limited; they really have to want it.

The major morbidity and potential mortality in these patients occur in the early postoperative period, but one must also keep in mind the long-term sequelae of the resection of lung parenchyma in these individuals. Paradoxically, there may be some improvement in lung function after pulmonary resection in these patients, especially if the lung parenchyma removed receives a minimal amount of the pulmonary perfusion. A quantitative ventilation–perfusion lung scan before pulmonary resection is useful in assessing the significance of the loss of lung parenchyma. An estimate of the predicted postoperative FEV_1 may be obtained by subtracting the percentage removed by the proposed resection based on the percentage of perfusion received by that area of lung parenchyma. A residual FEV_1 of less than 800 mL has been associated with an increased risk of postoperative morbidity and mortality.

In addition to pulmonary function studies, a functional assessment of a patient with compromised lung function may be appropriate in some circumstances (Table 3–3). This assessment may range from something as simple as having the patient climb one or two flights of stairs while oxygen saturation and pulse rate are monitored to formal exercise testing and calculation of maximal oxygen consumption ($\dot{V}O_{2\ max}$). It is reasonably certain that a patient who can walk up two flights of stairs can tolerate a lobectomy. For truly borderline patients, measurement of $\dot{V}O_{2\ max}$ may be the deciding test. A value of less than 15 mL/kg per minute has been associated with significantly increased postoperative morbidity and mortality. Patients in this category should be scrutinized closely before a decision is made to proceed with resection. It is this type of patient who may do better with a limited resection, albeit a compromise, such as a video-assisted wedge excision if the lesion is small and peripheral. It is highly unlikely that a patient with such severe pulmonary compromise could tolerate a pneumonectomy. Other variables

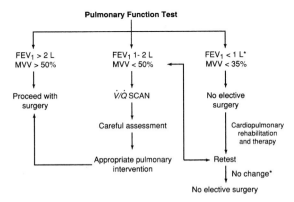

Figure 3–2. An algorithm suggesting the schema for evaluating pulmonary function.* The absolute numbers indicated are not absolute and depend on the individual in selected cases; FEV_1 may be as low as 0.6 L/min. (Adapted from Miller JI. Preoperative evaluation. *Chest Surg Clin North Am* 1992;4:701.)

TABLE 3–3 • *Interpretation of Risk in Patients with Pulmonary Disease*

Findings	Interpretation
Normal test	No increased risk demonstrated
Obstructive disorders	
$FEV_1 > 1.5$ L; MVV > 50% Normal blood gases	Little increased risk if special precautions taken in patient management
$FEV_1 = 1–1.5$ L; MVV = 35–50% Normal P_aCO_2; no more than slight hypoxemia; normal ECG	Definitely increased risk even with proper management; a relative contraindication to surgery
$FEV_1 = 1–1.5$ L; MVV = 35–50% Normal P_aCO_2; slight hypoxemia; abnormal ECG	Greatly increased operative risk; a contraindication to major elective surgical procedures
$FEV_1 = 1$ L; MVV < 35% Normal P_aCO_2; mild hypoxemia; normal ECG	Greatly increased operative risk; a contraindication to major elective surgical procedures; probably precludes extensive lung resection
$FEV_1 = 1$ L; MVV < 35% Elevated P_aCO_2; severe hypoxemia or abnormal ECG	Extremely high operative risk; only mandatory surgery justifiable; Probably precludes any pulmonary resection
Restrictive disorders	
VC >50%; $D_L > 50$% Normal blood gases	Little increased operative risk
VC = 35–50%; $D_L > 50$% Slight hypoxemia on exertion	Some increase in operative risk but not a serious contraindication to surgery, except extensive lung resection
VC < 35%; $D_L < 50$% or frank hypoxemia	Greatly increased operative risk, especially contraindicating extensive lung resection
Cardiopulmonary exercise testing	
$\dot{V}O_{2\,max} > 20$ mL/min/kg	Low operative risk
$\dot{V}O_{2\,max}$ 15–20 mL/min/kg	Moderate operative risk
$\dot{V}O_{2\,max}$ 10–15 mL/min/kg	High operative risk
$\dot{V}O_{2\,max} < 10$ mL/min/kg	Unacceptably high operative risk

D_L, diffusing capacity; ECG, electrocardiogram; FEV_1, forced expiratory volume at 1 sec; MVV, maximum voluntary ventilation; VC, vital capacity; $\dot{V}O_{2\,max}$, maximum oxygen consumption.
Modified from Burrows B, Knudson RJ, Kettel LJ. *Respiratory insufficiency*. Chicago: Year Book, 1975.

suggesting high risk include a PCO_2 of more than 45 mm Hg and elevated pulmonary artery pressures.

Postoperative Care

Successful postoperative care depends on aggressive preoperative preparation and continued respiratory and exercise therapy postoperatively (Box 3–2).

BOX 3–1 PREDICTORS OF POOR OUTCOME

- P_aCO_2 >46
- P_aO_2 <70
- D_LCO <50% predicted
- FEV_1 <0.8 (60% FVC)
- MVO_2 (maximum oxygen uptake) <10 mL/kg/min
- Maximum breathing capacity <50%.

Most patients who come to a thoracic surgeon have a history of smoking. Cessation of smoking prior to going to the operating room is mandatory. At least 1–2 weeks of smoking cessation can improve ciliary clearance and decrease secretions.

Adequate pain control is essential in the postoperative thoracic patient to ensure full respiratory effort. Pain control is best achieved by epidural analgesia. Use of an epidural analgesic minimizes the need for morphine and fentanyl, which depresses the respiratory drive. An epidural catheter can deliver local anesthesia such as bupivacaine. The main complication of local anesthetics administered via this route is cardiovascular depression. Decreased sympathetic output can drop peripheral vascular resistance, which can cause clinical hypotension.

Postoperative respiratory therapy is the cornerstone of rapid recovery of a thoracic patient. Careful induction of anesthesia avoids aspiration. Early chest physiotherapy, frequent ambulation, and bronchodilators minimize postoperative complications. Development of respiratory difficulty, particularly on postoperative day 2 or 3 is a harbinger of pneumonia or pulmonary edema. Signs of respiratory insufficiency must be treated aggressively at this point with incentive spirometry, ambulation, and nutritional support. Intravenous fluid should be minimized in the thoracic patient. Entry into the thoracic cage is not associated with the same fluid shifts as seen in abdominal cases. When pulmonary edema develops despite appropriate fluid management, diuretics should be instituted. Nasotracheal suctioning should be used as needed. Sputum cultures should be obtained and broad-spectrum antibiotics started early, even prior to the development of an infiltrate on chest radiographs. Atelectasis, although common in most surgical patients, can compromise a borderline thoracic patient. Early bronchoscopy may be necessary for compromised patients.

Mechanical Ventilation

Indications

Indications for mechanical ventilatory support are subjective and require clinical judgment (Figure 3–3). Support may be indicated secondary to problems with any component of the respiratory system: central nervous system, chest wall, airway, respiratory muscles, or alveoli. Patients with central nervous system depression secondary to narcotic overdose or closed head injury can require intubation to prevent aspiration and respiratory stimulation. Abnormalities in the chest wall such as flail chest, open pneumothorax, or marked scoliosis can require respiratory assistance. Respiratory muscle fatigue plays a role in respiratory failure requiring support in chronic obstructive pulmonary disease. Intubation is required in patients with facial trauma, anaphylaxis, or atelectasis from endobronchial masses or foreign bodies. Respiratory failure due to the alveolar component may be secondary to multiple causes, including cardiogenic or noncardiogenic pulmonary edema and extensive pneumonia. Mechanical support may be indicated in the setting of hypercapnia ($P_{CO_2} > 45$ mm Hg) or severe hypoxia ($P_{O_2} < 55$ mm Hg).

Modes (Figure 3–4)

Assist-controlled Ventilation

The standard method of positive-pressure mechanical ventilation involves volume-cycled lung inflation (i.e. each machine

---

BOX 3–2 PROPHYLACTIC MEASURES RECOMMENDED TO REDUCE POSTOPERATIVE COMPLICATIONS

Preoperatively

Education of patients to ensure optimal postoperative compliance and performance; cessation of smoking; training in proper breathing (incentive spirometry); bronchodilatation and control of infection and secretions when indicated; and weight reduction when appropriate

Intraoperatively

Reduction in time under anesthesia; control of secretions; prevention of aspiration; maintenance of optimal bronchodilatation; and intermittent hyperinflations

Postoperatively

Continuation of preoperative measure with particular attention to hyperinflation, mobilization of secretions, early ambulation, encouragement to cough, and control of pain, with attention to the effects of analgesia on the pattern of breathing

From Tisi GM. Preoperative evaluation of pulmonary function. *Am Rev Respir Dis* 1979;119:303.

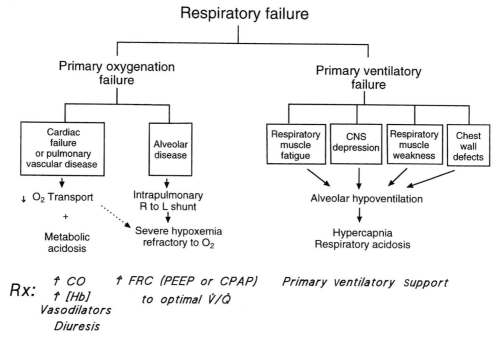

Figure 3–3. Modalities of respiratory failure. (CPAP, continuous positive airway pressure; PEEP, positive end-expiratory pressure.) (From Pearson FG, Cooper JD, Deslauriers J, *et al. Thoracic surgery*, 2nd ed. New York: Churchill Livingstone, 2002:156.)

breath delivers a preselected inflation volume; Figure 3–5). The patient can initiate each mechanical breath (assisted ventilation) but, when this is not possible, the ventilator provides machine breaths at a preselected rate. During conventional volume-cycled ventilation, the I:E ratio is maintained at 1:2 to 1:4. When the I:E ratio falls below 1:2, the lungs may not empty completely after each inflation. This can result in progressive hyperinflation.

An important note on assisted controlled ventilation is that the work of breathing can be considerable. This mode does not 'rest the diaphragm', as is often suggested. The contraction of the diaphragm continues as per the brainstem reflex. Patients on assist-controlled ventilation need to be watched for tachypnea. Increased frequency of machine breaths can lead to overventilation and severe respiratory alkalosis and the decreased time for exhalation can result in hyperinflation.

Intermittent Mandatory Ventilation

Intermittent mandatory ventilation (IMV) delivers periodic volume-cycled breathes at a preselected rate but allows spontaneous breathing between machine breaths. Because each spontaneous breath does not trigger a machine breath, there is reduced risk of respiratory alkalosis and hyperinflation with IMV. The principal disadvantages are an increase in the work of breathing and a tendency for the cardiac output to be reduced. The increased work of breathing during IMV could lead to respiratory muscle fatigue, which could further promote further ventilatory dependency. Positive-pressure mechanical ventilation can reduce cardiac output by impeding ventricular filling, and it can also increase cardiac output by reducing ventricular afterload.

Positive-controlled Ventilation

Positive-controlled ventilation (PCV) is pressure-cycled breathing that is controlled by the ventilator, without patient involvement (see Figure 3–5). Because peak airway pressure is lower in pressure-cycled than in volume-cycled machine breaths, there is less risk of barotrauma with PCV. The major advantage of PCV relates to the inspiratory flow pattern. In volume-cycled breathing, the inspiratory flow rate is constant throughout lung inflation, whereas, in pressure-cycled breathing, the inspiratory flow decreases exponentially dur-

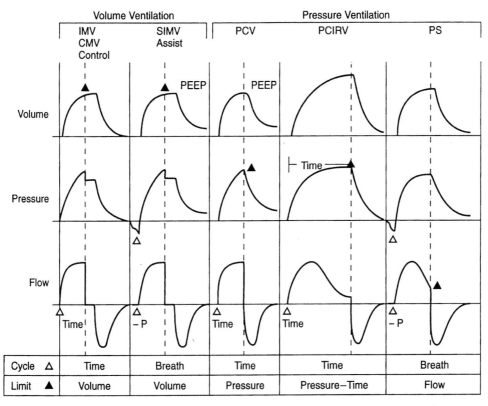

Figure 3–4. Patterns of airflow, airway pressure, and lung volume during mechanical ventilation. Gas flow is initiated (cycle Δ) by either patient effort (−P) or set time cycle. Inspiratory flow ceases (limit Δ) when a preset volume, pressure, or flow is achieved. (CMV, continuous mechanical ventilation; IMV, intermittent mandatory ventilation; PCIRV, pressure-controlled inverted-ratio ventilation; PCV, premature ventricular contraction; PEEP, positive end-expiratory pressures; PS, pressure support. (From Bartlett RH. Respiratory physiology and pathophysiology. In: Bartlett RH, ed. *Critical care physiology*. Boston: Little, Brown & Co., 1996.)

ing lung inflation. The decreasing inspiratory flow pattern reduces peak airway pressures and improves gas exchange. The major disadvantage of PCV is the tendency for inflation volumes to vary with changes in the mechanical properties of the lungs.

Pressure Support Ventilation

Pressure support ventilation (PSV) allows the patient to determine the inflation volume and respiratory cycle duration. This method of ventilation is used to augment spontaneous breathing, not to provide full ventilatory support. At the onset of each spontaneous breath, the negative pressure generated by the patient opens a valve that delivers the inspired gas at a preselected pressure (usually 5–10 cm H_2O). The patient's inspiratory flow rate is adjusted by the ventilator as needed to keep the inflation pressure constant. When the patient's inspiratory flow rate falls below 25% of the

peak inspiratory flow, the augmented breath is terminated. By recognizing the patient's inherent inspiratory flow rate, PSV allows the patient to dictate the duration of lung inflation and the inflation volume. The goal of PSV is not to augment the tidal volume but to provide enough pressure to overcome the resistance created by the tracheal tube and ventilator tubing.

Continuous Positive Airway Pressure

Continuous positive airway pressure (CPAP) maintains a positive pressure throughout a spontaneous breath. The patient does not need to generate a negative airway pressure to receive the inhaled gas. This eliminates the extra work involved in generating a negative airway pressure to inhale. CPAP may be used in intubated or non-intubated patients. CPAP masks are used to postpone intubation in patients with acute respiratory failure.

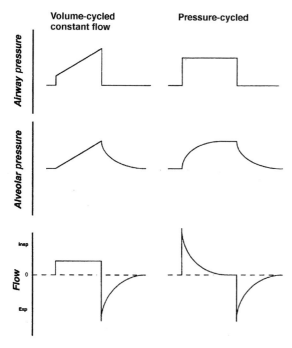

Figure 3–5. Idealized airway pressure, alveolar pressure, and flow tracings during volume-cycled ventilation (with constant inspiratory flow) and pressure-cycled ventilation. (From Marcy TW, Marini JJ. Control mode ventilation and assist/control ventilation. In: Stock MC, Perel A, eds. *Mechanical ventilatory support*. Philadelphia: Lippincott Williams & Wilkins, 1997.)

Positive End-Expiratory Pressure

Under normal circumstances, the volume of gas inhaled is exhaled completely. As a result, the expiratory airflow ceases by the end of expiration, and the alveolar pressure at end-expiration is equivalent to atmospheric pressure. When the alveolar pressure at end-expiration is above atmospheric pressure, it is referred to as positive end-expiratory pressure (PEEP). The distal air spaces tend to collapse at the end of expiration, and this tendency is exaggerated when the lungs are stiff. Alveolar collapse impairs gas exchange and makes the lungs stiffer. PEEP prevents the alveoli from collapsing. At the end of expiration, PEEP can open alveoli that have already collapsed. The improved oxygen exchange raises P_{O_2}, which allows the fractional concentration of inspired oxygen (F_iO_2) to be reduced to less toxic levels. Benefits of PEEP include increased functional residual capacity, increased lung compliance, increased arterial P_aO_2, and decreased pulmonary shunting. Disadvantages of PEEP ventilation include decreased cardiac output due to decreased venous return. Also, the risk of barotrauma is always present with PEEP (Table 3–4).

Acute Respiratory Distress Syndrome

Acute respiratory distress syndrome (ARDS) describes a syndrome of acute respiratory distress with diffuse interstitial edema, alveolar infiltrates, and decreased lung compliance (<50 mL/cm H_2O) with severe hypoxemia ($P_aO_2/F_iO_2 < 200$). Characteristically, hyperventilation is unresponsive to increasing oxygenation and is often associated with respiratory alkalosis. Cardiac-related pulmonary edema must be ruled out and chest radiographs will demonstrate bilateral lung infiltrates. ARDS carries a mortality of 30–40%.

The pathophysiology of ARDS has been widely studied but no consensus exists. It probably relates to increased pulmonary capillary permeability, which results from endothelial damage by toxins. The basic pathology is a diffuse inflammatory process that involves both lungs. Factors that probably contribute to the pathophysiology include complement activation, excessive activation of alveolar macrophages, release of inflammatory mediators and chemokines, and the production of oxygen free

TABLE 3–4 • *Beneficial and Detrimental Effects of Positive End-Expiratory Pressure*	
Beneficial Effects	**Detrimental Effects**
Alveolar recruitment	Alveolar overdistention (barotrauma)
Vascular derecruitment	Depression of cardiac output
Improvement of P_aO_2	Increased intracranial pressure (with high levels of PEEP)
Protection against ventilator-induced lung injury	Decreased renal and portal blood flow (related to decreased cardiac output)
Reduction of inspiratory workload	May increase inspiratory work of breathing
	Worsened hypoxemia (unilateral lung disease)

From Pearson FG, Cooper JD, Deslauriers J, *et al. Thoracic surgery*, 2nd ed. New York: Churchill Livingstone, 2002:165.

radicals. The alveolar spaces on both sides of the centrally located septum contain erythrocytes, leukocytes, and proteinaceous debris. Thus although ARDS is a type of pulmonary edema, ARDS is an inflammatory process, not an accumulation of watery edema fluid.

Many conditions predispose to ARDS, such as pulmonary contusion, pneumonia, cardiopulmonary bypass, use of blood products, sepsis, endotoxemia, gastrointestinal translocation, pancreatitis, and intracranial hypertension. The most common predisposing condition is sepsis, which is a systemic inflammatory response (such as fever or leukocytosis) due to infection.

Acute respiratory distress syndrome is clinically associated with increased dead space with decreased compliance and increased pulmonary vascular resistance. ARDS responds to PEEP, though not necessarily with increased F_iO_2. The earliest clinical signs of ARDS include tachypnea and progressive hypoxemia, refractory to supplemental oxygen. Within 24 hours, chest radiographs reveal bilateral pulmonary infiltrates. The principal concern is to differentiate ARDS from cardiogenic pulmonary edema. The severity of the hypoxemia can sometimes help to distinguish ARDS from cardiogenic pulmonary edema. If diagnostic recognition is a problem, Swan–Ganz catheters can be used to clinch the diagnosis. Pulmonary capillary wedge pressure (PCWP) greater than 18 mm Hg suggests cardiogenic pulmonary edema, whereas a pressure under 18 leans towards ARDS. Bronchoscopy is generally not warranted as a diagnostic tool in ARDS. However, bronchoscopy may be performed occasionally for other reasons in a patient with suspected ARDS (i.e. to identify infection).

Similarly, management of ARDS is controversial but basic principles of care include restricting fluids and treating the underlying condition (i.e. sepsis). A volume ventilator should be used to avoid high airway pressures, avoid high peak inspiratory pressures, and optimally avoid F_iO_2 above 50%. There is considerable evidence indicating that the large tidal volumes used during conventional mechanical ventilation (10–15 mL/kg) can damage the lungs.

The pathologic changes in ARDS are not distributed uniformly throughout the lungs. Rather, there are regions of lung infiltration interspersed with regions where the lung architecture is normal. These normal lung regions receive most of the delivered tidal volume. This results in overdistension of normal lung regions, which leads to alveolar rupture, surfactant depletion, and disruption of the alveolar–capillary interface. Recognition of the risk of lung injury at high inflation volumes and pressures has led to an alternative strategy where peak inspiratory pressures are kept below 35 cm H_2O by using tidal volumes of 7–10 mL/kg. The F_iO_2 should be kept at 50% or lower to minimize the risk of oxygen toxicity. Arterial oxygen saturation (S_aO_2) should be monitored instead of arterial PO_2 because S_aO_2 determines the oxygen content in arterial blood. An S_aO_2 above 90% should be sufficient to maintain oxygen delivery to peripheral tissues. If the F_iO_2 cannot be reduced to below 60%, external PEEP is added to help reduce the F_iO_2 to less toxic levels. The lung infiltration is ARDS is an inflammatory process, and diuretics do not reduce inflammation.

The ultimate goal of management in respiratory failure is an adequate level of oxygenation in the vital organs. Tissue oxygenation is considered to be inadequate if whole blood $\dot{V}O_2$ is less than 100 mL/min/m^2, venous lactate is greater than 4 mmol/L, or gastric intramucosal pH is less than 7.32.

Key Readings

Culver BH. Preoperative assessment of the thoracic surgery patient: pulmonary function testing. *Semin Thorac Cardiovasc Surg* 2001;13:92–104. *One view of what features should be evaluated in preparation for the operating room.*
Grippi MA. *Pulmonary pathophysiology.* Philadelphia: JB Lippincott, 1995. *Soft covered textbook that reviews the pathophysiology of several important lung disease processes.*
Tobin MJ. Advances in mechanical ventilation. *N Engl J Med* 2001;344:1986–1996. *Review of mechanical ventilation in this time of changing ventilators and various philosophies towards respirator management.*

Selected Readings

Azarow KS, Molloy M, Seyfer AE, Graeber GM. Preoperative evaluation and general preparation for chest-wall operations. *Surg Clin North Am* 1989;69:899–910.
Bisson A, Stern M, Caubarrere I. Preparation of high-risk patients for major thoracic surgery. *Chest Surg Clin North Am* 1998;8:541–555.
Brower RG, Ware LB, Berthiaume Y, Matthay MA. Treatment of ARDS. *Chest* 2001;120:1347–1367.
Celli BR. What is the value of preoperative pulmonary function testing? *Med Clin North Am* 1993;77:309–325.
Melendez JA, Fischer ME. Preoperative pulmonary evaluation of the thoracic surgical patient. *Chest Surg Clin North Am* 1997;7:641–654.
Stiller KR, Munday RM. Chest physiotherapy for the surgical patient. *Br J Surg* 1992;79:745–749.
West JB. *Pulmonary pathophysiology – the essentials*, 5th ed. Baltimore: Williams & Wilkins, 1998:198.

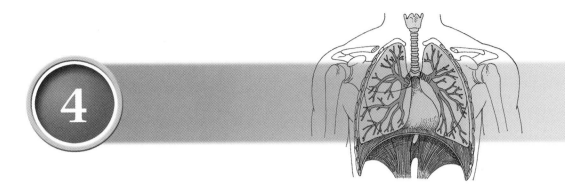

4

Diagnostic Procedures

RADIOGRAPHIC EVALUATION
OF THE CHEST

COMPUTED TOMOGRAPHY

MAGNETIC RESONANCE
IMAGING

RADIONUCLIDE STUDIES

BRONCHOSCOPY

MEDIASTINOSCOPY

THORACOSCOPY

Diagnostic Procedures: Key Points

- Develop an algorithm for reviewing a chest radiograph
- Appreciate the strengths of computed axial tomography
- Know when magnetic resonance imaging is the preferred modality over computed axial tomography
- Review the anatomy of the tracheobronchial tree as seen through a bronchoscope
- Appreciate the versatile function of thoracoscopic surgery

Radiographic Evaluation of the Chest

Chest radiographs remain a central part of the work up of a thoracic patient. Adequate examination of the chest necessitates at least two views, the posteroanterior (PA) and lateral projections. The upright PA view provides the best exposure of the lung fields and is the preferred initial study of the chest (Figure 4–1 on p. 68). The lateral view reveals mediastinal lesions, vertebral column lesions, pathology behind the heart and diaphragm, and small pleural effusions (Figure 4–2 on p. 69). Together

they provide a complete examination of the main features of the chest (Table 4–1 on p. 70).

Additional views such as lateral decubitus films are important in evaluating suspected pleural effusions or demonstrating air fluid levels in pulmonary cavities. As little as 50 cc can be identified in the lateral decubitus position. The most important way to assess abnormalities is to have serial x-rays over time to review changes.

A simple mnemonic (ABCDEFGHI) can be employed to remember to check for the important characteristics to be reviewed on rapid assessment of a chest film.

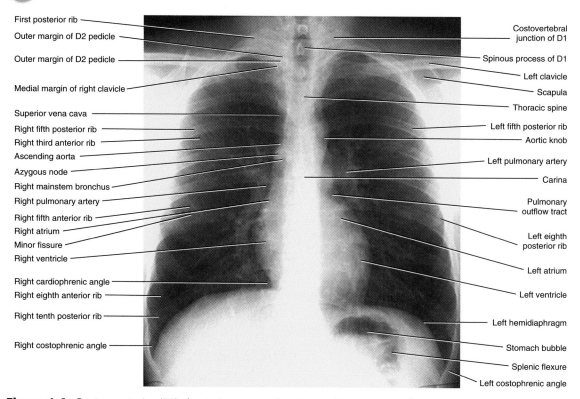

First posterior rib

Outer margin of D2 pedicle

Outer margin of D2 pedicle

Medial margin of right clavicle

Superior vena cava

Right fifth posterior rib

Right third anterior rib

Ascending aorta

Azygous node

Right mainstem bronchus

Right pulmonary artery

Right fifth anterior rib

Right atrium

Minor fissure

Right ventricle

Right cardiophrenic angle

Right eighth anterior rib

Right tenth posterior rib

Right costophrenic angle

Costovertebral junction of D1

Spinous process of D1

Left clavicle

Scapula

Thoracic spine

Left fifth posterior rib

Aortic knob

Left pulmonary artery

Carina

Pulmonary outflow tract

Left eighth posterior rib

Left atrium

Left ventricle

Left hemidiaphragm

Stomach bubble

Splenic flexure

Left costophrenic angle

Figure 4–1. Posteroanterior (PA) chest view: normal radiographic anatomy. The structures routinely seen are labeled. Note the specific markers for adequate positioning, e.g. trachea midline and equal left and right first rib pedicle-to-clavicle distances. With good PA technique, the scapulae remain outside the lung fields and the clavicles are below the upper two ribs. This is in contradistinction to the appearance on anteroposterior views. (From Meholic A, Ketai L, Lofgren R. *Fundamentals of chest radiology.* Philadelphia: WB Saunders, 1996:9.)

- *Airway.* The outlines of the trachea, carina, and bronchus can be established from a radiograph. The trachea is normally located slightly to the right of the midline because it is closely applied against the mass of the aortic arch. Matched with clinical knowledge about the patient, airway patency can be established.
- *Bone.* Begin with the scapula and then look at the humerus and shoulder joints. Inspect the clavicles and simultaneously note rotation and symmetry. Review the ribs in pairs from top to bottom. Always compare the two sides for symmetry (Figure 4–3 on p. 71). Concentrate on the posterior halves of the ribs then on the anterior sides of the ribs. The thoracic vertebrae are not well seen in a PA film, although you do appreciate some differences in the lateral films. A sense of the patient's age and nutritional status can be obtained by noting the density of the patient's bony structure.

- *Cardiac.* The heart is the largest of the mediastinal structures and all the profiles that bulge beyond the shadow of the spine represent parts of the heart or its great vessels (Figure 4–4 on p. 71). The simplest method of measuring the heart is to determine its relation to the width of the chest at its widest part near the level of the diaphragm. A typical cardiac profile should be 50% of the width of the chest. A larger profile and the appropriate clinical scenario should raise the suspicion of cardiac hypertrophy, dilated cardiomyopathy, or pericardial effusion.
- *Diaphragm.* The diaphragm should be viewed radiographically as two hemidiaphragms. Normally they are smooth curves originating from the midline at the origin of the 10th or 11th rib. The diaphragm may be elevated by large collections of fluid in the peritoneal space. In emphysema, with irreversible trapping of air in the lung and gradually increas-

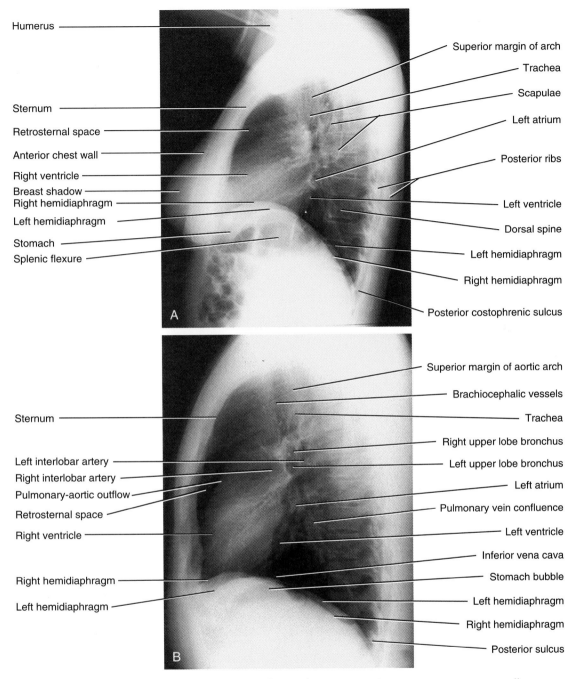

Figure 4–2. A, **B**, Lateral chest view: normal radiographic anatomy. Important structures usually seen are labeled. Note the specific position of the cardiac chambers, aortic and pulmonary outflow tracts, and hilar vasculature. (From Meholic A, Ketai L, Lofgren R. *Fundamentals of chest radiology.* Philadelphia: WB Saunders, 1996:10.)

ing overexpansion, the diaphragm is low and flat. Similarly, if there are large collections of pleural fluid or tumor masses in the lung, the diaphragm may be depressed.

• *Effusions.* The pleural space, although normally empty and collapsed, may contain either fluid or air or both. A massive collection of fluid on one side can displace the mediastinum toward

TABLE 4–1 • *Sites Examined in a Radiologist's Evaluation of the Chest Radiograph*

Frontal View	Lateral View
Bones	
Ribs: posterior ribs, anterior ribs, axillary margin	Spine
Spine	Sternum
Clavicles	
Mediastinum	
Aortic knob	Retrosternal space
Aortopulmonary window	Retrotracheal space
Pulmonary outflow tract	
Right paratracheal area	
Paraspinous lines	
Hilum	
Relative height and size of right and left hilum	Interlobar artery size and shape
Hilar angle	
Bronchial wall thickness and vascular distribution	
Heart	
Silhouette size	Posterior margin (including inferior vena cava junction)
Apex configuration (LV or RV)	Retrosternal space
Left atrium (carinal angle, double density, etc.)	
Calcifications	
Diaphragm/pleura	
Contour, including costophrenic angles	Pleural fissures
Upper abdomen	Contour, including costophrenic angles
Apices (thickening, pleural line, etc.)	Upper abdomen (free gas and surgical clips)
Parenchyma	
Entire lung field, including a repeat examination of the portions already seen at the sites listed above	Examine entire lung field, as on frontal view

From Meholic A, Ketai L, Lofgren R. *Fundamentals of chest radiology.* Philadelphia: WB Saunders, 1996:11.

the opposite side, depress the diaphragm, partially collapse the lung, and render the entire hemidiaphragm dense and white. Typically, 100–200 mL of fluid is not visible on a PA chest film; however, a lateral film is more sensitive for a small collection. Any air in the pleural space allows one to see the surface of the lung because of the air–tissue interface. The key to finding a pneumothorax is to look for the pleural margin of the lung, beyond which no lung markings extend (Figure 4–5 on p. 72). Obliteration of the costophrenic sinus indicates an effusion. As greater amounts of fluid collect, a rounded upward curving shadow forms across the chest wall. It never forms a horizontal fluid level unless there is also air present, opening up the pleural space. The best way to define an effusion is a follow-up study using a lateral decubitus view.

- *Fields (lung fields).* A normal lung will have several lines and shadows visible. These lung markings are vascular markings. The bronchial tree is air-filled and thin-walled and thus radiolucent. The largest vessels (hence the densest lung shadows) are at the hilum. The left hilum is higher than the right because of the higher takeoff of the left pulmonary artery, which hooks up over the left main stem bronchus. The range of parenchymal lung diseases is vast; however, it

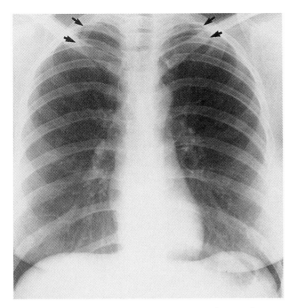

Figure 4-3. Posteroanterior chest radiograph: cervical ribs. Asymmetric development of rudimentary ribs (arrows) at the C7 level bilaterally, more prominent on the right. These are usually an incidental asymptomatic finding, but 5–10% of cervical ribs can be associated with thoracic outlet syndrome. (From Meholic A, Ketai L, Lofgren R. *Fundamentals of chest radiology.* Philadelphia: WB Saunders, 1996:223.)

is useful to recognize four common radiographic patterns: lung masses, air-space diseases, interstitial diseases, and atelectasis. Lung masses need to be approximately 1 cm before they can cast a shadow with enough resolution for assessment (Figure 4–6 on p. 72). Air-space diseases that cause alveolar filling will appear dense and radiopaque on the chest film. Interstitial lung diseases are diseases that affect the tissue surrounding the alveoli capillaries. The most common radiographic sign is Kerley B lines, which are short, horizontal lines that connect with the pleura along the lateral margins of the lung (Figure 4–7 on p. 72). Atelectasis is similar to air-space disease in that the air in the alveoli is lost. However, atelectasis occurs when the air in the alveoli is absorbed and not replaced by fluid or cells. This causes a loss of volume, which is the key radiographic finding.

- *Gastric bubble.* A typical gastric bubble shows a straight line marking the fluid level. The interposition of anything between the diaphragm and the fundus of the stomach will displace the bubble downward (Figure 4–8 on p. 73).
- *Hilum.* Compare the density of one hilum to another (Figure 4–9 on p. 73). The two focuses on inspection of the hilum are search for vascular abnormalities or significant adenopathy.
- *Intestines.* Free air under the diaphragm should always be checked for on a plain radiograph.

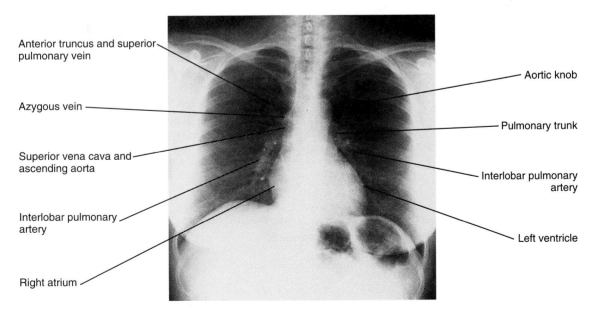

Anterior truncus and superior pulmonary vein

Azygous vein

Superior vena cava and ascending aorta

Interlobar pulmonary artery

Right atrium

Aortic knob

Pulmonary trunk

Interlobar pulmonary artery

Left ventricle

Figure 4-4. Normal posteroanterior chest with cardiovascular structures labeled. (From Meholic A, Ketai L, Lofgren R. *Fundamentals of chest radiology.* Philadelphia: WB Saunders, 1996:181.)

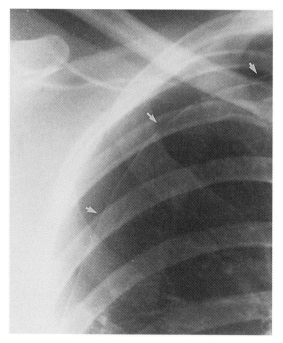

Figure 4–5. Posteroanterior chest radiograph: pneumothorax. Close-up demonstrates well the visceral pleural line (arrows) and also the lack of pulmonary vascular markings lateral to the pleural line. (From Meholic A, Ketai L, Lofgren R. *Fundamentals of chest radiology.* Philadelphia: WB Saunders, 1996:146.)

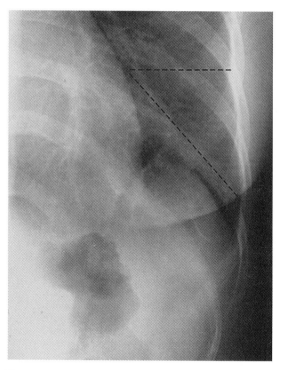

Figure 4–7. Posteroanterior chest view: Kerley B lines. A close-up of the left lower lung field shows multiple short, white, horizontal lines extending to the lateral pleural surface (within area defined by dotted lines), indicative of interstitial disease. Normal vessels do not extend to the pleural surface. (From Meholic A, Ketai L, Lofgren R. *Fundamentals of chest radiology.* Philadelphia: WB Saunders, 1996:67.)

Computed Tomography

Computed tomography (CT) scanning is the most convenient way to image the cross-sectional anatomy of the body (Figure 4–10 on p. 74, Table 4–2 on p. 75). Conventional chest CT is used to evaluate hilar and mediastinal masses and parenchymal lung nodules. Recently, new technology such as high-resolution CT and spiral CT have provided insight into clinical problems. Spiral–helical CT allows the thorax to be imaged in a single breath-hold.

Routine conventional CT of the thorax is displayed in the axial plane. The patient's right is imaged on the viewer's left. The images are usually displayed at 10 mm intervals, although thinner slices may be easily obtained. Density difference measurements allow for predicting tissue typing (Figure 4–11 on p. 76). CT has particularly increased sensitivity for small nodules in the order of 3 mm. Location of the mass is easily delineated

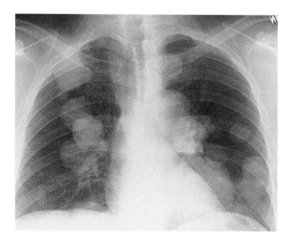

Figure 4–6. Posteroanterior chest radiograph: cannonball metastases – carcinoma of the esophagus. These hematogenous metastatic lesions vary from big to very big and are not 'too numerous to count.' Their size variation indicates different episodes of pulmonary parenchymal seeding. Large metastatic lesions are typically seen with soft tissue sarcomas, gastrointestinal metastases (especially colon carcinoma), testicular tumors, and uterine carcinoma. Lower lung field predominance of nodules is expected in metastatic disease but is not prominent in this picture. (From Meholic A, Ketai L, Lofgren R. *Fundamentals of chest radiology.* Philadelphia: WB Saunders, 1996:133.)

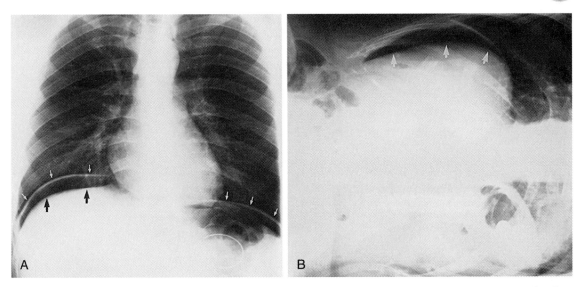

Figure 4–8. Upright chest and left lateral decubitus abdomen views: pneumoperitoneum. **A**, Upright chest x-ray in the postoperative patient demonstrates sickle-shaped lucencies shaped by the inferior contour of the diaphragms (white arrows). Usually, free intraperitoneal air is best seen above the liver edge (black arrows) beneath the diaphragm on the right side. **B**, The left lateral decubitus abdomen study (named for side down) demonstrates typical appearance of free air (arrows) above the dome of the liver. This is the best examination for identifying small amounts of pneumoperitoneum in patients who cannot be positioned upright. (From Meholic A, Ketai L, Lofgren R. *Fundamentals of chest radiology*. Philadelphia: WB Saunders, 1996:168.)

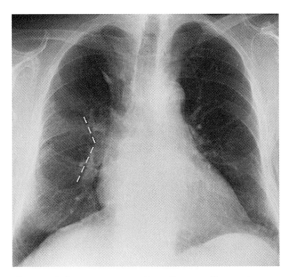

Figure 4–9. Posteroanterior chest radiograph: outline of hilar angle. The right superior pulmonary vein and right interlobar pulmonary artery cross, forming a shallow V (dotted lines), sometimes called the hilar angle. Masses or lymphadenopathy can blunt the apex of the V. Pulmonary edema can blur its outline. (From Meholic A, Ketai L, Lofgren R. *Fundamentals of chest radiology*. Philadelphia: WB Saunders, 1996:198.)

but determining invasion remains difficult. CT scanning is particularly useful in identifying mediastinal nodes when routine chest radiographs are equivocal or normal. Unfortunately, size criteria for enlargement do not allow complete separation of malignant from benign lymphadenopathy. In patients with primary neoplasms elsewhere, CT may be used to look for occult pulmonary metastasis.

The use of intravenous contrast allows separation of vascular from nonvascular mediastinal lesions and identification of vascular invasion by neoplasms (Figure 4–12 on p. 77). The technique is useful in investigating chest wall lesions or the extension of pulmonary or pleural tumors into the chest wall. CT is particularly useful in the detection of pleural-based neoplasms and can be used to identify pleural plaques (Figure 4–13 on p. 79). It can also be used to look at a pleural effusion that contains multiple locules or is loculated in a medial or subpulmonic location (Figure 4–14 on p. 80). CT can be used to identify bony destruction of chest wall tumors.

High-resolution CT is especially useful for investigating interstitial lung disease, bronchiectasis, and pulmonary emphysema. The very thin sections obtained with high-resolution CT allow for anatomically accurate depiction of fine structures of the lung parenchyma (Figure 4–15 on p. 81). However, the acquisition of noncontiguous sections

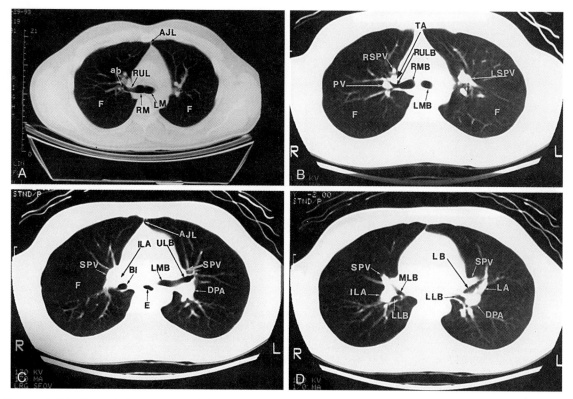

Figure 4–10. Normal CT anatomy of the chest using lung windows. **A,** Right and left upper lobe segments just below the level of the carina. Major fissures (F) appear as relatively avascular areas. ab, anterior segment bronchus; AJL, anterior junction line; RM/LM, right and left main stem bronchi; RUL, right upper lobe bronchus. **B,** Lobar bronchi and associated vascular structures 1 cm below carina. Note the well-defined upper lobe segmental anatomy, particularly on the right at this level. F, major fissures; LMB, left main stem bronchus; LSPV, left superior pulmonary vein and anterior segmental artery; PV, pulmonary vein, RMB, right main stem bronchus; RSPV, right superior pulmonary vein; RULB, right upper lobe bronchus; TA, truncus anterior. **C,** Axial image at the level of the bronchus intermedius and left upper lobe bronchi. Note the horizontal course of the left main stem bronchus (LMB) as it proceeds laterally and bifurcates at the upper lobe bronchus (ULB) level. AJL, anterior junction line; BI, bronchus intermedius; DPA, descending pulmonary artery; E, esophagus; F, fissure; ILA, interlobar artery; SPV, superior pulmonary vein. **D,** Axial CT scan at the level of the lingular and lower lobe bronchi. Note the bifurcation of the bronchus intermedius into the lower lobe bronchus (LLB) and middle lobe bronchus (MLB) on the right and similar appearance on the left of the left lower lobe bronchus and lingular bronchus (LB). DPA, descending pulmonary artery; ILA, interlobar artery; LA, lingular artery; SPV, superior pulmonary vein. (From Meholic A, Ketai L, Lofgren R. *Fundamentals of chest radiology.* Philadelphia: WB Saunders, 1996:19.)

means that large portions of the lung parenchyma are not imaged; thus, small nodules can be missed.

Computed tomographic angiography is emerging as an excellent tool for identifying pulmonary embolus. Requiring less time than conventional radionuclide studies, CT angiography has the advantage of rapid assessment of the critically ill patient. However, the same patients do risk renal injury because of the use of contrast agents with potentially nephrotoxic effects.

Magnetic Resonance Imaging

Although magnetic resonance imaging (MRI) will not replace CT, it is particularly useful for studying mediastinal structures, pulmonary vasculature, and particular situations involving bronchial carcinoma or chest wall, pleural, and diaphragmatic pathology (Box 4–1 on p. 81). Intravenous administration of gadolinium as a contrast agent allows better visualization of vascular structures. MRI provides a unique feature for investigating the thorax in that

TABLE 4–2 • *Indications for Chest Computed Tomography*

Conventional	High-Resolution CT	Spiral CT

Evaluation of masses
    Lung nodule or nodules
    Hilar/mediastinal mass*
	Evaluation of patients with
	    signs and symptoms of lung
	    disease but normal chest x-rays
		Evaluation of small lung
		    nodules

Evaluation of pleural disease
    Malignant
	Immunocompromised patients
	    (AIDS)
		Evaluation of lesions adjacent
		    to the diaphragm

Empyema*	Dyspnea of unknown origin
	Characterization of diffuse
	    infiltrative pulmonary disease
		Evaluation of suspected
		    vascular lesion of the
		    mediastinum or hilum*

Staging/treatment/follow-up
    for neoplastic disease
	Evaluation of disease activity
	    and response to therapy, e.g.
	    usual interstitial pneumonitis
		Hemoptysis

Aortic dissection (special
    protocol)†
	Early identification of drug
	    toxicity, e.g. bleomycin	

	Evaluation of need for and
	    optimum site/method for lung
	    biopsy	

*Contrast agent optimal. † Contrast agent required.
From Meholic A, Ketai L, Lofgren R. *Fundamentals of chest radiology.* Philadelphia: WB Saunders, 1996:17.

the images obtained can be reconstructed in several anatomic planes: sagittal versus coronal images (Figure 4–16 on p. 82). Thoracic MRI is poorly suited for an unfocused survey. MRI does not image lung parenchyma as well as CT. Conventional and high-resolution CT provides superior anatomic detail of lung parenchyma and air spaces (Figure 4–17 on p. 84).

Magnetic resonance imaging is particularly strong in delineating mediastinal pathology. In the anterior mediastinum, MRI is excellent for focused studies of the thymus, ectopic parathyroids, and germ cell tumors. The multiplanar imaging capabilities of MRI provide an advantage over CT in accurately depicting extraglandular extension of thymic pathology (Figure 4–18 on p. 84). MRI is also excellent at locating ectopic parathyroid adenomas because they exhibit low T1 signal, high T2 signal, and avid contrast enhancement. CT scanning is inaccurate in distinguishing solid tumors and cysts in the mediastinum, whereas MRI with gadolinium can reliably demonstrate differences (Figure 4–19 on p. 85). The middle mediastinum contains blood vessels, lymph nodes, lymphatics, the trachea, the esophagus, and a variety of neural structures. MRI and CT are comparably sensitive in detecting mediastinal lymph nodes. However, MRI has an advantage in distinguishing them from adjacent vascular structures (Figure 4–20 on p. 86).

Magnetic resonance imaging does provide some advantages over CT in imaging bronchial carcinoma. MRI can identify tumor infiltration of rib bone marrow. It is particularly valuable in determining the resectability of superior sulcus tumors and assessing tumor invasion of mediastinal structures, chest wall, and spine, especially with the coronal reconstruction. In patients who cannot receive iodinated contrast media for CT, MRI should be used as the primary imaging modality for staging cancer. MRI and CT have similar accuracy in evaluating a hilar mass and adenopathy. Occasionally on CT it is difficult to distinguish a hilar mass from an adjacent pulmonary vessel. In these instances, MRI may have some value. Tumors in the hilum can cause postobstructive atelectasis and pneumonitis. CT is superior to MRI for identifying obstructive endobronchial lesions. However, MRI can often differentiate atelectasis or pneumonitic lung from an obstructing tumor.

Pleural pathology is adequately examined by CT but MRI can be useful in selected situations. MRI can classify pleural fluid collections as transudative, exudative, or complex. The high soft-tissue contrast of MRI with gadolinium is helpful in distinguishing complex fluid collections from solid neoplasms (Figure 4–21 on p. 87).

The complex shape of the diaphragm makes it difficult to assess on conventional axial images using CT. MRI in the sagittal and

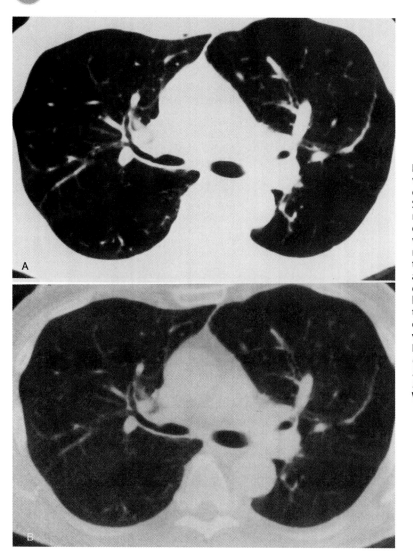

Figure 4–11. Effect of varying window level and width on the caliber of pulmonary vessels. Scans are with 5 mm collimation. **A,** At a window level of –500 Hounsfield units (H) and width of 750 H the larger pulmonary vessels are shown but the smaller peripheral vessels are not seen. **B,** With the window level unchanged at –500 H but the window width increased to 2000 H, the gray scale changes but the caliber of the vessels remains constant. (From Moss AA, Gamsu G, Genant HK. *Computed tomography of the body with magnetic resonance imaging,* 2nd ed. Philadelphia: WB Saunders, 1992:162.)

coronal planes can determine if a mass is above or below the diaphragm or invades the diaphragm.

Radionuclide Studies

For completeness sake, nuclear medicine imaging for pulmonary embolism will be discussed, chiefly as a modality that is used to assess ventilation–perfusion abnormalities. However, the reader should note that, with the rapid improvement of CT scanning, isotope studies are becoming obsolete for many pulmonary diagnostics.

Ventilation–perfusion scans have typically been useful for the diagnosis of pulmonary embolus. In a perfusion scan, the lung tissue

peripheral to an arterial block is not perfused with tagged radioactive particles so a defect is produced on the scan. When the perfusion scan is abnormal, a ventilation scan is performed by inhalation of a radioactive gas. A patient who is clinically suspected of having a pulmonary embolus who has a perfusion scan defect but a normal ventilation scan probably does have an embolus. In addition, postoperative function after lobectomy can be calculated from the ventilation and perfusion scans by studying the unilateral function of the tumor-bearing lung or the regional pulmonary function of the affected lobe.

Several alternative nuclear medicine scans are becoming part of thoracic disease management. Radioactive iodine (iodine-131)

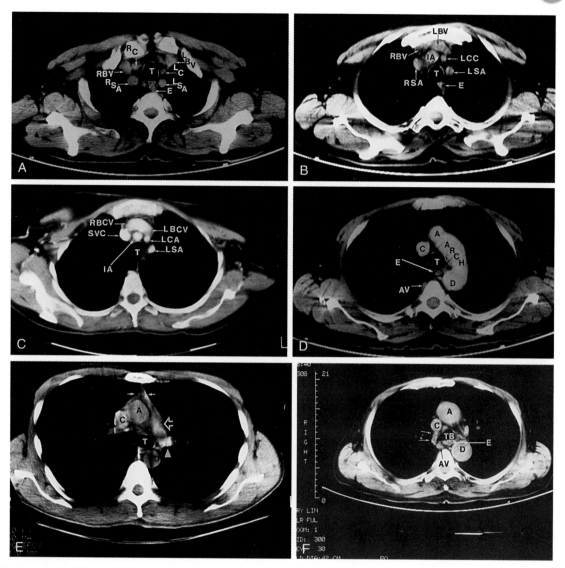

Figure 4–12. Normal CT anatomy of the chest using mediastinal windows. Mediastinal and cardiovascular anatomy is well-defined with this window. Key anatomic levels are selected from thoracic inlet to diaphragm.

A–C, Inlet to arch. **A,** Non-contrast-enhanced CT demonstrates right and left brachiocephalic veins (RBV and LBV) lateral to right and left common carotid arteries (RC and LC) and subclavian arteries (RSA and LSA). E, esophagus; T, trachea. **B,** Contrast-enhanced CT demonstrates right and left brachiocephalic veins converging, although the superior vena cava is not yet formed. The left common carotid artery (LCC), innominate artery (IA), and right and left subclavian arteries (RSA and LSA) are visible at this level. LBV, left brachiocephalic vein; RBV, right brachiocephalic vein. **C,** Contrast-enhanced CT with excellent bolus – vessels with increased intensity (white) compared with **A.** At this level, just above the arch, there is confluence of the right and left brachiocephalic veins (RBCV and LBCV) into the superior vena cava (SVC). Also visualized are the innominate artery (IA), left subclavian artery (LSA), and left common carotid artery (LCA). T, trachea.

D, Arch. Non-contrast-enhanced CT demonstrating ascending (A) and descending (D) segments of aorta with the arch in between. Other structures identified at this level are the superior vena cava (C), trachea (T), esophagus (E), and azygous vein (AV).

E–H, Infra-arch. **E,** Non-contrast-enhanced CT at the level of the aorticopulmonary (AP) window. Structures seen include the thymus (arrows), superior portion of left pulmonary artery (solid arrowhead), and inferior portion of the aortic arch (open arrow). The last finding shows evidence of partial volume averaging. The area between the ascending (A) and descending (D) aorta is the AP window, so named because it is normally void of vessels and lymph nodes. **F,** Contrast-enhanced CT at the tracheal bifurcation (TB). Major structures seen at this level are the azygous arch (arrows) as the azygous vein (AV) turns forward and empties into the superior vena cava (C). A, ascending aorta; D, descending aorta; E, esophagus.

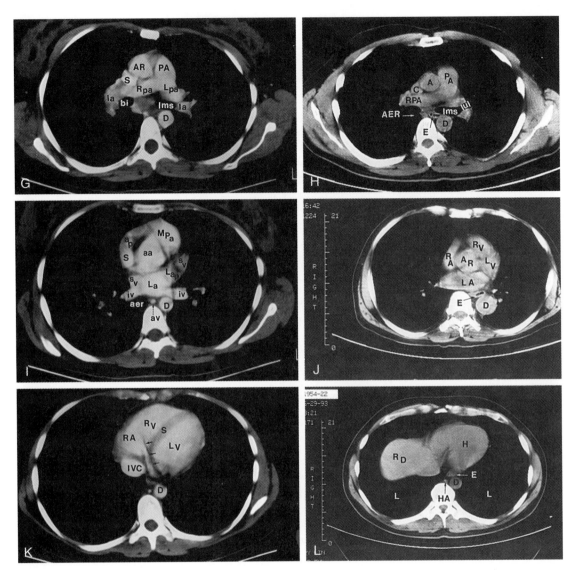

Figure 4–12. Continued. **G**, Contrast-enhanced CT at this subcarinal level demonstrates the main pulmonary artery (PA) and the root of the aorta (AR). The main pulmonary artery bifurcates into the right and left pulmonary arteries (Rpa and Lpa). On sections proceeding from superior to inferior through the hilum, the left pulmonary artery is encountered first. bi, bronchus intermedius; D, descending aorta; Ia, interlobar arteries; Ims, left main stem bronchus; S, superior vena cava. **H**, Non-contrast-enhanced CT at 1 cm below **part G**. The left main pulmonary artery is not visible. The azygoesophageal recess (AER) is concave, which is normal. A, ascending aorta; C, superior vena cava; D, descending aorta; E, esophagus; Ims, left main stem bronchus; lul, left upper lobe bronchus; PA, main pulmonary artery; RPA, right pulmonary artery.
I–K, Pericardiac level. **I**, Contrast-enhanced CT at the level of the left atrium. The left atrium (La) is the highest and most posterior cardiac chamber, seen here accepting bilateral inferior (iv) and superior (sv) pulmonary venous inflow. Also seen are the left atrial (Lap) and right atrial (ap) appendages, the superior vena cava (S), the ascending aorta (aa), and the main pulmonary outflow tract (MPa). aer, azygoesophageal recess; av, azygous vein; D, descending aorta. **J**, Contrast-enhanced CT at the level of the 'five-chambered heart.' Five major chambers are seen: left atrium (LA), right atrium (RA), left ventricle (LV), right ventricle (RV), and aortic root (AR). D, descending aorta; E, esophagus. **K**, Contrast-enhanced CT at the level of the coronary sinus (arrows), seen posterolateral to the right ventricle (RV) and medial to the right atrium (RA) and inferior vena cava (IVC). D, descending aorta; LV, left ventricle; S, interventricular septum.
L, M, Diaphragm level. **L**, Non-contrast-enhanced CT at the upper right diaphragm level. At this level, the right dome of the diaphragm (RD) is encountered at the same level as the apex of the heart (H) on the left. D, descending aorta; E, esophagus; HA, hemiazygous vein; L, lung bases.

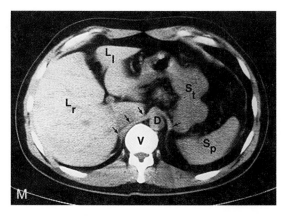

Figure 4–12. Continued. **M**, Non-contrast-enhanced CT at the level of the diaphragmatic crura: Seen at this level are segments of liver – right lobe (Lr), left lobe (Ll) – stomach (St), spleen (Sp), and the diaphragmatic crura (arrows) as they descend to attach to the lower vertebral bodies. The crura demarcate the lowest intrathoracic space (medial) from the subdiaphragmatic spaces (retroperitoneal/intra-abdominal) laterally. D, descending aorta; V, vertebral body. (From Meholic A, Ketai L, Lofgren R. *Fundamentals of chest radiology*. Philadelphia: WB Saunders, 1996:20, 22.)

may be taken up by a functional thyroid tumor or substernal goiter. Gallium-67 scans may aid in the diagnosis of emphysema and interstitial lung diseases (Figure 4–22 on p. 87). Indium 111-labeled leukocytes can identify localized infections within the mediastinum. Positron emission tomography (PET) scans take advantage of the propensity of tumor cells to take up more glucose than normal tissues. Radioactive glucose can be injected into a patient with a known neoplasm and PET scanning can identify regions of metastasis by increased utilization and intracellular trapping of glucose.

Bronchoscopy

Bronchoscopy has several diagnostic and therapeutic uses in the management of pulmonary disease. Bronchoscopy permits direct visualization of the airway, biopsy of suspicious masses, washings for cytological examination, and removal of small masses (Box 4–2 on p. 88). Stenting of diseased airways and control of intraluminal bleeding has also been used in select patients.

Flexible bronchoscopy is performed from the right side of the patient with the operator facing the head of the bed. The endoscope can be passed transnasally or transorally. Once past the vocal cords, the trachea consists of C-shaped cartilaginous strips anteriorly and a membranous flexible portion posteriorly. The trachea is approximately 10–12 cm long before reaching the bifurcation. The trachea is crossed anteriorly by the innominate vein. The innominate artery and carotid artery lie along the anterolateral wall of the trachea. The aortic arch lies to the left of the trachea and the superior vena cava to the right. Posterolaterally lie the right and left paratracheal lymph node chains.

At the carina, the right bronchus can be identified because it tends to drop more vertically (Figure 4–23 on p. 89). The first branch of the right bronchus is the right upper lobe, which branches within 1 cm of the carina.

Figure 4–13. Asbestos-related pleural plaques. Prone high-resolution CT scan shows pleural plaques (straight white arrows) separated by a layer of extrapleural and subcostalis muscles (black arrows). (From Moss AA, Gamsu G, Genant HK. *Computed tomography of the body with magnetic resonance imaging*, 2nd ed. Philadelphia: WB Saunders, 1992:272.)

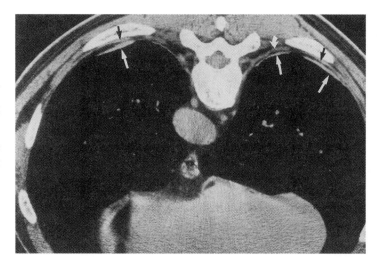

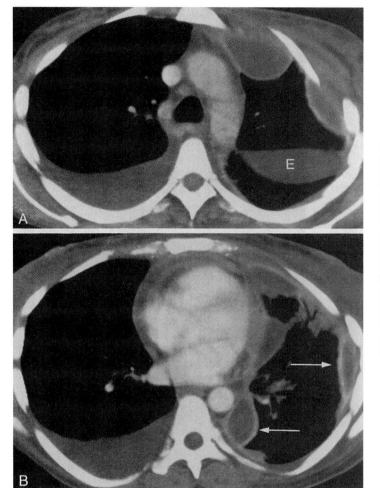

Figure 4–14. Multiple loculated pleural effusions with an empyema. **A**, CT scan at the level of the aortic arch demonstrates bilateral pleural effusions. The effusion on the right is free flowing and the one on the left is loculated at multiple sites. Effusion (E) is present in the left major fissure. **B**, CT scan at a level of the heart again shows the free-flowing right pleural effusion. On the left side, two empyema cavities (arrows) are visible laterally and paraspinously. Lung consolidation with air bronchograms is seen in the lingula. (From Moss AA, Gamsu G, Genant HK. *Computed tomography of the body with magnetic resonance imaging*, 2nd ed. Philadelphia: WB Saunders, 1992:270.)

This branch comes off at a 90° angle and comes out laterally. The remainder of the right bronchus, the bronchus intermedius, extends 2 cm before dividing into the right middle segment and the basilar bronchial segment. The right pulmonary artery crosses anteriorly to the right main stem bronchus at its origin and lies on the anterolateral surface of the bronchus.

The right upper lobe bronchus divides into three segmental bronchi (apical, posterior, and anterior). The middle lobe divides into the medial and lateral segments. The lower lobe divides into the superior segment and four basilar segments (anterior, medial, lateral, and posterior basal).

The left main stem bronchus extends 3 cm from the tracheal bifurcation to the division into the upper and lower lobes. The left bronchus passes inferior to the aortic arch. The first branch is the left upper lobe bronchus, which comes off at a 110° angle from the left main stem. The continuation becomes the lower lobe segment.

The left upper lobe bronchus divides into an upper division and a lower division. The upper division gives rise to the apicoposterior and anterior segments. The lower division is the lingual and gives rise to the superior and inferior lingular segmental bronchi. The left lower lobe bronchus divides into the anteromedial basal segment, the lateral basal segment, and the posterior basal segment.

After initial inspection, brushings, washings, and biopsy may be performed as indicated (Figure 4–24 on p. 90). A diagnostic bronchoscopy may include brushings and biopsy of suspected mucosal abnormalities, bronchoalveolar lavage of a segment, and transbronchial lung biopsy (Figure 4–25 on p. 90).

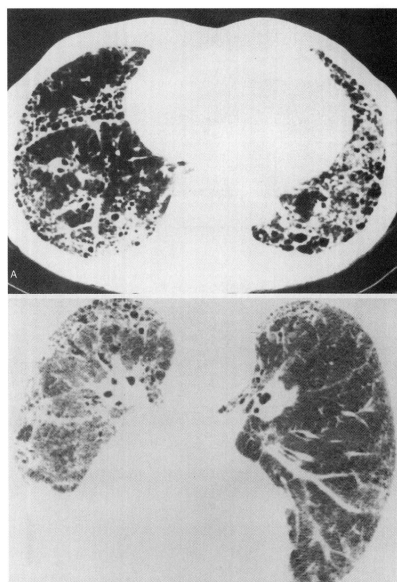

Figure 4–15. Idiopathic pulmonary fibrosis with honeycombed lung in three patients. **A**, High-resolution CT scan through the lower lungs demonstrates the typical subpleural distribution of honeycomb lung in a patient with idiopathic pulmonary fibrosis. Honeycombing in the right middle lobe is subpleural, adjacent to the major fissure. More extensive abnormalities are present on the left. **B**, Prone high-resolution CT scan in another patient demonstrates subpleural honeycombing at both lung bases. The ground-glass appearance in the left lower lobe suggests an active alveolitis. (From Moss AA, Gamsu G, Genant HK. *Computed tomography of the body with magnetic resonance imaging*, 2nd ed. Philadelphia: WB Saunders, 1992:210.)

BOX 4–1 CHEST PATHOLOGY FOR WHICH MRI IS PREFERABLE TO CT

- Evaluation of mediastinum for vascular abnormality in patient who cannot receive intravenous contrast agent
- Evaluation of coarctation or aortic dissection
- Evaluation for chest wall invasion by tumor
- Most cardiac imaging other than detection of coronary artery calcifications

From Meholic A, Ketai L, Lofgren R. *Fundamentals of chest radiology*. Philadelphia: WB Saunders, 1996:26.

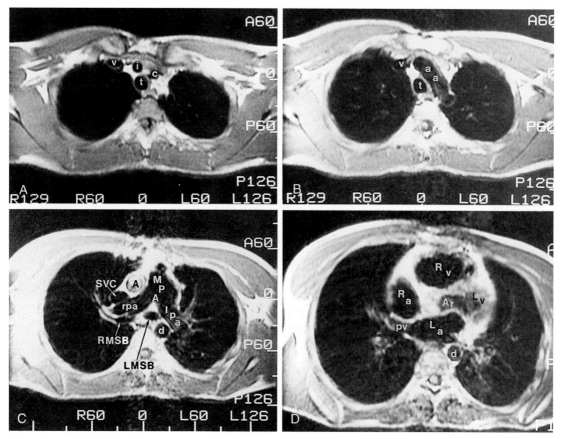

Figure 4–16. MRI of the chest and heart: normal anatomy using T1 spin echo technique. On T1 images (best for MR anatomy), fat is white (increased signal), blood/air/calcium is black (decreased signal), and muscle/fascia is gray (intermediate signal). Axial images corresponding to the CT images shown in Figures 4–10 and 4–12 were taken at the thoracic inlet (**A**), aortic arch (**B**), right and left pulmonary tracts (**C**), and five-chambered heart (**D**). **A**, The anatomy is not always as easily seen as with CT. Only the right brachio-cephalic vein (v), innominate artery (i), left carotid artery (c), and trachea (t) are seen on this image. **B**, At the level of the aortic arch (aa), the right superior vena cava (v) and trachea (t) are seen. **C**, At the level of the main pulmonary outflow tract (MPA), the right and left pulmonary arteries (rpa and lpa), superior vena cava (SVC), aortic root (A), descending aorta (d), left main stem bronchus (LMSB), and right main stem bronchus (RMSB) are seen. **D**, At the level of the five-chambered heart, the right and left ventricles (Rv and Lv), right and left atria (Ra and La), aortic root (Ar), a right pulmonary vein (pv), and descending aorta (d) are seen.

The diagnostic yield from fiberoptic bronchoscopy varies from 20% to 80%, but a specific benign diagnosis is made only 10% of the time. Recognizing this, it is hard to justify the performance of a bronchoscopy if one is looking to make a diagnosis of benign disease. Unfortunately, percutaneous needle aspiration biopsy does not fare much better. Although its sensitivity in making the diagnosis of malignancy is high, a specific benign diagnosis can be made only about as often as the rate achieved bronchoscopically. A 'negative' needle biopsy is of no help and necessitates a further diagnostic procedure, while a diagnosis of malignancy essentially tells us

what we already know – the lesion has to be excised.

Mediastinoscopy

Mediastinoscopy is the definitive invasive procedure to stage the superior mediastinal lymph nodes. It is reliable in assessing pretracheal, paratracheal, subcarinal, and tracheobronchial lymph nodes (2R and L, 4R and L, 7, and 10R; Figure 4–26 on p. 91). Because the lymphatic system is sampled and some areas are beyond reach, there is a false-negative incidence of approximately 10%.

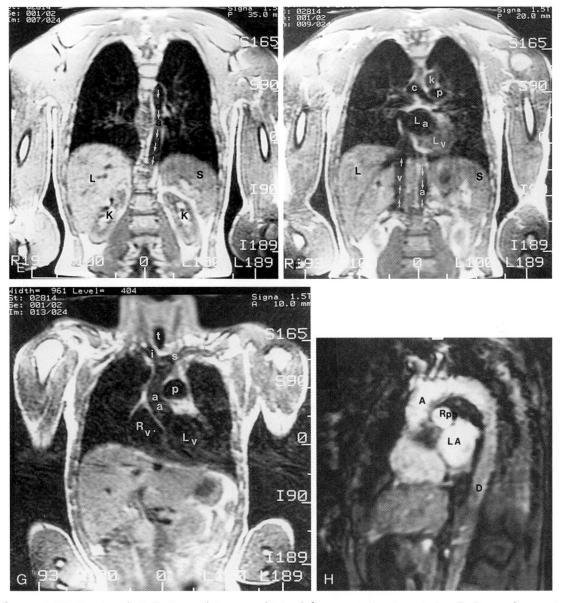

Figure 4–16. Continued. **E–G**, Coronal images obtained from posterior to anterior. **E**, Descending aorta (da and arrows). L, liver; K, kidneys; S, spleen. **F**, View in the plane of the left atrium (La) shows the left ventricle (Lv), aortic knob (k), pulmonary artery (p), carina (c), aorta (a with arrows). L, liver; S, spleen. **G**, The most anterior level of the right and left ventricles (Rv and Lv) demonstrate the ascending aorta (aa) with two of three main branches. i, innominate; p, main pulmonary artery; s, subclavian; t, trachea. **H**, Sagittal MRI. A, ascending aorta; D, descending aorta; LA, left atrium; RPA, right pulmonary artery. (From Meholic A, Ketai L, Lofgren R. *Fundamentals of chest radiology*. Philadelphia: WB Saunders, 1996:24–25.)

The decision to perform mediastinoscopy is based on a review of the chest CT scan and the documentation of enlarged mediastinal lymph nodes. The definition of what constitutes nodal enlargement varies among centers, but lymph nodes 1.5 cm or more in diameter arouse enough suspicion to be considered enlarged by most.

The standard cervical mediastinoscopy involves creating a pretracheal tunnel through a small single cervical incision (Figure 4–27 on p. 92). The patient's neck should be hyperextended by placing a roll beneath the scapulae. A transcervical incision just above the sternal notch should be made and continued down through the platysma. The strap

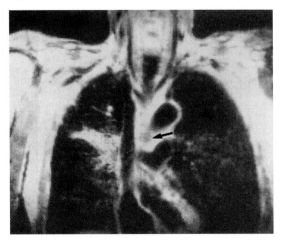

Figure 4–17. Contralateral N3 nodes in the aortic-pulmonic window. Coronal MR demonstrates atelectasis of the anterior segment of the right upper lobe due to an endobronchial tumor. A contralateral N3 node (arrow) is visible deep in the aortic–pulmonic window. Biopsy of this node demonstrated metastatic tumor, making the tumor nonresectable. (From Moss AA, Gamsu G, Genant HK. *Computed tomography of the body with magnetic resonance imaging*, 2nd ed. Philadelphia: WB Saunders, 1992:104.)

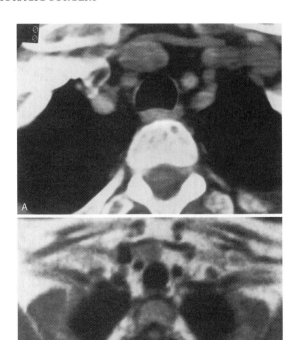

Figure 4–18. Superior mediastinal parathyroid adenoma in a patient with recurrent hyperparathyroidism following neck exploration. **A**, CT scan demonstrates a 2 cm mass immediately in front of the trachea. **B**, T1-weighted MRI at the same level demonstrates the mass, which is low in signal intensity and can be readily distinguished from mediastinal fat. (From Moss AA, Gamsu G, Genant HK. *Computed tomography of the body with magnetic resonance imaging*, 2nd ed. Philadelphia: WB Saunders, 1992:97.)

muscles are separated in the midline and pretracheal fascia is entered. With blunt finger dissection, the mediastinal plane is created anterior to the trachea. The mediastinoscope can then be inserted after finger palpation for enlarged, firm lymph nodes. Dissection is carried out using a suction cautery with the tip of the mediastinoscope providing the countertraction.

The anterior mediastinotomy or 'Chamberlain procedure' was developed to assess lymph nodes in the aortopulmonary window and left para-aortic area. The procedure can be used on either side to obtain tissue from an anterior mediastinal mass or a centrally located mass within the hilum. Access to the mediastinum is gained by excising the second costal cartilage in a subperichondrial plane. The internal mammary vessels are either protected or ligated and the pleura is reflected laterally so that the surgeon remains extrapleural, although entry into the pleural space is not problematic (Figure 4–28 on p. 93).

Thoracoscopy

The term video-assisted thoracic surgery (VATS) encompasses all procedures performed with the thoracoscope, including those that are purely 'thoracoscopic.' The bony thorax, as opposed to the abdomen, provides its own space once the lung is collapsed, so insufflation of gas, used in the abdomen to create a working space, is unnecessary and even slightly dangerous. The space in the chest is created simply by placing an endobronchial tube and collapsing the ipsilateral lung. This requires a general anesthetic but certain procedures typically involving the parietal pleura may be performed with only regional anesthesia and intravenous sedation since the lung collapses in the spontaneously breathing patient once the negative, intrathoracic pressure is lost.

The patient is placed on the operating table in the lateral decubitus position, and the chest

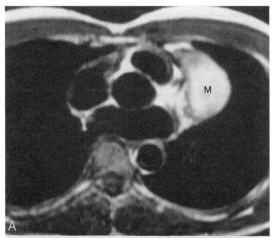

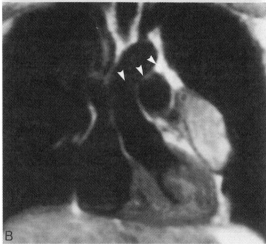

Figure 4–19. Congenital thymic cyst in an asymptomatic adult male. **A,** Cardiac-gated MR image demonstrates a mass to the left of the base of the heart. The mass (M) is homogeneous and appears not to be infiltrating the mediastinum. **B,** Coronal MR image shows a plane of cleavage (arrowheads) between the mass and the heart, probably representing the pericardium. (Courtesy of Clark Carrol, MD, Houston, TX.)

is prepared and draped as for a thoracotomy (Figure 4–29 on p. 95). Incision placement depends somewhat on the procedure to be performed, but the location of the incision for insertion of the videothoracoscope remains constant in the seventh or eighth intercostal space aligned with the anterior superior iliac spine. A 1 cm incision is made and deepened to the intercostal muscles, as if one were inserting a chest tube; indeed, it is through this incision that the chest tube is placed at the conclusion of the surgical procedure. Entry into the chest is made with the index

finger, to assure absolute safety. Occasionally, the lung is adherent to the chest wall, and these adhesions must be broken up with the index finger to allow for placement of the trocar sheath. Additional incisions are made as needed – usually arrayed in a triangular fashion, which facilitates instrument placement and allows one to work in coordination with an assistant (Figure 4–30 on p. 95). It is best to work with two video monitors, which are placed at the head of the table on each side, so that both the operator and the assistant have an unobstructed view of the surgical field.

The instrumentation available for thoracoscopy has been slowly improving. Instruments designed specifically for laparoscopy proved to be poor for this application. Grasping the lung without tearing the parenchyma proved to be especially difficult with these instruments. The most significant development in instrumentation, one that markedly expanded the utility of thoracoscopy, was the introduction of the endoscopic linear stapler. This instrument, more than any other, propelled thoracoscopy out of the realm of pure diagnostics into the mainstream of therapeutic applications.

The major but certainly not the only indication for thoracoscopy in the management of pleural disease remains the undiagnosed pleural effusion (Table 4–3 on p. 96). In the past, the patient with an empyema often was forced to undergo thoracotomy for debridement and decortication to rid the space of infection and allow the lung to re-expand. With thoracoscopic techniques, many of these patients may now avoid thoracotomy, especially if they are seen early in the course of their disease. Thoracoscopic debridement and decortication are indicated in the febrile patient with a pleural effusion in whom tube thoracostomy provides incomplete drainage. The fibrinous nature of the exudate precludes complete drainage with a tube alone and mechanical debridement is required. Likewise, videothoracoscopic techniques have proved useful in the management of the organized posttraumatic hemothorax in which a chest tube is unable to effectively drain the organized clot and debris.

Benign pleural tumors, specifically solitary fibrous tumors, commonly arise from the visceral pleural surface and, depending upon size, are ideal lesions for thoracoscopic resection. Videothoracoscopy also has increased our ability to deal successfully with malignant pleural effusions, especially those in

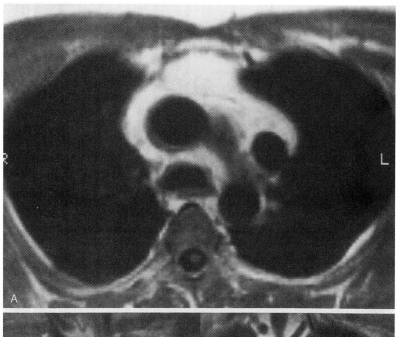

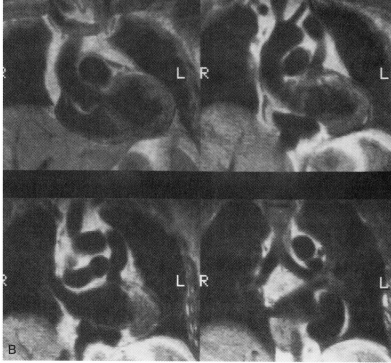

Figure 4–20. Persistent left superior vena cava. **A,** Cardiac-gated MR image demonstrates a large anomalous vessel to the left of the aortic-pulmonic window. The right superior vena cava is absent. **B,** Cardiac-gated coronal MR image confirms the persistent left superior vena cava coursing lateral to the main pulmonary artery and posterior to the left atrium to join the coronary venous system. (From Moss AA, Gamsu G, Genant HK. *Computed tomography of the body with magnetic resonance imaging*, 2nd ed. Philadelphia: WB Saunders, 1992:66.)

which loculations are present. When tube thoracostomy results in incomplete drainage or one attempt at chest tube pleurodesis has failed, thoracoscopy – whereby the chest is evacuated under direct vision and talc is insufflated – is the procedure of choice. Patients sclerosed with talc seemed to have less pain following the procedure. The ability to perform thoracoscopic talc pleurodesis under local anesthesia may make the technique attractive for most patients with malignant effusions (Figure 4–31 on p. 96).

Transbronchial lung biopsy often is successful in providing diagnostic material in

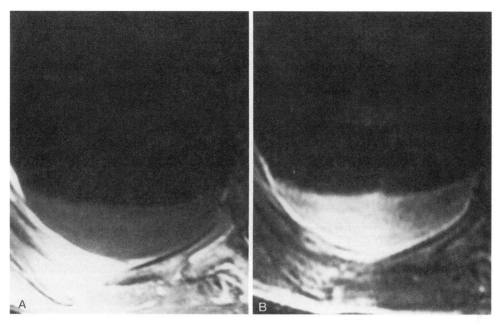

Figure 4–21. MRI scan of pleural effusion. On the T1-weighted image (**A**), the pleural effusion is lower than muscle in signal intensity. On the T2-weighted image (**B**), the pleural effusion shows a marked increase in signal intensity. (From Moss AA, Gamsu G, Genant HK. *Computed tomography of the body with magnetic resonance imaging*, 2nd ed. Philadelphia: WB Saunders, 1992:266.)

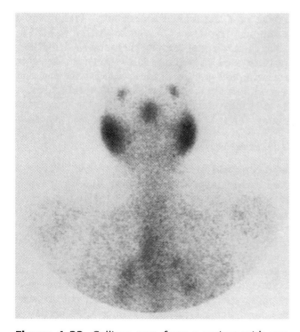

Figure 4–22. Gallium scan from a patient with sarcoidosis. Note the increased uptake of gallium in the conjunctival tissue, parotid glands, and hilar and mediastinal lymph nodes. (From Pearson FG, Cooper JD, Deslauriers J, *et al. Thoracic surgery*, 2nd ed. New York: Churchill Livingstone, 2002:665.)

patients with diffuse pulmonary infiltrates. In situations in which a transbronchial biopsy fails to provide diagnostic material, a VATS procedure is indicated. Before the advent of videothoracoscopy, many of these patients were treated empirically, usually with steroids. Lung biopsy, which required a thoracotomy, albeit a 'mini' one, was reserved for patients who either failed empiric therapy or were desperately ill and in intensive care. The empiric approach probably is warranted and may, in fact, be preferred in the non-neutropenic cancer patient with acute pneumonitis, for whom broad-spectrum antibiotic therapy is usually the treatment of choice. In the nonimmunocompromised patient, usually with a chronic interstitial process, serious consideration must be given to obtaining a piece of lung tissue. VATS lung biopsy will always provide diagnostic material.

Before the introduction of videothoracoscopy, a thoracotomy was required solely for the purpose of obtaining a piece of lung tissue. The thoracotomy usually consisted of a small inframammary incision into the chest through the fourth or fifth intercostal space, a procedure that can be done expeditiously

BOX 4–2 AMERICAN THORACIC SOCIETY GUIDELINES FOR FLEXIBLE FIBEROPTIC BRONCHOSCOPY

Diagnostic Uses

- To evaluate lung lesions of unknown etiology that appear on the chest x-ray
- To assess airway patency
- To investigate unexplained hemoptysis, unexplained cough, localized wheeze, or stridor
- To search for the origin of suspicious or positive sputum cytology
- To investigate the etiology of unexplained paralysis of a vocal cord or hemidiaphragm, superior vena cava syndrome, chylothorax, or unexplained pleural effusion
- To evaluate problems associated with endotracheal tubes, such as tracheal damage, airway obstruction, or tube placement
- To stage lung cancer preoperatively and subsequently to evaluate, when appropriate, the response to therapy
- To obtain material for microbiologic studies in suspected pulmonary infections
- To evaluate the airways for suspected bronchial tear or other injury after thoracic trauma
- To evaluate a suspected tracheoesophageal fistula
- To determine the location and extent of respiratory tract injury after acute inhalation of noxious fumes or aspiration of gastric contents
- To obtain material for study from the lungs of patients with diffuse or focal lung diseases

Therapeutic Uses

- To remove retained secretions or mucous plugs not mobilized by conventional noninvasive techniques
- To remove foreign bodies
- To remove abnormal endobronchial tissue or foreign material by use of forceps or laser techniques
- To perform difficult intubations
- To aid in the delivery of brachytherapy
- To aid in the deployment of expandable wire stents

Conditions Involving Increased Risk

- Lack of patient cooperation
- Recent myocardial infarction or unstable angina
- Partial tracheal obstruction
- Unstable bronchial asthma
- Respiratory insufficiency associated with moderate to severe hypoxemia or any degree of hypercarbia
- Uremia and pulmonary hypertension (possible serious hemorrhage after biopsy)
- Lung abscess (danger of flooding the airway with purulent material)
- Obstruction of the superior vena cava (possibility of bleeding and laryngeal edema)
- Debility, advanced age, malnutrition
- Unstable cardiac arrhythmia
- Respiratory failure requiring mechanical ventilation
- Disorders requiring laser therapy, biopsy of lesions obstructing large airways, or multiple transbronchial lung biopsies

The danger of a serious complication is especially high in the following conditions

- Malignant arrhythmia
- Profound refractory hypoxemia
- Severe bleeding diathesis that cannot be corrected when biopsy is anticipated

BOX 4–2 AMERICAN THORACIC SOCIETY GUIDELINES FOR FLEXIBLE FIBEROPTIC
BRONCHOSCOPY (CONT'D)

Contraindications

- Absence of consent from the patient or his or her representative
- Bronchoscopy by an inexperienced person without direct supervision
- Bronchoscopy without adequate facilities and personnel to care for emergencies such as cardiopulmonary arrest, pneumothorax, or bleeding
- Inability to adequately oxygenate the patient during the procedure

Adapted with permission from the guidelines for fiberoptic bronchoscopy in adults. Accepted as official position paper by the American Thoracic Society Board of Directors, November 1986; from Sokolowski RW, Burgher LW, Jones FL, *et al.* Guidelines for fiberoptic bronchoscopy in adults. *Am Rev Respir Dis* 1987;136:1066.

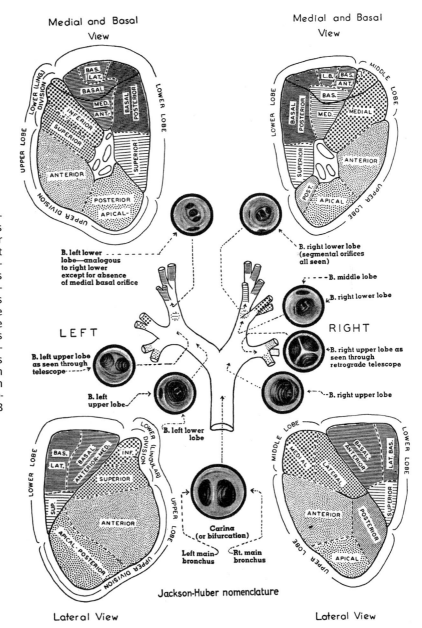

Figure 4–23. Drawings showing the pulmonary segments and the lobal bronchi and their segmental branches. The inset circles show the schematic representation of the landmarks seen endoscopically at the various points. The bronchial tree is shown 'upside down,' because it is desired to represent the structures in the same relations observed by the bronchoscopist when the patient is examined in the usual position of dorsal recumbency. (From Jackson C, Jackson CL. *Bronchoesophagology.* Philadelphia: WB Saunders, 1950.)

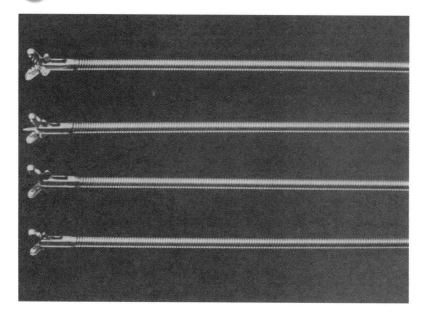

Figure 4–24. A selection of flexible biopsy forceps for use through the flexible fiberoptic bronchoscope. (From Pearson FG, Cooper JD, Deslauriers J, *et al. Thoracic surgery*, 2nd ed. New York: Churchill Livingstone, 2002:86.)

and allows one to obtain enough lung parenchyma to make a diagnosis. There should be minimal morbidity with this approach, and it still represents the best approach to lung biopsy in the critically ill, hemodynamically fragile patient who is ventilator-dependent (requiring high peak airway pressures and high inspired oxygen concentration), for whom transport to the operating room represents a substantial risk. The 'mini' anterior thoracotomy does not require single-lung ventilation and thus avoids the potential morbidity and mortality associated with exchange of the endotracheal tube for an endobronchial tube in these

high-risk patients. However, the surgical exposure achieved by this approach can significantly limit the area of lung that may be accessible for biopsy. It is also difficult to obtain tissue from more than one site of the lung with this approach.

In most patients, however, VATS wedge lung biopsy represents the best alternative to the 'mini' thoracotomy. It offers the advantage of excellent visualization of the entire lung so that suspect areas can be biopsied under direct vision and all areas of the lung can be reached with relative ease. The technique avoids spreading of the ribs, which seems to be one of the factors responsible

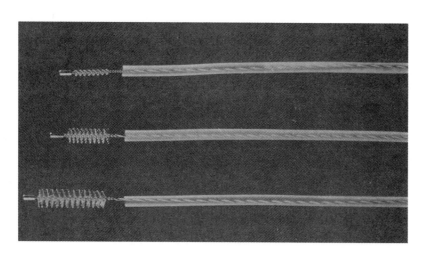

Figure 4–25. Bronchial brushes in protective plastic catheter sheaths can be used to obtain protected samples from the distal airways for culture. (From Pearson FG, Cooper JD, Deslauriers J, *et al. Thoracic surgery*, 2nd ed. New York: Churchill Livingstone, 2002: 86.)

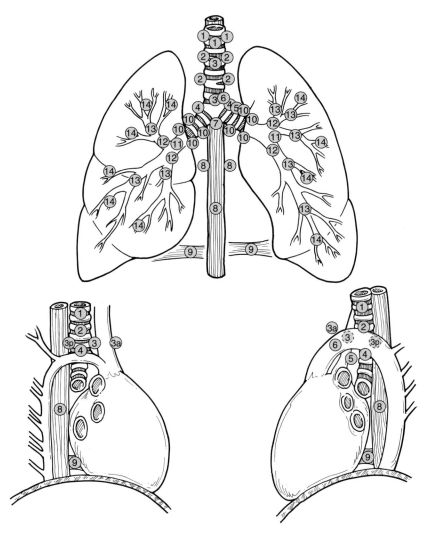

1. Superior mediastinal or highest mediastinal
2. Paratracheal
3. Pretracheal
   3a. Anterior mediastinal
   3p. Retrotracheal or posterior mediastinal
4. Tracheobronchial
5. Subaortic or Botallo's
6. Paraaortic (ascending aorta)

7. Subcarinal
8. Paraesophageal (below carina)
9. Pulmonary ligament
10. Hilar
11. Interlobar
12. Lobar—upper lobe, middle lobe, and lower lobe
13. Segmental
14. Subsegmental

Figure 4–26. Lymph node stations recommended by the American Joint Committee on Cancer. (Redrawn from Naruke T, Suemasu K, Ishikawa S. Lymph node mapping and curability at various levels of metastasis in resected lung cancer. *J Thorac Cardiovasc Surg* 1978;76:832.)

for the pain that results following thoracotomy, including anterior thoracotomy. It may be that thoracoscopic biopsy causes less postoperative pain, which may be important in weaning patients from a ventilator in the immediate postoperative period, and results in a shorter hospital stay. When lung biopsy

is indicated, thoracoscopic biopsy is our procedure of choice for nonventilated patients. For patients requiring mechanical ventilation we prefer a limited anterior thoracotomy with minimal rib spreading. This is a simple procedure that can be performed expeditiously and avoids the need for single-lung ventilation.

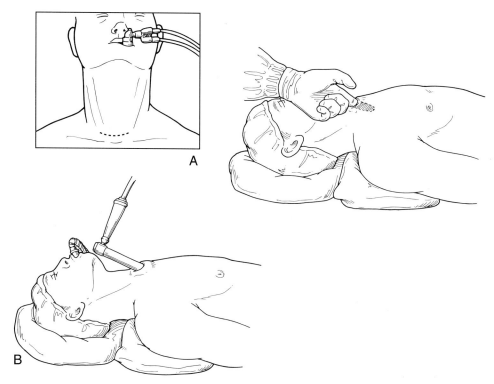

Figure 4–27. Cervical mediastinoscopy. **A,** The endotracheal tube is positioned at the left corner of the mouth, with the anesthesia equipment to the patient's left side. The shoulders are elevated on an inflatable pillow, the top of the head is aligned with the top of the operating table, and the occiput rests on a ring cushion. The incision is positioned one finger-breadth superior to the clavicular heads. Following transverse division of the subcutaneous fat and platysma, the balance of the dissection is carried out vertically in the midline plane. The strap muscles are separated. The thyroid isthmus is retracted superiorly and the dissection is carried down to the anterior surface of the trachea at the level of the second or third tracheal ring. Once the pretracheal plane is reached, and the last areolar tissue has been dissected from the anterior surface of the trachea, the index finger is inserted into the mediastinum, staying on the anterior surface of the trachea. **B,** The mediastinoscope is inserted and advanced along the pretracheal plane. Dissection of the pretracheal and paratracheal spaces is facilitated with the use of an insulated sucker, which can also be used to cauterize bleeding points following nodal biopsy. A long length of gauze packing should always be available, as should a sternal saw or Lubschke knife for the rare occasion when emergency sternotomy might be necessary for control of bleeding.

The solitary indeterminate pulmonary nodule is a problem routinely confronted by the thoracic surgeon. In light of the emergence of VATS as a minimally invasive procedure that can be performed with low morbidity even in compromised patients, we must examine closely the current management of a patient who presents with an indeterminate nodule. Whereas in the past definitive management required open thoracotomy, with its attendant morbidity, this is no longer the case. Thoracoscopy offers the opportunity both to definitively make the diagnosis and to treat many of these lesions and, therefore, causes a refocus in our thinking.

Certain lesions are not considered for VATS excision. For lesions greater than 3 cm in diameter, the likelihood of malignancy is so high (>90%) that, in the absence of metastatic disease, thoracotomy and anatomic resection – i.e. lobectomy – should be the first procedure undertaken. The CT scan aids greatly in localizing the nodule, and we have found it to be the only localizing study required. Even deep-seated lesions may be palpated and located, a technique that becomes easier with experience. Our technique relies heavily on instruments specifically designed for thoracoscopy that greatly facilitate the procedure, especially in grasping or moving the lung to the palpating finger.

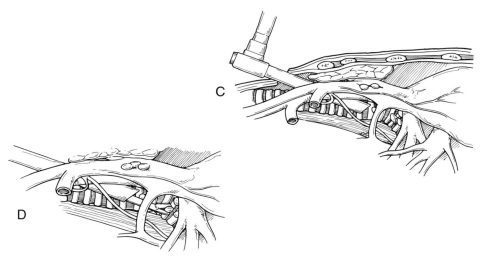

Figure 4–27. Continued. **C**, This lateral 'cut out' view shows the mediastinoscope passing down the right side of the trachea. Dissection with a sucker tip aids in unroofing the nodes. **D**, Each time the mediastinoscope is inserted, care must be taken to ensure its insertion immediately adjacent to the trachea. Biopsies are routinely taken from right peritracheal, bronchial, and subcarinal lymph node areas. Dissection along the left peritracheal and tracheobronchial angle regions must be done with extreme care to avoid injury to the adjacent left recurrent laryngeal nerve. Prior to biopsying the lymph node, it should be mobilized as much as possible to ensure that it is the lymph node and not a major vessel. Particular care must be taken to avoid mistaking the azygos vein for a right tracheobronchial angle lymph node. Even when the operator is quite experienced, a long aspirating needle should be placed in the lymph node and suction applied to the attached syringe, to confirm that the structure to be biopsied is not a vessel, or a flattened lymph node closely applied to the surface of a major vessel. (Redrawn from Urschel HC Jr, Cooper JD. *Atlas of thoracic surgery.* New York: Churchill Livingstone, 1995:61, 63.)

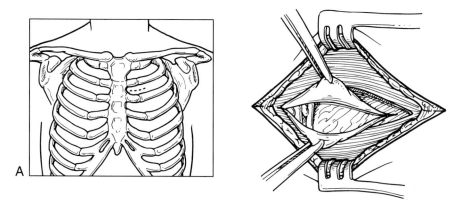

Figure 4–28. A, B, Anterior–second interspace mediastinoscopy. Left upper lobe tumors may metastasize to subaortic lymph nodes or to anterior mediastinal lymph nodes along the course of the left phrenic nerve. These areas are not accessible by standard cervical mediastinoscopy. To access these regions, a left anterior mediastinotomy may be performed, if the preceding cervical mediastinoscopy has been negative. The anterior mediastinoscopy is carried out prior to closure of the cervical incision. **A,** A 3 cm incision is made over the second interspace just lateral to the sternum. Fibers of the pectoralis muscle are separated and dissection is carried down to the intercostal membrane, which is incised, with care taken to stay lateral to the internal mammary vessels. The tip of the index finger is inserted down to the pleura, directed immediately behind the sternum to the midline. The index finger is used to displace the pleura to the left, providing extra pleural access to the ascending aorta and subaortic space. Alternatively, a transpleural route may be used.

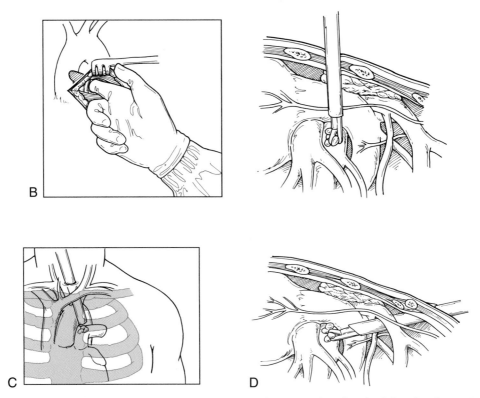

Figure 4–28. Continued. **B**, With the surgeon standing at the patient's right, the left index finger is inserted into the cervical mediastinoscopy incision and positioned posterior to the aortic arch. The right index finger is then placed through the anterior mediastinotomy incision and directed to the anterior portion of the aortic arch and the subaortic space, which can then be palpated between the two fingertips. If any abnormality is palpated either in the anterior mediastinal space or in the subaortic space, the mediastinoscope can be inserted and biopsies obtained. A metastatic tumor in subaortic lymph nodes has a less ominous prognosis than positive lymph nodes in the superior mediastinal space. The anterior mediastinotomy not only allows for a biopsy of such nodes but allows the determination as to the degree of extranodal extension or fixation, which does affect both prognosis and resectability. **C, D**, Extended cervical mediastinoscopy. An alternative to the use of anterior mediastinotomy for evaluation of subaortic and anterior mediastinal lymph nodes is the extended cervical mediastinoscopy. If the standard cervical mediastinal lymph node biopsy is negative, a plane is developed anterior to the aortic arch, down to the subaortic space. To do this, the index finger is placed through the cervical incision, and down to the left side of the innominate artery at its origin from the aortic arch. The tip of the index finger is curved anteriorly and used to create a plane anterior to the aorta angling obliquely down toward the left sternal border. In most cases, the mediastinoscope can then be placed along this tract, anterior to the aortic arch and down to the subaortic space. However, this is not advisable if there is palpable aortic calcification or atherosclerosis. Furthermore, this maneuver may not be technically feasible in some patients due to enlargement of the aorta, or anterior displacement of the aortic arch due to tortuosity. **C**, Through a transverse cervical incision, 3 cm in length and one finger-breadth above the sternal notch, similar to that for standard cervical mediastinoscopy, the mediastinoscope is passed anterior to the trachea. It passes posterior to the innominate vein, slightly to the right of the left carotid artery, and anterolaterally to the aortic arch. **D**, The lateral view shows the mediastinoscope inserted through the cervical incision posterior to the innominate vein and anterior and lateral to the aortic arch. The subaortic nodes in the aortopulmonary window are dissected bluntly and biopsied through the mediastinoscope. Hemostasis is secured. (Redrawn from Urschel HC Jr, Cooper JD. *Atlas of thoracic surgery*. New York: Churchill Livingstone, 1995:65, 67.)

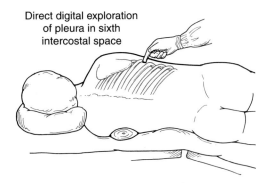

Figure 4–29. The patient is placed in the lateral decubitus position for video-assisted thoracoscopy. (Redrawn from Hanke I, Douglas JM Jr. General approach to video-assisted thoracoscopic surgery. In: Sabiston DC Jr, ed. *Atlas of cardiothoracic surgery*. Philadelphia: WB Saunders, 1995.)

Centrally located lesions, which lie in close proximity to hilar structures, are not suitable for VATS wedge excision and require open thoracotomy.

Video-assisted thoracic surgery has proved useful as an adjunct to more conventional procedures used in the invasive staging of lung cancer. Mediastinoscopy, as mentioned earlier, remains the gold standard for invasive staging of the mediastinum, but lymph nodes in the posterior subcarinal space (level 7) and in the aortopulmonary window (level 5) are not accessible. VATS offers an unmatched ability to visualize the aortopulmonary window and sample lymph nodes in this region; the same is true for the subcarinal space when it is approached from the right side. A VATS staging procedure is not a substitute for mediastinoscopy, but in certain situations directed by findings on the chest CT scan, it may add valuable staging information. This is particularly important because of the interest in preoperative therapy (neoadjuvant) for patients proven to have N2 (mediastinal) lymph node disease.

The utility of VATS is limited for assessing resectability, especially if one is trying to

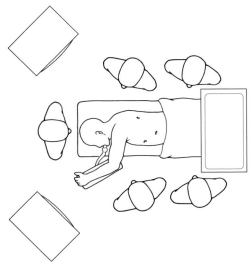

Figure 4–30. Organizational set-up in the operating room. The patient is usually placed in the lateral position with an axillary roll under the 'down' side. A double-lumen endotracheal tube is employed to collapse the 'up' side lung (CO_2 is not necessary). Monitors are placed on each side of the table so that the surgeon, who usually stands on the right side of the table if right-handed, and the assistant, standing on the opposite side, may both follow the activity in the chest by looking straight ahead. The nurse and the camera holder are placed in position on each side of the Mayo stand, with the anesthesiologist in the usual position at the head of the table. Variations of this may be instituted in abnormal situations. All the thoracoscopy instruments are laid out ahead of time. The camera is placed in the most inferior position through the port farthest away from the area to be visualized and operated. It is usually in the midaxillary line through approximately the eighth interspace. An anterior port in the midclavicular line is made usually in the fourth interspace and one in the posterior part lateral to the angle of the scapula in the fourth interspace. The camera is inserted first in the usual fashion and the other ports are placed under direct vision through the camera. Care is taken to use the thoracentesis needle and not to injure the lung. If there is pleurosynthesis, this procedure is more precarious and thoracotomy may be necessary. (Redrawn from Urschel HC Jr, Cooper JD. *Atlas of thoracic surgery*. New York: Churchill Livingstone, 1995:225.)

TABLE 4–3 • *Current Applications of VATS*	
Indications generally accepted and commonly performed (Diagnostic)	Excision of indeterminate pulmonary nodule Lung biopsy for interstitial disease in nonventilated patients Biopsy of pleural lesion Biopsy of mediastinal mass Biopsy of lymph nodes in aortopulmonary window
(Therapeutic)	Pleurodesis for malignant pleural effusion Debridement and drainage of loculated empyema or hemothorax Excision of benign pleural lesions Excision of benign pulmonary lesions Excision of blebs with pleurodesis for spontaneous pneumothorax Bullectomy for giant bullae with compressed lung Sympathectomy for hyperhidrosis and upper extremity pain syndromes
Indications not generally accepted but commonly performed	Excision of mediastinal tumors Pericardial window Wedge excision of early lung cancer as definitive treatment in patients with poor pulmonary reserve "Volume reduction" for diffuse bullous lung disease Treatment of disease of the thoracic spine
Indications not generally accepted and not commonly performed	Lobectomy Esophageal myotomy for achalasia Excision of benign tumors of the esophagus Total esophagectomy for esophageal cancer Biopsy of mediastinal lymph nodes for esophageal cancer staging Ligation of thoracic duct for chylothorax Excision of mediastinal parathyroid adenoma Closure of patent ductus arteriosus

From Meholic A, Ketai L, Lofgren R. *Fundamentals of chest radiology.* Philadelphia: WB Saunders, 1996:17.

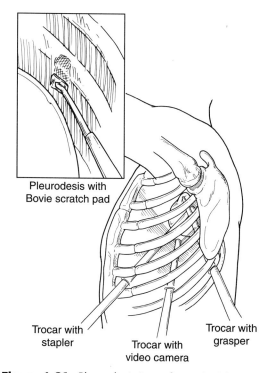

Pleurodesis with Bovie scratch pad

Trocar with stapler

Trocar with video camera

Trocar with grasper

Figure 4–31. Pleurodesis is performed with a Bovie scratch pad. (Redrawn from Hanke I, Douglas JM Jr. Thoracoscopic resection of blebs and pleurodesis. In: Sabiston DC Jr, ed. *Atlas of cardiothoracic surgery.* Philadelphia: WB Saunders, 1995.)

document direct invasion of mediastinal structures (either T3 or T4), but it is occasionally of use. Dissection often proves difficult and potentially hazardous, and there is no substitute for putting one's hand on a lesion of questionable resectability. VATS proves extremely useful, however, in documenting the absence of diffuse pleural metastatic disease if this possibility has been raised (usually by the presence of a pleural effusion).

Many primary lesions of the mediastinum prove to be ideal for VATS management. Lesions in all compartments of the mediastinum are easily accessible, and whether biopsy only or complete excision is the intent, VATS techniques save many patients from having to undergo thoracotomy. To approach a lesion in the anterior mediastinum, the patient is positioned with the side to be operated on, tilted up at approximately 30° instead of in the full lateral position. Often a small inframammary incision is employed.

The patient with a large, diffuse mediastinal mass from which tissue is required for diagnosis may also, at times, benefit from a VATS approach. Many of these lesions are more readily accessed for biopsy through an

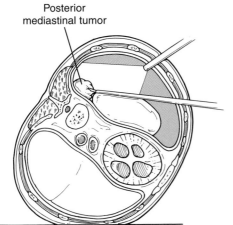

Posterior
mediastinal tumor

Access around lung assisted with gravity
and 45° forward rotation of
patient from lateral position

Figure 4–32. A cross-sectional view shows the mediastinum, tumor, and instruments. The patient is rotated to facilitate access to the tumor. (Redrawn from Hsu C-P, Douglas JM Jr. VATS for posterior mediastinal tumors. In: Sabiston DC Jr, ed. *Atlas of cardiothoracic surgery*. Philadelphia: WB Saunders, 1995.)

extrapleural, parasternal approach by excision of the costal cartilage (usually the second). Lesions that are not close to the anterior chest wall may be approached and readily sampled with a VATS approach.

The posterior mediastinum is also the site of either solid or cystic lesions that are amenable to VATS resection. Incisions used to approach these posterior mediastinal lesions differ slightly from those used for access to the anterior mediastinum (Figure 4–32).

Key Readings

Kaiser LR, Daniel TM. *Thoracoscopic surgery.* Boston: Little, Brown & Co., 1993. *Best description of the field of laparoscopic surgery of the chest in print.*

Wagner M, Lawson T. *Atlas of chest imaging: correlated with anatomy with MRI and CT.* New York: Raven Press, 1992. *An excellent primer on learning how to read CT and MRI scans of the chest.*

Selected Readings

Allen MS, Deschamps C, Jones DM, *et al.* Video-assisted thoracic surgical procedures: the Mayo experience. *Mayo Clin Proc* 1996;71:351–359.

Burt ME, Flye MW, Webber BL, Wesley RA. Prospective evaluation of aspiration needle, cutting needle, transbronchial, and open lung biopsy in patients with pulmonary infiltrates. *Ann Thorac Surg* 1981;32:146–153.

Freundlich IM, Bragg DG. *A radiologic approach to diseases of the chest.* Baltimore: Williams & Wilkins, 1997.

Lillington GA. *A diagnostic approach to chest diseases: differential diagnoses based on roentgenographic patterns.* Baltimore: Williams & Wilkins, 1987.

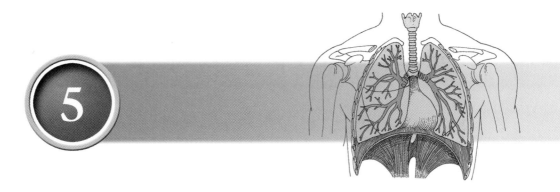

5

Thoracic Trauma

Thoracic Trauma: Key Points

- Develop an algorithm for rapid assessment and management of the thoracic trauma patient
- Develop clear indications for emergent thoracic procedures, including establishing a surgical airway, performing a tube thoracostomy, and initiating a thoracotomy
- Diagnosis and management of thoracic wall injuries (rib fractures, flail chest, sternal fractures)
- Diagnosis and management of lung-space injuries such as pneumothorax and hemothorax
- Basic understanding of the principles for specialized thoracic trauma scenarios (tracheobronchial injuries, esophageal injuries, and diaphragmatic injuries)

Overall thoracic trauma mortality is 10%, with chest injuries accounting for 25% of all trauma related deaths, and complications of chest trauma contribute to another 25% of all deaths. Injuries to the chest can occur by blunt trauma and penetrating trauma. Penetrating trauma is usually produced by a knife or bullet, whereas the majority of blunt trauma comes from motor vehicle deceleration injuries. Less than 10% of blunt chest traumas and only about 15–30% of penetrating chest injuries require thoracotomy.

Considering immediate deaths after motor vehicle accidents, the most frequent injuries leading to a fatal outcome include blunt cardiac injuries with chamber disruption and injuries to the thoracic aorta. Early deaths are caused by airway obstruction, major respiratory problems, such as tension pneumothorax, massive hemothorax, and cardiac tamponade (Figure 5–1).

These clinical situations are easily managed if recognized promptly. Chest wall trauma is the most frequent injury after blunt thoracic trauma. Most thoracic injuries are managed with simple procedures such as clinical observation, thoracentesis, respiratory support, and adequate analgesia. The remaining 15–20% of patients sustaining chest trauma require a thoracotomy for definitive repair of major intrathoracic injuries (Table 5–1).

Stab and gunshot wounds are responsible for the majority of penetrating chest wall trauma. The pathophysiology of chest trauma includes three factors: hypoxia, hypercarbia, and acidosis. Hypoxia can be caused by airway obstruction, changes in intrathoracic pressure (e.g. tension pneumothorax, open pneumothorax), ventilation-perfusion mismatches (e.g. contusion, hematoma, alveolar collapse), and hypovolemia (e.g. blood loss). Hypercarbia is

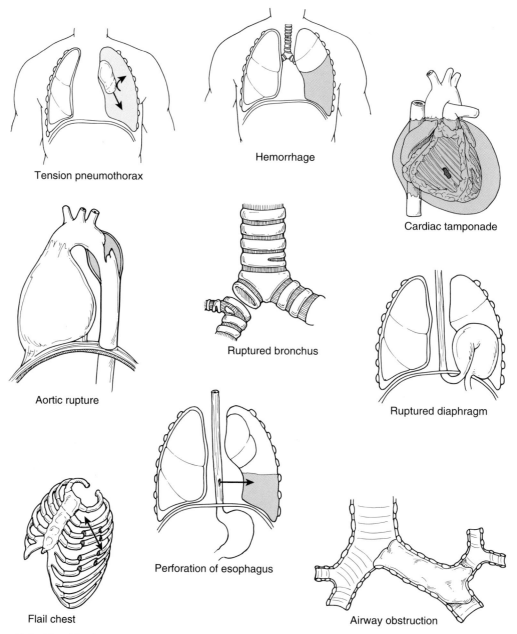

Tension pneumothorax

Hemorrhage

Cardiac tamponade

Aortic rupture

Ruptured bronchus

Ruptured diaphragm

Flail chest

Perforation of esophagus

Airway obstruction

Figure 5–1. The life-threatening lesions of chest trauma. (Redrawn from Hood RM, Boyd AD, Culliford AT. *Thoracic trauma.* Philadelphia: WB Saunders, 1989:36–37.)

caused by inadequate ventilation resulting from the presence of a collapsed lung, associated head injuries with altered mental status, or exogenous intoxication (drugs and alcohol). Acidosis is caused mainly by hypoperfusion from blood loss.

Initial Assessment (Figure 5–2)

The first priority is the maintenance of a patent airway (Figure 5–3). This may be obtained by simply mobilizing the mandible forward (chin lift and jaw thrust) and removing foreign bodies from the oropharynx. An oral or nasal airway may suffice, but patients with more severe injuries or with severe head injuries require tracheal intubation, either by a nasal or oral route or by means of a surgical airway. A cervical collar must be used to maintain strict alignment of the spinal column because of the risk of aggravating neurologic injuries. Tracheostomy or cricothyroidotomy may be indicated as an emergency procedure when an upper airway

TABLE 5–1 • *The Lethal Lesions of Thoracic Trauma*

Lesion	Symptoms	Physical Findings	Portable Chest X-ray	Diagnostic Procedure	Surgical Management
Tension pneumothorax	Dyspnea	Absent breath sounds; dyspnea; mediastinal shift; cyanosis; subcutaneous emphysema (maybe)	Pneumothorax; mediastinal shift; interstitial air in tissues	Thoracentesis; chest x-ray	Chest tube insertion
Intrathoracic hemorrhage	Dyspnea; shock-like state; apprehension	Absent breath sounds; dullness to percussion; hypotension	Opacification of hemithorax	Chest film; thoracentesis	Thoracotomy
Cardiac tamponade	Dyspnea; apprehension	Hypotension; venous distention; distant heart sounds	Slight enlargement of heart shadow; bottle-shaped cardiac silhouette	CVP measurement over 15 cm	Thoracotomy
Deceleration aortic injury	Nonspecific	Nonspecific	Widened mediastinum; narrowed trachea; left main bronchus; pleural fluid; fracture of ribs 1 and 2	Aortogram	Thoracotomy; prosthetic graft
Tracheobronchial rupture	Nonspecific dyspnea; hemoptysis	Nonspecific; may have pneumothorax or tension pneumothorax. Mild hemoptysis; subcutaneous emphysema	Not consistent: tension pneumothorax, pneumothorax, rib fractures; Air bronchogram absent	Bronchoscopy	Thoracotomy; primary repair
Rupture of the diaphragm with gastric herniation	None or progressive respiratory distress	None; absent breath sounds; mediastinal shift; bowel sounds heard over chest	Gastric air bubble above diaphragm; lower rib fractures; mediastinal shift	Nasogastric tube; contrast studies of stomach; look for paralysis of diaphragm	Nasogastric tube; early thoracotomy or laparotomy

TABLE 5–1 • *The Lethal Lesions of Thoracic Trauma (Continued)*

Lesion	Symptoms	Physical Findings	Portable Chest X-ray	Diagnostic Procedure	Surgical Management
Massive flail chest with pulmonary contusion	Dyspnea; shock-like state	Destabilized chest wall dyspnea; rales, cyanosis, hypertension	Rib fractures evident; pulmonary contusion; pneumothorax	Serial ABC+ observation	Chest tube; intercostal block; stabilize chest wall; intubate; ventilate; restrict fluids; control secretions
Esophageal perforation	Pain; dysphagia; fever; history of etiologic injury	Swelling of cervical area; auscultate for mediastinal air	Mediastinal air; widened retrotracheal space; widened mediastinum; pleural fluid; pneumothorax	Contrast study of esophagus	Immediate operative repair
Airway obstruction					
Upper	Dyspnea; wheezing	Stridor; dyspnea; cyanosis	Nonspecific	Observation only	1) Oral or nasal airway 2) Endotracheal tube 3) Cricothyroido-tomy 4) Tracheostomy
Lower	Dyspnea; wet cough; history of aspiration	Rales; wheezing; cyanosis; absent breath sounds	Absent air bronchogram; pulmonary infiltrate; atelectasis	Auscultate; ABC; chest x-ray if necessary	Bronchoscopy; intubate; ventilate

obstruction exists or when an endotracheal tube cannot be inserted.

The second priority is hemodynamic control, which in a trauma setting refers to control of all life-threatening hemorrhage. This includes establishing two large-bore intravenous lines and rapid infusion of isotonic colloids and blood products.

The history of the mechanism of injury is important in predicting potential thoracic trauma. Information about patients having requiring extrication from behind steering wheels, crushed automobiles, and rapid deceleration can focus the surgeon's search. The physical examination of the chest is extremely important in identifying life-threatening situations that require immediate attention (Box 5–1). In evaluating the thorax, note should be made of the status of the neck veins and tracheal deviation (both of which may often be obscured by the cervical collar), obvious lacerations or penetrating trauma, examination of the back of the torso, decreased or absent breath sounds, and muffled heart sounds. These can indicate the presence of a tension pneumothorax, massive hemothorax, open pneumothorax, flail chest, or cardiac tamponade.

The chest x-ray is of the utmost importance in thoracic trauma. However, life-threatening injuries override the necessity for a chest x-ray for diagnosis and should be identified clinically (Box 5–2). On chest x-ray the features to examine are an obliteration of the aortic knob, tracheal deviation, obscured view of the AP window (loss of the space between the pulmonary artery and the aorta), depression of the left main stem bronchus, deviation of the esophagus (nasogastric tube), widened paratracheal stripe, widened paraspinal interfaces, presence of a pleural

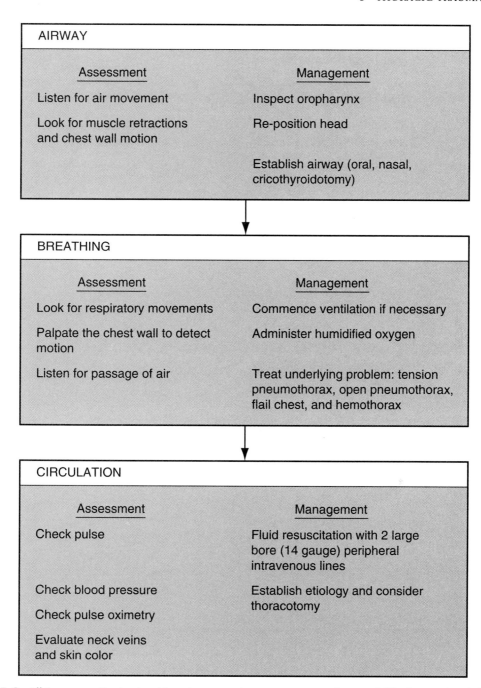

Figure 5-2. All trauma patients should undergo a primary survey to rule out all life-threatening injuries.

or apical cap, loss of costophrenic angles, and rib fractures. The chest x-ray is useful to identify a pneumothorax, hemothorax, rib fractures, widened mediastinum, pneumomediastinum, and clavicular and scapular fractures. Arterial blood gas can provide additional important information about the status of the respiratory system.

Emergency Procedures

Surgical Airway

The two choices for a surgical airway, cricothyroidotomy and tracheostomy (Figures 5–4, 5–5), may be indicated in selected patients with thoracic injury. If there is difficulty intubating

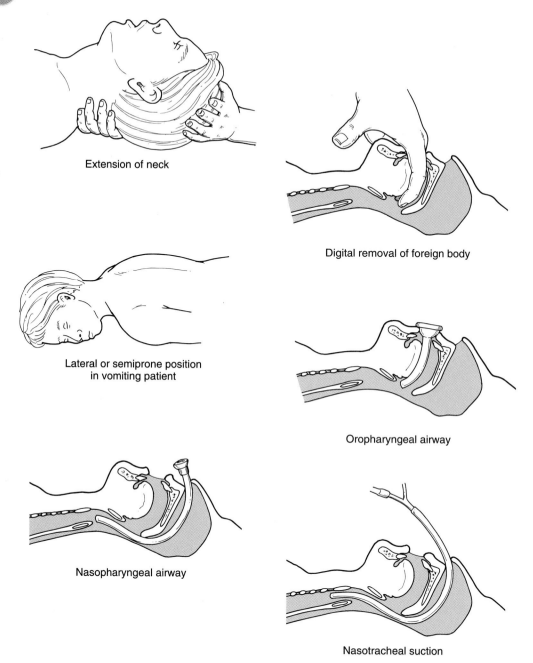

Figure 5–3. Diagrammatic representation of techniques of relief of acute airway obstruction. Some are simple and often overlooked. The method will vary, depending on the cause and severity of the obstruction. (Redrawn from Hood RM, Boyd AD, Culliford AT. *Thoracic trauma*. Philadelphia: WB Saunders, 1989:16–17.)

the trachea or the patient has massive facial trauma, the surgeon should be prepared for immediate cricothyroidotomy in the trauma bay. The surgeon should simply call for an antiseptic solution, a scalpel, and a No. 6 tracheostomy tube. Further dissecting instruments beyond his index finger can often be a luxury in the trauma bay.

Tube Thoracostomy

Tube thoracostomy is the most common procedure performed in the management of thoracic trauma. Approximately 85% of patients sustaining chest injuries require only clinical observation or tube thoracostomy. A large-bore (36–40F) chest tube should be used in adoles-

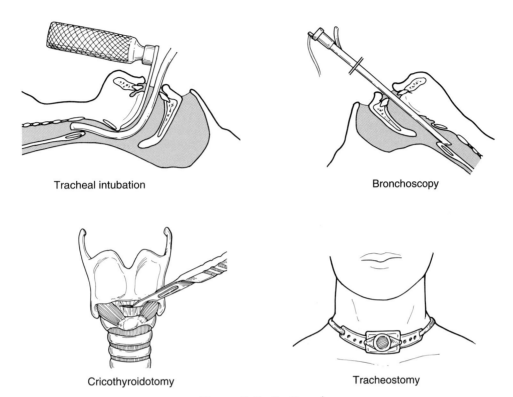

Tracheal intubation

Bronchoscopy

Cricothyroidotomy

Tracheostomy

Figure 5–3. Continued.

BOX 5–1 RAPID PHYSICAL EXAMINATION OF A PATIENT TO RULE
OUT THORACIC INJURY

Look
- Examine anterior and posterior chest for lacerations and bruises
- Examine oropharynx
- Check for neck vein distention
- Rule out tracheal deviation

Palpate
- Palpate neck and chest to rule out crepitus
- Rule out bony injuries

Listen
- Evaluate breath sounds
- Evaluate heart sounds

cents and adult patients. The proper site of insertion is in the fifth or sixth intercostal space in the midaxillary line aligned with the anterior superior iliac spine (Figure 5–6). The index finger should be inserted into the pleural space before tube placement to be sure that the pleural cavity has been entered and is free of adhesions and that intra-abdominal organs have not herniated through the diaphragm. The tube should be advanced posteriorly and superiorly in the pleural cavity. Following insertion, the tube should be secured in the skin of the chest wall and connected to a collection system under suction (Figure 5–7). A chest x-ray is usually obtained after chest tube insertion to confirm adequate placement and positioning. General criteria for chest tube removal include absence of air leak and less than 100 mL of fluid drainage over a 24-hour period (Figure 5–8).

Thoracotomy

An emergency thoracotomy is indicated after chest trauma in the following situations:

- Cardiac arrest (resuscitative thoracotomy)
- Massive hemothorax (>1500 mL blood through the chest tube acutely or >200–300 mL/h after initial drainage)
- Penetrating injuries of the anterior chest with cardiac tamponade
- Large open wounds of the thoracic cage
- Major thoracic vascular injuries in the presence of hemodynamic instability

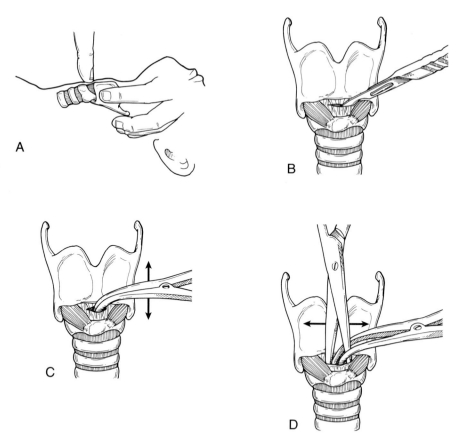

Figure 5–4. Cricothyroidotomy. **A,** With the patient in position with the neck extended, the thyroid cartilage is held with one hand and the forefinger is used to palpate the space between the thyroid and cricoid cartilages. **B,** The skin is incised over the thyrocricoid membrane. The membrane is incised and the lumen entered. **C,** A tracheal spreader is introduced. **D,** The opening is enlarged to the point that a tracheostomy tube can be introduced. (Redrawn from Hood RM. *Techniques in general thoracic surgery.* Philadelphia: WB Saunders, 1985:40.)

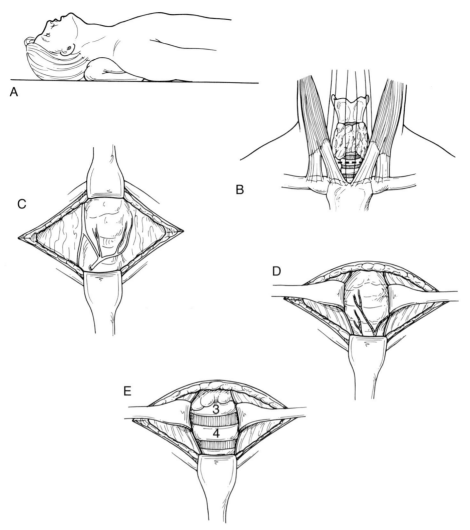

Figure 5–5. Tracheostomy. The basic steps in tracheostomy. (Redrawn from Hood RM. *Techniques in general thoracic surgery*. Philadelphia: WB Saunders, 1985:42.)

- Major tracheobronchial injuries
- Evidence of esophageal perforation (Box 5–3).

The anterolateral thoracotomy is an important procedure to a thoracic surgeon in the acute setting (Figure 5–9). The incision can be made quickly in less than a minute, requiring little special equipment. Exposure is usually adequate for relief of tamponade and repair of most penetrating cardiac injuries. Exposure of the left lung is only fair but is usually adequate. The incision can be extended across the sternum and converted into a bilateral anterior thoracotomy.

Non-emergency indications for thoracotomy in a trauma patient who over the course of several weeks to months develops thoracic complications include:

- Empyema not resolved with tube thoracostomy
- Clotted hemothorax
- Lung abscess
- Thoracic duct injuries
- Tracheoesophageal fistulas
- Chronic sequelae of vascular injuries (pseudoaneurysms and arteriovenous fistulas).

These patients often require operative management if they fail conservative treatment initially.

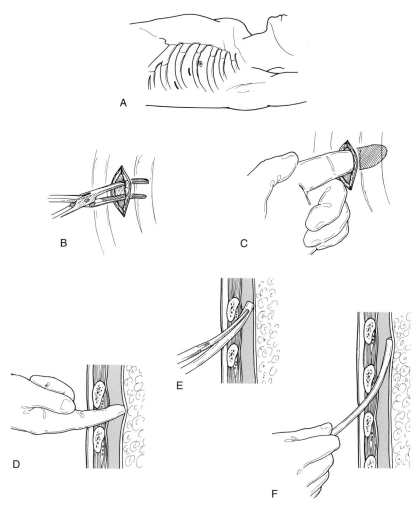

Figure 5–6. Chest tube insertion. **A,** Two sites for chest tube insertion. The upper site is in the anterior axillary line in the fourth interspace and is the site preferred for pneumothorax. The lower site is the fifth or sixth interspace in the posterior axillary line. A tube for drainage of hemothorax or a pleural effusion would use this site. **B,** A skin incision has been made and a sharp hemostat (tonsil or Crile) is used to enlarge the wound, penetrate the musculature, and enter the pleural space. **C,** A finger is introduced to explore and further widen the wound. **D,** A 2–3 cm wound has been made and a finger is introduced into the pleural space to widen the opening and to ascertain that the lung is not adherent to the chest wall. **E,** The chest tube is being introduced into the pleural space using a large hemostat for guidance. **F,** The trocar chest tube has been bent to an angle of about 30° and is being gently introduced and guided into position. **G–I,** A technique of suturing the chest tube to the skin and leaving a suture to tie when the tube is removed. **J,** The chest tube has been inserted, sutured in place, and connected to one of the available drainage systems. These drainage systems consist of a collection area, a waterseal apparatus, and a suction-regulating system (on the right). (Redrawn from Hood RM. *Techniques in general thoracic surgery.* Philadelphia: WB Saunders, 1985:36.)

Thoracic Wall Injuries (Box 5–4)

Rib Fractures

Rib fractures are the most common blunt chest injury. Ribs 4–10 are usually fractured. Multiple rib fractures are the hallmark of severe trauma caused by high-energy transfer. Patients with multiple rib fractures should have intrathoracic and abdominal injuries investigated. Fractures of the lower ribs (9–12) are associated with an increased incidence of hepatic and splenic injuries. Fractures of the upper ribs (1–3), clavicle, or scapula often are associated with major neurovascular

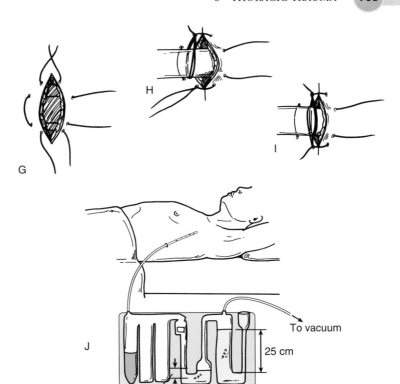

Figure 5-6. Continued.

injuries. Any evidence of a neurologic defect of the brachial plexus, an absent radial pulse, a pulsating supraclavicular mass, and a widened mediastinum are findings that require computed tomography (CT) aortography. In the elderly, because of their decreased bone density, reduced chest wall compliance, increased incidence of underlying parenchymal disease, and rib fractures, this may lead to decreased ability to cough, reduced vital capacity, and infectious complications.

One or two rib fractures without pleural or lung involvement are usually treated on an outpatient basis. Cough assistance and intratracheal suction may be necessary for several days. Unless there is sufficient rib-cage injury to cause structural instability, the majority of treatment is directed towards pain relief. Pain on inspiration is usually the primary clinical manifestation after rib fractures. Other clinical signs associated with rib fractures include tenderness to palpation and crepitus. Rib fractures are confirmed by chest x-ray.

Poor pain control contributes significantly to complications such as atelectasis and pneumonia. Pain control is attempted initially with oral or intravenous analgesics. Intercostal nerve blocks with bupivacaine are effective for pain control; however, they are not feasible for multiple fractures and require frequent injections. The intercostal block sites should be at the posterior angle of the rib but not medial to this point (Figure 5–10). Epidural analgesia is adequate for patients with multiple or bilateral fractures, providing adequate pain control and appropriate pulmonary toilet, decreasing the number of complications. Alternative pain control mechanisms include intrapleural regional analgesia with a catheter in the pleural cavity and transcutaneous electric nerve stimulation.

Flail Chest

By definition, a flail chest occurs in the presence of two or more fractures in three or more consecutive ribs, causing instability of the chest wall; however, it can also occur after costochondral separation. It is characterized by paradoxical motion of the chest wall (inward with inspiration and outward with expiration). Fractures can be located in the anterior, lateral, or posterior chest wall (Figure 5–11). Flail chest occurs in 10–15% of patients sustaining major chest trauma, and the chance of having an intrathoracic injury in this situation increases severalfold. Pulmonary contusion should be assumed until proved otherwise in any injury

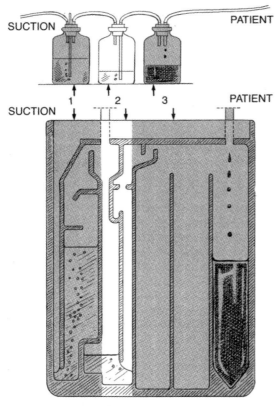

Figure 5–7. Water and drainage apparatus, three-bottle system. 1, Pressure-regulating devices. 2, Water seal devices. 3, Collecting chambers. (Modified with permission of Deknatel, Inc., Floral Park, NY, from Hood RM, Boyd AD, Culliford AT. *Thoracic trauma.* Philadelphia: WB Saunders, 1989:139.)

that is severe enough to destabilize the chest wall. Closed head injury is the most frequent associated extrathoracic injury, contributing to higher morbidity and mortality rates. Isolated flail chest carries a low mortality rate in younger patients.

The paradoxical motion increases the work of breathing, and the most important consequence of flail chest is respiratory failure. Until recently, it was believed that ineffective air movement between the lungs caused by the paradoxical motion of the chest wall was the main cause of respiratory distress. It has come to be understood that underlying pulmonary contusion and pain during inspiration are the most important components in the pathophysiology of respiratory failure. Sequential measurements of forced vital capacity, tidal volume, and inspiratory force are useful to predict which patients will require ventilatory support. The pathophysiological effects may be present immediately or may progress over

several hours and present as late respiratory decompensation.

Prophylaxis and early intervention must be the guiding principle, with adequate pain control the key. There are many methods of stabilizing the chest wall. Endotracheal intubation with the use of a volume ventilator stabilizes the thoracic wall in an expanded position that tends to minimize late chest wall collapse and later disability. Intermittent mandatory ventilation (IMV) with humidified oxygen at a rate of 10–16 breaths per minute, associated with moderate levels of positive end-expiratory pressure or continuous positive airway pressure, is usually used. It is maintained until pain control permits vigorous pulmonary hygiene and early mobilization of the patient and may be the most important therapeutic maneuver. Patients are given aggressive pulmonary physiotherapy with incentive spirometry, deep coughing, suctioning, humidification of the air, and chest percussion with postural drainage. Bronchoscopy is used liberally to remove retained secretions promptly and to expand areas of collapse. Within 5–10 days, chest-wall stability can be restored. Rarely is open reduction and fixation warranted in correcting chest wall instability.

Care should be taken not to fluid-overload these patients because it may impair respiratory function even further. Patients without evidence of respiratory distress can be managed with analgesia only. Pain control can be provided by intercostal nerve block or more adequately by epidural anesthesia. If respiratory distress develops, endotracheal intubation and mechanical ventilation with peak-end expiratory pressure are usually indicated, as long as pain control is adequate. Open reduction and internal fixation of sternal or rib fractures is rarely needed.

Sternal Fractures

Although rare, sternal fractures may occur after motor vehicle accidents, most commonly in older patients and front-seat vehicle occupants. The presence of a fractured sternum implies significant trauma to the anterior chest wall with high-energy transfer. The fracture is usually linear in the midportion of the body of the sternum (Figure 5–12).

Signs and symptoms include chest pain, particularly over the sternum, and crepitus. A hematoma over the sternum may be seen (caused by the steering wheel) or across the chest (seat belt sign). A lateral x-ray should be

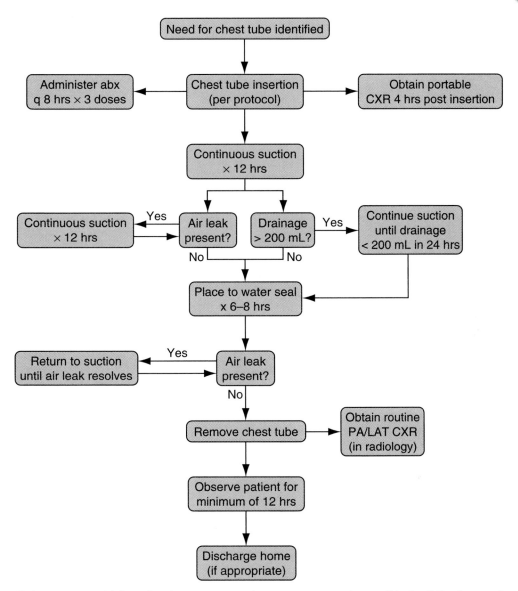

Figure 5–8. Practice guidelines for thoracostomy tube management. abx, antibiotic; CXR, chest radiograph; LAT, lateral; PA, posteroanterior. (From Andrales G, Huynh T, Broering B, *et al.* A thoracostomy tube guideline improves management efficiency in trauma patients. *J Trauma* 2002;52:210–216.)

obtained in these circumstances and usually confirms the diagnosis. Special sternal views may be required. Sternal fractures also constitute a marker for serious associated injuries, including myocardial contusion, myocardial rupture, esophageal perforation, airway injury, and thoracic aortic rupture.

Treatment is usually conservative, although patients with significant chest wall instability may require open reduction and internal fixation with stainless steel wire (Figure 5–13).

Scapular Fracture

Fractures of the scapula are uncommon and are due to significant force of impact (Table 5–2). There is a high incidence of concomitant brachial plexus injuries, which should be ruled out. Treatment consists of shoulder immobilization with subsequent early range of motion exercises. Surgical repair may be indicated when glenohumeral joint function is impaired.

BOX 5–3 INDICATIONS FOR CHEST THORACOTOMY

Emergency Indications
- Witnessed cardiac arrest
- Massive hemothorax
- Penetrating chest trauma with suspicion of tamponade
- Large open wound to thoracic cage
- Major thoracic vascular injury with hemodynamic instability
- Tracheobronchial injury
- Esophageal perforation

Non-Emergency Indications
- Nonresolving empyema
- Clotted hemothorax
- Lung abscess
- Thoracic duct injury
- Tracheoesophageal fistula
- Sequelae of vascular injury (pseudoaneurysm, arteriovenous fistula)

Clavicular Fracture

Clavicular fractures are quite common. Isolated fractures rarely compromise ventilation and treatment by stabilization and a figure-of-eight dressing splint plus analgesia is effective. Only rarely is operative repair necessary for severely displaced fractures. Damage to the underlying subclavian vessels or the brachial plexus is rare.

Pulmonary Injuries

Pneumothorax

A pneumothorax occurs when air from an injured lung or airway is trapped within the pleural cavity, increasing the normal negative intrapleural pressure. It may be caused by penetrating or blunt mechanisms. These conditions may be the result of external penetration with disruption of the parietal pleura, but consideration should be given to disruption of the visceral pleura secondary to injury to the lung caused by internal trauma or barotrauma; or to disruption of the mediastinal pleura secondary to injury of the esophagus or tracheobronchial tree.

Pneumothoraces are classified according to the volume of lung loss or collapse identified on chest x-ray or by respiratory and systemic signs. The three types of pneumothorax, partial, tension, and open pneumothorax, all follow the same principle of decompression.

Partial Pneumothorax

In a small pneumothorax, the volume loss is one third of the normal lung volume. In a large pneumothorax, the lung is completely collapsed but there is no mediastinal shift or associated hypotension. Following blunt trauma, partial pneumothorax is caused by rib fractures penetrating the lung parenchyma, or by lung injuries without chest wall involvement. Deceleration injuries and sudden increases in intrathoracic pressure also may cause a pneumothorax. Clinical findings suggestive of a pneumothorax include decreased breath sounds, hyperresonance to percussion, and decreased expansion of the affected lung during inspiration. The presence of subcutaneous emphysema is alarming in appearance but is relatively harmless. This is not in itself an indication for chest-tube insertion. However, most traumatic pneumothoraces should be managed with a chest tube. Delayed increase in the volume of a pneumothorax may occur at any time and may become life-threatening.

Tension Pneumothorax

A tension pneumothorax is characterized by complete lung collapse, tracheal deviation, mediastinal shift leading to decreased venous return to the heart, hypotension, and respiratory distress (Figure 5–14). It usually occurs in patients with parenchymal lung injury under positive pressure ventilation. Clinical signs and symptoms include dyspnea, tachypnea, hypotension, diaphoresis, and distended neck veins. It is diagnosed clinically, constituting a life-threatening emergency. Chest x-rays are not necessary to confirm the diagnosis and delays to definitive treatment significantly increase the risk of circulatory collapse and cardiorespiratory arrest.

This is a true surgical emergency and treatment includes chest decompression, initially with a large-bore needle inserted in the second intercostal space on the midclavicular line and subsequent tube thoracostomy. Re-expansion

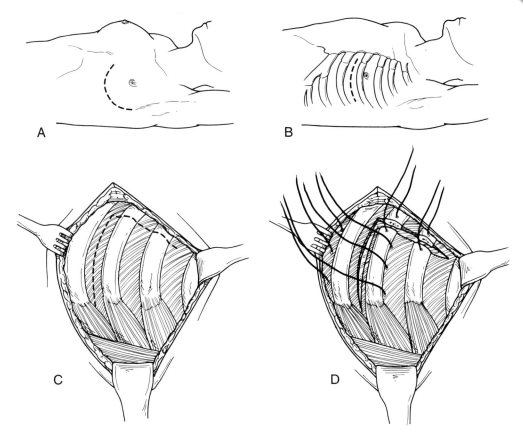

Figure 5–9. Left submammary thoracotomy. **A,** The incision usually employed in female patients. **B,** Incision usually employed in male patients. The fourth interspace is usually the interspace of choice. **C,** Rib cartilages above the incision may be incised and also the inferior cartilage may be severed. **D,** The basic method by which the chest wall is reconstructed prior to wound closure. (Redrawn from Hood RM. *Techniques in general thoracic surgery.* Philadelphia: WB Saunders, 1985:78.)

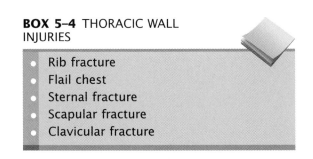

BOX 5–4 THORACIC WALL INJURIES

- Rib fracture
- Flail chest
- Sternal fracture
- Scapular fracture
- Clavicular fracture

of the lung and re-approximation of the pleural surfaces usually seal the lung defect. All patients with a pneumothorax, regardless of its size, who will undergo positive-pressure ventilation should be considered for chest tube placement before starting mechanical ventilation.

Open pneumothorax

Open pneumothorax, also known as sucking chest wound, occurs when there is a significant defect in the chest wall (e.g. large-caliber gunshot wounds, traumatic thoracotomy) large enough to exceed the laryngeal cross-sectional area, allowing the air to enter from the exterior into the pleural cavity and leading to lung collapse as a result of a rapid equilibration between the intrathoracic (pleural) pressure and the atmospheric pressure. The increased intrathoracic pressure also causes mediastinal shift and decreased venous return. Signs and symptoms include hypoxia, hypercarbia, hypotension, and respiratory and circulatory failure. Management of an open pneumothorax includes applying an occlusive dressing and placement of a chest tube before closure of the

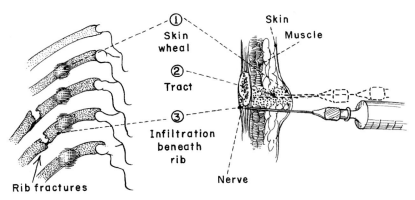

Figure 5-10. The technique of intercostal nerve block. Note that the infiltrating needle is 'walked' under the lower rib margin, unlike the technique of thoracentesis. (From Zuidema GD, Rutherford RB, Ballinger WF. *The management of trauma*, 4th ed. Philadelphia: WB Saunders, 1985:402.)

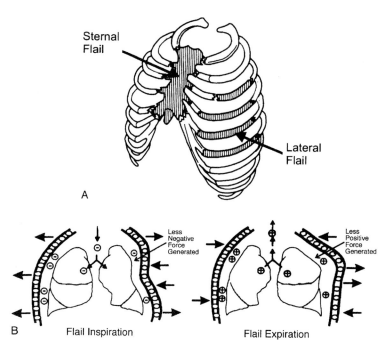

Figure 5-11. A, Anatomic drawing indicating flail segments involving four ribs fractured at two locations with and without sternal flail. **B,** Drawing of the chest in **A** illustrating the paradoxical movement of the chest during respiration. (From Pearson FG, Cooper JD, Deslauriers J, *et al. Thoracic surgery*, 2nd ed. New York: Churchill Livingstone, 2002:1834.)

chest wall defect to avoid the development of a tension pneumothorax.

Hemothorax

Blood may accumulate in the pleural cavity after blunt or penetrating injuries. Depending on the nature of the injury, bleeding may vary from minor to massive. The pleural space can accumulate up to 3 liters of blood. Most often, hemothorax occurs from intercostal arteries or the internal mammary artery. Sudden massive hemothorax is usually the result of major pulmonary vascular injury or major arterial wounds, while minor lung injuries may only cause a small hemothorax.

Symptoms depend on the amount of blood that has accumulated in the pleural space. On physical examination, breath sounds may be decreased on the side of the injury. A chest x-ray obtained in the upright position may reveal accumulations of blood greater than 200 mL; however, a supine film may demonstrate a diffuse haziness or none at all (Figure 5-15).

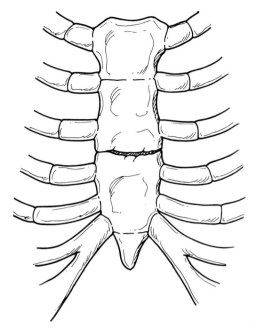

Figure 5–12. Transverse fracture of the sternal body. (Redrawn from Cuschieri J, Kralovich KA, Patton JH, *et al.* Anterior mediastinal abscess after closed sternal fracture. *J Trauma* 1999;47: 551–554.)

Management is directed at correcting the hypovolemia and at evacuating the blood from the pleural cavity (Figures 5–16, 5–17) Hemothoraces are initially treated by placement of large-bore chest tubes (36F) and, in approximately 85% of cases, the bleeding will stop as the lung is re-expanded because of the low pressure in the systemic circulation. Two chest tubes may be placed, one anteriorly and one posteriorly, to prevent blood accumulation and its subsequent complications. Clotted hemothorax, when not managed early and when several weeks have passed, may result in organized fibrin deposition on the pleural surfaces and lung entrapment. This may require decortication.

A small number of cases will have continued bleeding and will require a thoracotomy. These usually result from injuries in systemic arteries (intercostal arteries or internal mammary artery), veins, or major pulmonary vessels, or are cardiac in origin. Autotransfusion should be considered in these circumstances. As previously described, indications for emergency thoracotomy are initial chest tube output of 1500 mL of blood or persistent drainage of 200–300 mL per hour.

Pulmonary Contusion

Pulmonary contusion occurs more frequently after blunt chest trauma; however, penetrating injuries may also cause significant contusions of the lung parenchyma. This has been defined as a pathologic state in which hemorrhage and edema of the lung parenchyma cause consolidation of large areas of pulmonary tissue, without parenchymal disruption.

Pathophysiology involves decreased lung compliance and the development of ventilation–perfusion mismatch, leading to hypoxemia and increased work of breathing. Respiratory failure occurs more often in patients with large contusions, in the elderly, and in those with underlying chronic lung disease, aggravated by inadequate pain control.

Diagnosis is confirmed by low P_aO_2 and by a chest x-ray demonstrating a well-defined infiltrate underlying the contused area on the chest wall (Figure 5–18). In some cases, radiologic findings may not be present upon admission and may develop 24–48 hours after the initial injury. Pulmonary contusion may be confused with the adult respiratory distress syndrome or may even be associated with it.

Management is directed toward maintaining good oxygenation and adequate pulmonary toilet. Judicious crystalloid infusion is important to avoid fluid overload and pulmonary edema; however, intravascular volume depletion also should be avoided to decrease the risk of global ischemia and multiple organ failure. Patients with persistent low P_aO_2 levels who do not respond to supplemental oxygen, pulmonary toilet, and pain control should be intubated and mechanically ventilated. Correction of acute anemia and coagulopathy, by means of transfusing packed red blood cells and blood products, is important to minimize blood loss and increase oxygen-carrying capacity and delivery to the tissues. No benefits have been demonstrated for the use of prophylactic antibiotics or steroids.

Pneumonia is the most frequent complication, particularly in the elderly, aggravating chronic lung diseases, increasing ventilator days, and significantly contributing to mortality rate. Mortality rates vary according to age, associated injuries, and chronic underlying lung disease.

Pulmonary Laceration

Simple lacerations of the lung are common after penetrating injuries and rare after blunt trauma. Patients usually have variable degrees of

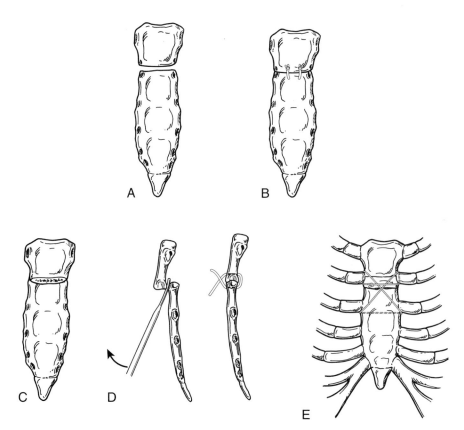

Figure 5–13. Diagrams of various fractures. **A, B**, Common sternal fracture at the junction of the manubrium with the lower sternum. Widely separated or mobile fragments may be stabilized with simple wire sutures. **C, D**, A displaced or sublimated transverse fracture necessitates reduction and stabilization. **E**, Wire stabilization may be useful when fractures are oblique or comminuted or when there is too much osteoporosis for simple sutures to hold the fragments securely. (Redrawn from Hood RM. *Techniques in general thoracic surgery.* Philadelphia: WB Saunders, 1985:217.)

pneumothorax and hemothorax. Management usually includes chest tube placement to drain blood in the pleural space and re-expand the lung. Occasionally, major and persistent air leaks develop. This situation is sometimes identified immediately after chest tube place-

TABLE 5–2 • *Mechanism of Injury for 57 Patients with Scapulothoracic Disassociation*	
Motorcycle crash	25
Motor vehicle crash	20
Pedestrian	4
Fall from height	3
Snowmobile	2
Machinery entrapment	2
All-terrain vehicle	1

Damschen et al., 1997.

ment, but it may be more evident when mechanical ventilation with positive pressure is started. Massive air leaks should raise suspicion for major tracheobronchial injuries.

In most cases, pulmonary lacerations heal promptly after chest tube insertion. Massive hemorrhage from extensive lung injuries can be treated by oversewing or stapling the wound or, more rarely, by performing wedge or lobar resections. Gunshot wounds causing through-and-through injuries to the lung can be managed by opening up the missile trajectory (tractotomy) and exploring both entrance and exit wounds to obtain hemostasis (Figure 5–19). Wedge resections of peripheral injuries to the lung parenchyma that are actively bleeding can be accomplished by using a straight stapler. Complications associated with large injuries in the lung parenchyma, as well as after tractotomy, include increased bleeding and air embolism, which may be

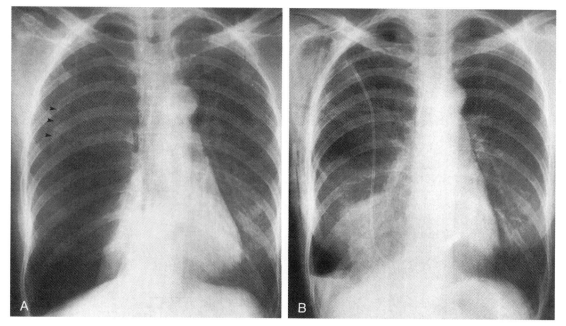

Figure 5-14. Tension pneumothorax. **A,** Posteroanterior (PA) radiograph demonstrates airless right lower and middle lobes, with volume loss in the right upper lobe caused by a large pneumothorax. Note the sharp white line demarcating the edge of the pleura (arrowheads). Despite the degree of atelectasis, the right hemidiaphragm is depressed and the heart and mediastinal structures are shifted toward the contralateral side, indicative of a tension pneumothorax. **B,** PA radiograph following placement of a chest tube shows that there is reduction in the size of the right pneumothorax with a small amount of fluid now present within the right pleural space. Note the air–fluid level present inferiorly. Diminished diaphragmatic depression and mediastinal shift is apparent. The air-space process in the right lower lobe presumably is secondary to rapid inflation pulmonary edema. (From Hood RM, Boyd AD, Culliford AT. *Thoracic trauma.* Philadelphia: WB Saunders, 1989:73.)

controlled by stapling the lung parenchyma. Air embolism can be minimized by decreasing the peak inspiratory pressure and cross-clamping the pulmonary hilum.

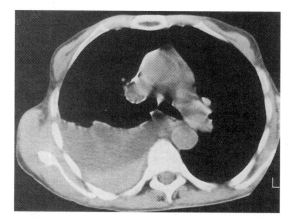

Figure 5-15. Hemohydrothorax. CT scan at the level of the carina demonstrates a blood–fluid level within the right pleural space, with the high-density blood layering posteriorly. (From Hood RM, Boyd AD, Culliford AT. *Thoracic trauma.* Philadelphia: WB Saunders, 1989:72.)

Tracheobronchial Injuries

Tracheobronchial injuries are uncommon. Most patients with these injuries die at the scene or during transport as a result of poor ventilation and associated injuries. Tracheal injuries usually occur after direct compression of the airway with a closed glottis related to clothesline-type trauma or after being thrust forward and striking the anterior cervical area on a steering wheel. Tears to the airway following blunt trauma usually occur within 2 cm of the carina. Decelerating injuries cause partial or complete avulsion of the right main stem bronchus. Penetrating wounds may cause tracheobronchial injuries at any level.

Several mechanisms have been described, including linear rupture of the membranous portion of the trachea following an abrupt increase in large airway pressures due to thoracic compression in a patient with a closed glottis; also disruption of the trachea at points of fixation – at the carina and the cricoid – due to the shearing forces seen with rapid deceleration. Transection of the trachea near the carina

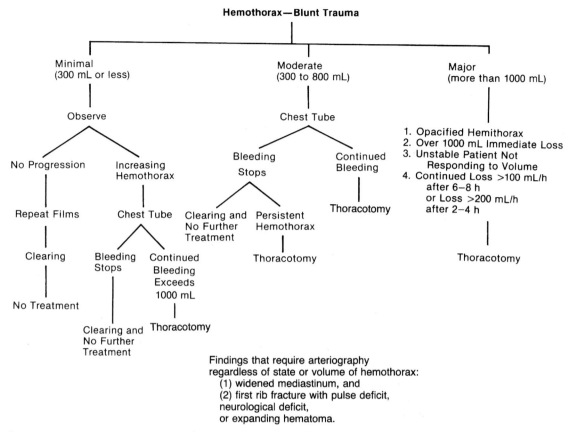

Figure 5–16. Algorithm for the management of hemothorax due to blunt trauma. (From Hood RM. *Surgical diseases of the pleura and chest wall.* Philadelphia: WB Saunders, 1986:222.)

can be due to lateral traction on the lungs with crushing chest injuries, which acutely decreases the anterior–posterior diameter of the thoracic cavity.

Patients may have pneumothorax, massive air leak, subcutaneous emphysema, voice impairment, hemoptysis, pneumomediastinum, and respiratory distress (Figure 5–20). Bronchial injuries may be missed initially and can often present late. Hemoptysis, pneumothorax, and hemothorax are not common. One third of the patients are not diagnosed in the first 24 hours. Isolated pneumomediastinum, which can be quite trivial, can be present with injury to the trachea, main stem bronchus, or esophagus. Bronchoscopy is always required if one of the aforementioned signs is present, and it should ideally be performed before intubation. On bronchoscopy, the initial clue may be the inability to discern the usual tracheal and endobronchial landmarks.

Small injuries usually heal spontaneously; however, late complications such as stricture formation at the injury site, recurrent pulmonary infection, and atelectasis may occur. Minor injuries of the upper airway after blunt trauma should be treated by placing the endotracheal tube beyond the injury. If this is not possible, a tracheostomy should be performed. More extensive wounds – i.e. greater than one third of the circumference of the airway – are primarily repaired after the contralateral bronchus has been selectively intubated (Figure 5–21). When complete tracheal separation has occurred, a cervical incision must be made rapidly, although usually the patient may be intubated over a bronchoscope. Once into the neck and superior mediastinum, the distal tracheal segment must be visualized, grasped, and delivered into the wound. Intubation should then be performed endotracheally and stainless steel wire or monofilament suture should be used to repair the trachea. Should the injury extend down deeper into the mediastinum, a median sternotomy or a partial sternotomy with a trap door to expose

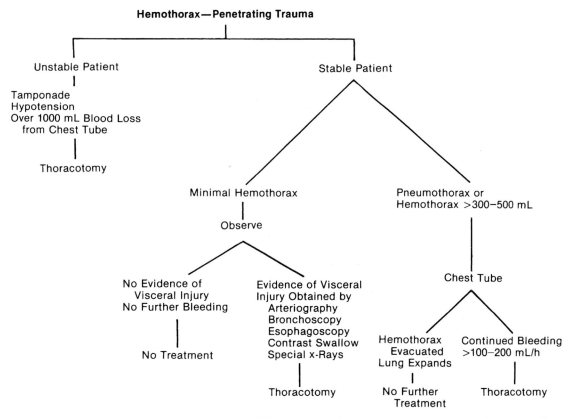

Figure 5–17. Algorithm for the management of hemothorax due to penetrating trauma. (From Hood RM. *Surgical diseases of the pleura and chest wall.* Philadelphia: WB Saunders, 1986:224.)

the proximal intrathoracic trachea should be performed.

With a severe major bronchial injury, a posterolateral thoracotomy is made on the injured side. The mediastinal pleura is widely opened. The open trachea or bronchus is occluded digitally while the endotracheal tube is guided into the uninjured bronchus and the cuff is inflated. Re-anastomosis can then be attempted. Considerable effort should be made to clear the distal bronchus of mucus and the ends should be excised so anastomosis can be performed. The mucosa should be approximated with a 3-0 or 4-0 interrupted absorbable suture. Following completion of a repair, a strip of pleura, an intercostal muscle pedicle, or an omentum pedicle should be used to buttress the suture line. It is best to avoid using any periosteum from the ribs when mobilizing the intercostal muscle pedicle because this can recalcify and lead to stenosis of the airway. Interposing a strip of viable tissue between the trachea and esopha-

gus is especially important when both structures are injured.

Esophageal Injuries

Most esophageal injuries are secondary to penetrating trauma and may occur at any level. The esophagus is well protected in the posterior mediastinum and injuries after blunt trauma are rare. Sudden increases in intra-esophageal pressure as a result of a direct blow to the epigastrium may cause rupture of the distal esophagus. Associated injuries are the rule. One needs to maintain a high level of suspicion in order to avoid missing an esophageal injury.

Esophageal injury after blunt trauma should be considered in patients with a pleural effusion without rib fractures, pain out of proportion to the clinical findings, subcutaneous emphysema, or pneumomediastinum without an obvious source, and gastric contents in the

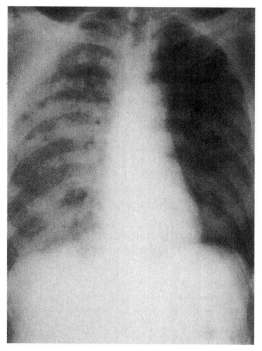

Figure 5–18. This anteroposterior supine chest x-ray film of a patient with blunt trauma demonstrates diffuse patchy infiltrate of the entire right lung field, which represents a massive pulmonary contusion. (From Tomlanovich MC. Pulmonary parenchymal injuries. *Emerg Med Clin North Am* 1983;1:379.)

chest tube. All mediastinal traversing gunshot wounds or stab wounds near the posterior midline should be evaluated for possible esophageal injury.

The diagnosis is confirmed with esophagography and esophagoscopy, with esophagoscopy being the most definitive. These tests have a reported sensitivity that varies from 50% to 90%.

Treatment consists of early debridement, primary repair, and drainage if identified within 24 hours after injury. Injuries diagnosed after 24 hours are usually accompanied by mediastinal contamination but mostly may be repaired primarily as long as there is complete drainage and debridement of the mediastinum and pleural space.

Diaphragmatic Injuries

Diaphragmatic injuries are often caused by penetrating injuries. Patients sustaining penetrating injuries below the nipples and above the costal margins should be investigated to rule out diaphragmatic injury. Surgeons should recall that the diaphragm is 3–5 cm higher during expiration and that, during the Valsalva maneuver, the diaphragm may reach as high as the third anterior rib. Two prospective series performed where all patients with penetrating left thoracoabdominal trauma underwent surgical evaluation (either by laparoscopy, thoracotomy, or laparotomy) established the incidence of occult diaphragmatic injuries in stable patients at around 25%. With crushing blunt chest injury, rupture of the diaphragm should be suspected when there are lateral rib fractures over the lower rib cage. Following blunt trauma, injury to the diaphragm involves both sides equally, as reported in autopsy and CT scan studies, although, in clinical practice, left-sided injuries are more frequent (Table 5–3).

Only a minority of patients will have respiratory distress, cardiac disturbances, deviated trachea, and bowel sounds in the chest. Symptoms are usually related to other organ system injuries or the presence of hypovolemic shock (Table 5–4). The diagnosis is suspected

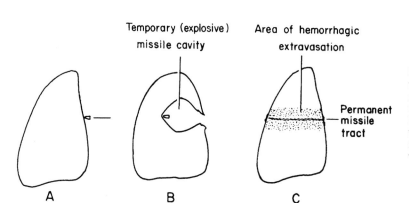

Temporary (explosive) missile cavity   Area of hemorrhagic extravasation

Permanent missile tract

A   B   C

Figure 5–19. Schematic illustration of the effects of high-velocity missile wounding of the pulmonary parenchyma. (From Fischer RP. Pulmonary resections for severe pulmonary contusions secondary to high-velocity missile wounds. *J Trauma* 1974;14:293.)

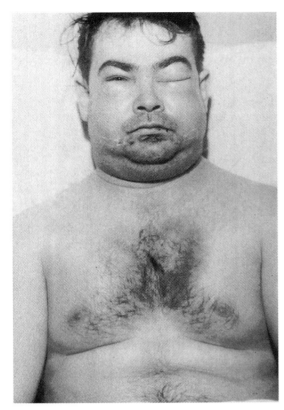

Figure 5–20. A photograph of a young man weighing only 114 pounds who sustained a tracheal laceration from a steering wheel injury. The extent of subcutaneous emphysema is apparent; in this patient it occurred without pneumothorax. (From Hood RM, Sloan HE. *J Thorac Cardiovasc Surg* 38:460, 1959.)

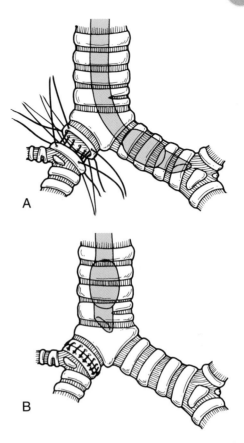

Figure 5–21. Repair of traumatic rupture of the bronchus. **A,** The technique of re-anastomosis of the right main bronchus, in which the endotracheal tube is advanced into the left main bronchus. Interrupted full-thickness sutures are used. **B,** The suture line is complete and the endotracheal tube has been withdrawn back into the trachea. (Redrawn from Hood RM. *Techniques in general thoracic surgery.* Philadelphia: WB Saunders, 1985:51.)

when respiratory distress develops after a severe blow to the abdomen without apparent chest injury or when an upright chest film demonstrates visceral herniation. In fact, herniation of intra-abdominal contents may not occur immediately, or may not be evident on initial chest x-ray, delaying the diagnosis. Herniation occurs as a result of the pressure differential between the thoracic and the abdominal cavity. If missed on initial hospitalization, this diagnosis has presented as late as 20 years after the initial insult. The stomach is the most frequent organ to herniate, followed by the transverse colon, spleen, and other viscera (Figure 5–22). Because the proximal stomach is tethered by the mesenteric and vascular attachments, the gastric herniation can resemble a para-esophageal hernia. The herniated stomach can become partially obstructed and begin to dilate. Massive dilatation of the stomach can

cause collapse of the lung and shifting of the mediastinum.

The evaluation includes peritoneal lavage in those with stab wounds to the epigastrium, thoracoscopy in patients with hemothorax or pneumothorax, or laparoscopy in those with a normal chest film and an external wound in the thoracoabdominal transition. Chest and abdominal x-rays should be obtained in hemodynamically stable patients who have sustained a gunshot wound in an attempt to determine the trajectory of the missile. Chest radiography may demonstrate elevation or irregularity of the diaphragm and show viscera in the chest (Figure 5–23).

Every stable patient with a stab wound or gunshot wound to the left thoracoabdominal

TABLE 5–3 • *Classification of Traumatic Diaphragmatic Hernia*

Right Side

Immediate herniation	With injury to liver or other viscera
	With obstruction of the colon or small bowel
	Asymptomatic
Delayed herniation	Liver
	Colon or small intestine
	Asymptomatic
	With obstruction or strangulation

Left Side

Immediate herniation	With injury to hollow viscus, liver, or spleen
	With limited visceral herniation
	With extensive herniation of multiple viscera and respiratory embarrassment
	Asymptomatic
Delayed herniation	Obstruction of the stomach, with or without perforation
	Obstruction or strangulation of small bowel or colon
	Asymptomatic

Herniation into the Pericardium

Rupture Through the Esophageal Hiatus

Disruption of Surgical Wounds of the Diaphragm

From Hood RM. Traumatic diaphragmatic hernia. *Ann Thorac Surg* 1971;12:315.

TABLE 5–4 • *Associated injuries with diaphragmatic trauma: review of 32 patients (Brasel et al., 1996)*

Injury	n (%)
Spleen	16 (50)
Liver + hepatic artery	15 (47)
Pelvic fracture	13 (41)
Other orthopedic	16 (50)
Head injury	13 (41)
Bowel	12 (38)
Rib fracture	10 (31)
Other thoracic	10 (31)
Other intra-abdorninal	7 (22)
Kidney	5 (16)
Bladder	2 (6)

region, between the nipple and costal margin, should be considered for laparoscopy. If the bullet is in the abdomen, the patient will undergo an exploratory laparotomy and the diagnosis of a diaphragmatic injury will be made intraoperatively. Acute diaphragmatic rupture is usually repaired through a midline abdominal incision because of the increased incidence of associated intra-abdominal injuries. Chronic defects discovered months or years after the initial injury can be treated through a transthoracic, abdominal, or combined approach. At the time of surgical exploration, the entire diaphragm should be inspected. All diaphragmatic injuries should be repaired. Perforations fail to heal without surgical intervention because the positive intra-abdominal pressure keeps the tear patent and results in blood, bile, or contaminated fluid collecting in the pleural space. Rents are repaired with interrupted horizontal sutures. Larger defects may eventually require use of a prosthetic material.

Patients with diaphragmatic injuries tend to have high mortality and morbidity. Even when the abdomen is surgically explored, surgeons fail to notice diaphragmatic injures. The result may be herniation of viscera several months or years later.

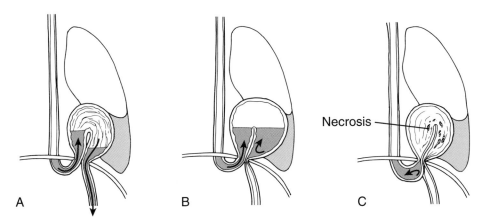

Figure 5–22. This diagram demonstrates the possible sequelae when the stomach herniates through the ruptured diaphragm. **A,** When neither afferent nor efferent loops are obstructed, the stomach does not dilate and respiratory distress does not occur. **B,** If there is efferent loop obstruction, which is the most common situation, rapid gastric dilatation occurs. **C,** If both loops are obstructed, this becomes a closed loop obstruction, which will progress to necrosis and perforation. Note that the greater curvature lies uppermost. (Redrawn from Felson BF. *Chest roentgenology*. Philadelphia: WB Saunders, 1973.)

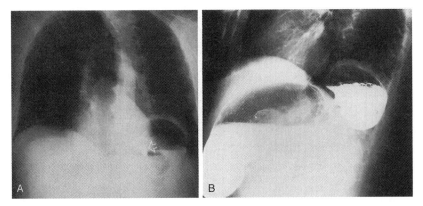

Figure 5–23. Diaphragmatic rupture. **A,** Oblique film of the chest shows an air-containing viscus above the level of the left hemidiaphragm. A bullet is present within the left upper quadrant of the abdomen (arrow). **B,** Lateral film from an upper gastrointestinal examination demonstrates partial herniation of the stomach into the left hemithorax. (From Hood RM, Boyd AD, Culliford AT. *Thoracic trauma*. Philadelphia: WB Saunders, 1989:90.)

Key Readings

American College of Surgeons. Thoracic trauma. In: *Advanced trauma life support for doctors*, 6th ed. Chicago: American College of Surgeons Committee on Trauma, 1997:125–141. *Up-to-date recommendations by the American College of Surgeons on the current management of thoracic trauma and need-to-know information for all trainees in thoracic surgery.*

Hood RM, Boyd AD, Culliford AT. *Thoracic trauma*. Philadelphia: WB Saunders, 1989. *Excellent review of all aspects of thoracic trauma and the etiology, pathophysiology, and management of key injuries that confront a thoracic surgeon.*

Selected Readings

Adrales G, Huynh T, Broering B, *et al*. G. A thoracostomy tube guideline improves management efficiency in trauma patients. *J Trauma* 2002;52:210–214.

Brasel KJ, Borgstrom DC, Meyer P, Weigelt JA. Predictors of outcome in blunt diaphragm rupture. *J Trauma* 1996;41:484–487.

Cohn SM. Pulmonary contusion: review of the clinical entity. *J Trauma* 1997;42:973–979.

Cuschieri J, Kralovich KA, Patton JH, *et al*. Anterior mediastinal abscess after closed sternal fracture. *J Trauma* 1999;47:551–554.

Damschen DD, Cogbill TH, Siegel MJ. Scapulothoracic dissociation caused by blunt trauma. *J Trauma* 1997;42:537–540.

Feliciano DV, Rozycki GS. Advances in the diagnosis and treatment of thoracic trauma. *Surg Clin North Am* 1999;79:1417–1429.

Greenberg MD, Rosen CL. Evaluation of the patient with blunt chest trauma: an evidence based approach. *Emerg Med Clin North Am* 1999;17: 41–62.

Kshettry VR, Bolman RM III. Chest trauma. Assessment, diagnosis, and management. *Clin Chest Med* 1994;15:137–146.

Lowdermilk GA, Naunheim KS. Thoracoscopic evaluation and treatment of thoracic trauma. *Surg Clin North Am* 2000;80:1535–1542.

Zinck SE, Primack SL. Radiographic and CT findings in blunt chest trauma. *J Thorac Imag* 2000;15: 87–96.

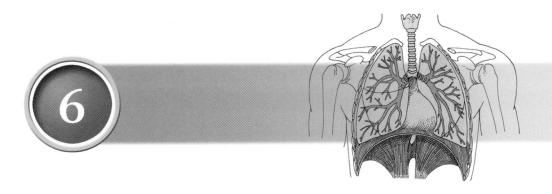

6

Pulmonary Resections

Pulmonary Resections: Key Points

- Understand the anatomical features that make each segmental resection unique
- Understand the key aspects that make operating on the lungs unique: meticulous closure of stapled edges, careful dissection of pulmonary vessels, and care of the bronchial stump
- Appreciate what situations require a complete pneumonectomy
- Review the intraoperative decisions that affect postoperative management

During the first four decades of the 20th century, carcinoma of the lung was an uncommon disease and most pulmonary resections were performed for inflammatory disease or tuberculosis. Most lung cancers were treated with pneumonectomy when they were deemed operable. Lesser resections were performed for benign disease processes. It took a number of years before surgeons recognized that resection of less than an entire lung could be adequate treatment for lung cancer.

Preoperative Considerations

Recognizing that surgery is the best treatment for early-stage disease, it is important that the appropriate procedure is performed. Lobectomy remains the definitive resection for most lung cancers, since it is an anatomic resection that removes the regional lymph nodes located along the lobar bronchus. Doing less than a lobectomy must be considered a compromise, although it is tempting to consider a non-anatomic wedge excision for small primary tumors. There are patients in whom lobectomy is not feasible because of compromised pulmonary function, and a lesser resection offers the best alternative. Whenever possible, the lesser resection should be an anatomic segmental resection, which takes the segmental artery and vein as well as the segmental bronchus with its accompanying lymph nodes. Wedge resection, a non-anatomic form of resection in that bronchovascular structures are not isolated and taken separately along with regional lymph nodes, is another alternative, although not ideal for most patients with primary lung cancers.

Some patients may undergo invasive staging before pulmonary resection. The decision to perform mediastinoscopy may be based on computed tomography (CT) scan findings of enlarged mediastinal lymph nodes or positron-emission tomography (PET) scan results. The criteria for defining 'enlarged' varies, and the sensitivity and specificity of the technique vary depending on the size that is set. We perform mediastinoscopy when lymph nodes more than 1.5 cm in diameter are seen on the CT scan. Others perform mediastinoscopy on all patients before pulmonary resection, recognizing that the majority of procedures will reveal only nodes without evidence of metastatic disease.

Whether mediastinoscopy is used selectively or routinely, the key point is accurate staging of the mediastinum in a patient with lung cancer. This mandates either complete mediastinal lymph node staging at thoracotomy or lymph node dissection. The problem with lymph node staging alone is the issue of how lymph nodes are chosen to be sampled, a problem not present when a complete lymph node dissection is carried out. Mere palpation of a node or an assessment of nodal size will miss lymph nodes harboring intranodal or microscopic disease. It is not clear what percentage of nodal disease is missed with a staging procedure because of the variability in the selection of nodes to be sampled and the lack of a study in which nodes are first sampled followed by a complete lymph node dissection. From our own experience, 10–20% of resections in which lymph node disease is not suspected result in positive lymph nodes being identified by the pathologist. An operation without lymph node staging information must be considered incomplete. Accurate staging allows the surgeon to discuss prognosis realistically with the patient and allows the patient the opportunity to either participate in a trial of postoperative adjuvant therapy or be evaluated for treatment outside of a protocol setting.

Right-Sided Pulmonary Resections

Exploration of the right chest has several unique anatomic features related to pulmonary resection. The right main pulmonary artery is relatively long and courses posterior to the superior vena cava and across the carina. This extra length of the artery, at times, is an advantage for some proximal lesions that in a similar location on the left side would not be resectable because of the short length of the left main pulmonary artery relative to the bifurcation. There has to be enough length of artery distal to the bifurcation so that a clamp can be placed and the artery divided and sutured. The distance between the carina and the origin of the right upper lobe bronchus usually is less than 2 cm, and the carina is readily mobilized from the right side. Access to the proximal left main stem bronchus is significantly easier from the right side compared with the left side, where the aortic arch limits access both to the origin of the left main bronchus and the carina. Mobilization of the carina is not possible from the left chest, and even visualization of the carina from the left is difficult. Carinal resections are preferentially performed through a right thoracotomy or a median sternotomy.

The superior mediastinum, the space accessed by the mediastinoscope, is well visualized from the right side. The area bounded by the azygos vein (inferior), the trachea (posterior), the subclavian vein (superior), and the superior vena cava (anterior) delineates this compartment, whose lymph-node-bearing contents may be removed *en bloc* through the right side. No such access exists on the left side, where the left paratracheal nodes are relatively inaccessible because of the location of the aortic arch. As mentioned above, with the access afforded to the carina from the right side, it follows that the subcarinal space is readily dissected for lymph node removal.

On the right side, the azygos vein is an important anatomic landmark. The vein courses from posterior to anterior across the main stem bronchus to empty into the superior vena cava. Just inferior to where it crosses the bronchus is the origin of the upper lobe bronchus, which is a key anatomic feature. Rarely is it necessary to divide the azygos vein but it may be taken with impunity if involved by tumor or if it limits access to the lymph node bearing area.

Right Upper Lobectomy

The long right main pulmonary artery with the apical-anterior branch and the discrete take-off of the upper lobe bronchus makes this an ideal resection to begin learning techniques in thoracic surgery. The so-called truncus anterior, the apical-anterior branch of the pulmonary artery, also facilitates segmental resections of the right upper lobe. Once this branch is divided, the segmental bronchi are easily visualized.

Once the patient is positioned on the left side (left lateral decubitus position), the chest is entered through either a standard posterolateral thoracotomy incision or a vertical axillary muscle-sparing incision. The chest is entered through the fifth intercostal space for the posterolateral incision or the fourth intercostal space for the muscle-sparing incision. The hilum and mediastinum are palpated to assess the extent of involvement and determine resectability.

The lung is retracted posteriorly with the surgeon's left hand and the hilar pleura is incised anteriorly and superiorly. The superior pulmonary vein is identified and dissected distally toward the lung parenchyma and proximally to the pericardial reflection. The vein is encircled with a finger once the appropriate plane of dissection is entered. Care must be taken to avoid injury to the pulmonary artery, which lies directly posterior to the superior pulmonary vein (Figure 6–1). The middle lobe venous branch, which usually enters the superior pulmonary vein, is identified and preserved. This vein almost always drains to the superior pulmonary vein but occasionally may be found entering the inferior pulmonary vein. Lying just superior and posterior to the vein is the right main pulmonary artery. The artery is dissected circumferentially and followed proximally, where it is observed as it courses posterior to the superior vena cava. The artery is easily encircled with a finger once the appropriate plane of dissection is entered. After the artery is encircled, an umbilical tape is passed and a Rumel tourniquet is placed. Should the artery be inadvertently entered, it is a simple matter to snug down on the tourniquet and control the bleeding. The artery is dissected distally and the so called truncus anterior, the apical-anterior arterial branch, is

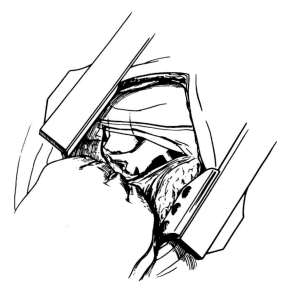

Figure 6–1. View of the right hilum as seen from the right side of the table. The hilar pleura has been incised and the right main pulmonary artery and superior pulmonary vein are well seen. Note the middle lobe vein draining into the superior pulmonary vein. This vein must be preserved when performing a right upper lobectomy. The continuation of the artery distal to the apical-anterior trunk passes posterior to the superior pulmonary vein.

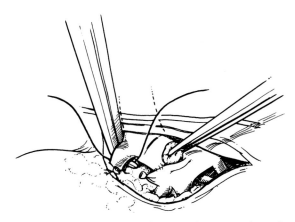

Figure 6–2. At times, the apical venous branch obscures the origin of the apical-anterior arterial trunk and must be divided before the arterial branch is divided. Here the venous branch has been divided in preparation for division of the apical-anterior trunk. The right-angle clamp is around the arterial branch. The artery is divided between carefully placed 0 silk ligatures.

identified (Figure 6–2). This usually occurs as a common trunk, but the individual segmental branches may arise separately from the main artery, with the branch to the anterior segment coming off the artery as the most proximal branch.

Once the pulmonary artery has been identified, the dissection proceeds superiorly along the hilum to enter the plane of the bronchus. The azygos vein is a significant landmark. This vein crosses the right main stem bronchus just superior to the origin of the right upper lobe bronchus. The vein courses from posterior to anterior and the bronchus lies medial to the vein. It is rarely necessary to divide the azygos vein unless it is involved by tumor. Once the artery is dissected away from the bronchus, it is possible to encircle the upper lobe bronchus at this point if deemed necessary. At times, it is advantageous to divide the bronchus first, especially if the primary tumor or lymph nodes involve the branches of the pulmonary artery.

The lung is retracted anteriorly by the assistant to reveal the posterior aspect of the hilum. To facilitate upper lobectomy, dissection is begun in the bifurcation formed by the upper lobe bronchus and the bronchus intermedius by incising the overlying pleura (Figure 6–3). With care taken to coagulate small bronchial vessels that are present in this 'crotch,' the pleura is incised. A lymph node is a constant finding in this location, and the dissection frees this node anteriorly away from the bifurcation. The bronchus may be encircled at this point and taken, if desired (see Figure 6–3).

Just anterior to this lymph node, however, lies the branch of the pulmonary artery to the superior segment of the lower lobe, which is easily visualized from this posterior approach. Once this arterial branch is identified, the posterior portion of the major fissure may be completed with a firing of the linear stapler (Figure 6–4). The lower lobe superior segment arterial branch is the most posterior branch of the artery within the fissure, and the stapler may be safely passed just posterior to the branch. The pleura within the fissure needs to be incised, and the appropriate location for placement of the stapler may be found by placing the forefinger in the 'crotch' just dissected posteriorly and the thumb in the fissure. The fissure at the appropriate spot is quite thin and may be further thinned out by finger dissection of the parenchyma held between the thumb and forefinger. This move is safe because the location of the artery is known and it has been dissected free. The move also avoids extensive dissection in the fissure in a search for the pulmonary artery. Until the location of the artery is known, firing a stapler across the fissure, as is commonly done, adds little; it really brings you no closer to the artery. Taking advantage of the ana-

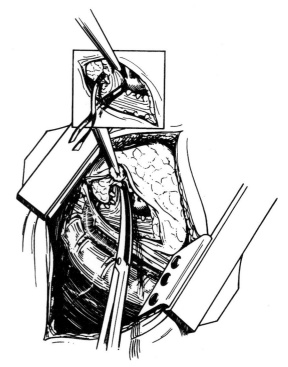

Figure 6–3. One of the most important concepts in pulmonary surgery is visualization of the anatomy in three dimensions. Much of the dissection may be done from behind, or from the posterior aspect of, the hilum. Here the bifurcation between the bronchus intermedius and upper lobe bronchus is being dissected and the upper lobe bronchus skeletonized. There is the constant finding of a lymph node at this 'crotch.' Incision at the bifurcation and elevating the lymph node out of the area reveals the pulmonary artery within the fissure. **Inset,** Once the bifurcation is dissected, the bronchus may be encircled. Surprisingly, if the artery has been dissected, the bronchus may be taken at this point.

tomy posteriorly allows easy identification of the artery in the fissure without actually dissecting in the fissure and thus avoiding air leaks. Once the artery is identified and dissected in the correct plane, the posterior portion of the major fissure is very simple to complete.

Alternatively, the upper lobe bronchus may be encircled and divided at this point, which allows complete visualization of the artery from behind the fissure. This is the preferable move when there is nodal involvement in the fissure that makes dissection on the artery difficult. The arterial branch to the posterior segment of the upper lobe is adjacent (superior) to the superior segmental branch and occasionally may arise from this branch (Figure 6–5). The arterial supply to the middle lobe usually arises just opposite the takeoff of the superior segmental branch. There is usually one middle lobe arterial branch, but two branches are not uncommon.

The superior pulmonary vein is divided between rows of staples laid down by a vascular stapler, or alternatively the vein may be ligated and suture-ligated (Figure 6–6). Alternatively, a vascular clamp may also be placed, the divided vein sutured with a horizontal mattress stitch, the clamp removed, and the suture run as a simple stitch anterior to the mattress stitch back to where it began.

Once the vein is divided, the continuation of the pulmonary artery is identified as it lies posterior to the vein. The middle lobe arterial branch is readily identified from the anterior aspect of the hilum and, to facilitate division of the fissure and separation of the middle lobe from the upper lobe, the branch should be mobilized for a short distance. The arterial branch to the posterior segment of the upper lobe may be seen through an anterior exposure or an additional anterior segmental branch may be identified. Once the artery is identified from this anterior approach and the middle lobe artery is seen, the minor fissure, which is usually incomplete and poorly formed, may be divided with an application of the linear stapler.

The posterior segmental branch of the artery is ligated and divided within the fissure. With the lung again retracted anteriorly, the origin of the upper lobe bronchus is well seen, and a stapler is used to close the bronchus (Figure 6–7). The bronchus is taken as close as possible to its

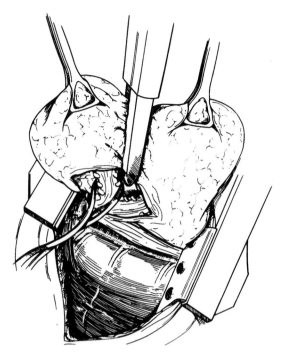

Figure 6–4. Once the artery is identified and the branch to the superior segment of the lower lobe defined, the posterior aspect of the major fissure may be divided with a linear stapler. There are no arterial branches that occur posterior to the superior segmental branch thus allowing the fissure to be defined and divided. Here placement of the stapler has been facilitated by the upper and lower lobes being grasped with Duval lung clamps.

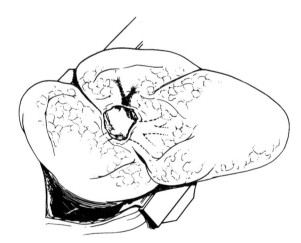

Figure 6–5. View of the pulmonary artery from within the fissure showing the position of the arterial branch to the posterior segment of the upper lobe in relation to the middle lobe branch and the superior segmental branch. If the fissure is well developed, the overlying pleura may be incised and dissection carried down directly on the vessel. If the fissure is poorly developed, it is easier to divide the bronchus, identify and divide the posterior segmental branch, and then complete the fissure with several firings of the linear stapler.

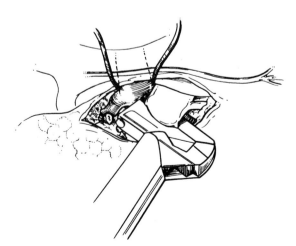

Figure 6–6. Proximal control of the artery has been obtained by placing an umbilical tape around the artery. The superior pulmonary vein, with the middle lobe vein left behind, is divided between rows of vascular staples. Here the stapler is being applied to the vein.

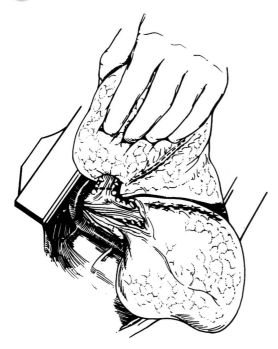

Figure 6–7. The right upper lobe bronchus is divided as close to its origin as possible *(dotted line)*. The point of division should not be so close that it compromises the lumen of the main bronchus or bronchus intermedius. It is safest to approach the bronchus from this posterior approach since its origin is very visible.

origin without compromising the right main stem bronchus. The bronchus is divided and the upper lobe removed if the minor fissure has been divided. If the minor fissure remains, it is completed with a firing of the linear stapler. To obtain definitive staging information, a complete mediastinal lymph node dissection is performed.

After the minor fissure is divided and the right upper lobe removed, the middle lobe is left without tether, since the oblique fissure is usually complete. Postoperatively, this situation may predispose to torsion and infarction of the middle lobe. To prevent this very significant complication, the middle lobe is 'reattached' to the lower lobe, either by placement of several absorbable sutures in a figure-of-eight fashion or by placing a row of staples between the two lobes. The middle lobe must be properly oriented when it is attached to the lower lobe.

There are several potential pitfalls to avoid when performing a right upper lobectomy. For the most part, it is one of the most straightforward of the pulmonary resections, but problems may occur. The middle lobe vein

must be identified and preserved when the superior pulmonary vein is divided. Once the superior pulmonary vein has been divided, great care must be taken to avoid injury to the middle lobe artery, especially when the minor fissure is divided. Traction exerted on the upper lobe while it is still attached to the middle lobe by the intact minor fissure may result in an avulsion injury to the middle lobe artery. As already mentioned, the right main bronchus may be narrowed if the upper lobe bronchus is taken too close to its origin. This usually occurs when the lobe is retracted upward, tenting the main stem bronchus before the stapler is placed. If the main bronchus has been injured, it is best to proceed with sleeve resection instead of trying to 'repair' the damage. Waiting for a stricture to become symptomatic creates far more difficulties.

Right Middle Lobectomy

Frequently, the right middle lobe must be removed for a variety of diseases. The middle lobe is a common site for inflammatory disease and bronchiectasis. It is also a common location for mycobacterial infections other than tuberculosis. Middle lobectomy is thought by many to be the most difficult lobectomy because of the problems presented by the fissures. This is an erroneous concept, since it is possible to accomplish the bronchovascular dissection and division from an anterior approach if the fissures are problematic.

If the major fissure is well developed and the pulmonary artery can be visualized easily within the fissure, the overlying pleura is incised. If the artery is not visible, the fissure overlying the artery must be divided in order to identify the artery. This creates air leaks and is generally messy and time-consuming. Significant dissection in the fissure is required to proceed with this 'standard' approach, and it is safest to gain proximal control of the pulmonary artery by incising the hilar pleura overlying the main pulmonary artery with the lung retracted posteriorly. Within the fissure, the middle lobe arterial branch is identified as it originates from the pulmonary artery, usually just opposite the branch to the superior segment of the lower lobe (see Figure 6–5). Most commonly, there is a single arterial branch to the middle lobe, but occasionally two branches are identified. The arterial supply to the middle lobe is ligated with silk ligatures and divided.

Once the arterial supply is divided, the middle lobe bronchus may be seen lying deep to the artery and slightly inferior, as viewed from within the fissure. The bronchus is dissected back to its origin from the bronchus intermedius, stapled, and divided. Alternatively, the bronchus may be divided and closed with interrupted sutures of braided or monofilament absorbable material of size 3–0 or 4–0.

With the lung retracted posteriorly, the anterior hilar pleura over the superior pulmonary vein is incised. The middle lobe venous branch or branches most commonly drain into the superior pulmonary vein but can drain into the inferior vein on rare occasions (see Figure 6–1). To ensure that a branch is coming from the middle lobe, the lobe may be grasped with a lung clamp and retracted laterally (upward towards the incision). This will avoid division of small branches coming from the upper lobe. The venous branch is then divided after it is ligated with silk ligatures and secured with a suture ligature.

Once the bronchovascular structures have been divided, the minor fissure is completed with a firing of the linear stapler. The major fissure is likely to be well developed and is easily completed, and the lobe is removed.

An alternative technique for middle lobectomy is also illustrated and is likely to be more useful and versatile. This technique does not rely on the pulmonary artery being visible within the fissure and does not require extensive dissection in the fissure to identify the artery.

The lung is retracted posteriorly. The hilar pleura overlying the superior pulmonary vein is incised and the middle lobe vein identified. The vein is ligated and divided, and immediately posterior to the vein lies the middle lobe bronchus (Figure 6–8). The bronchus is surrounded by connective tissue, which is divided, care being taken to coagulate any bronchial arterial branches that are encountered. The bronchus should be followed back to its origin from the bronchus intermedius. The middle lobe arterial branch lies just posterior and slightly superior to the middle lobe bronchus but may not be visible before the bronchus is divided.

Staying close to the bronchial wall, the surgeon encircles the bronchus with a right-angled clamp to avoid damage to the adjacent arterial branch (Figure 6–9). The bronchus is divided with a scalpel, using a right-angled clamp as a guide. The bronchial stump is closed with interrupted sutures. Alternatively, a stapler may be applied to close the middle lobe bronchus.

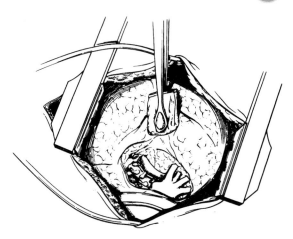

Figure 6–8. View of the right hilum from the left side of the table. The superior pulmonary vein has been dissected out and the middle lobe vein identified, ligated, and divided. The ligated stump of the middle lobe vein is seen. Immediately posterior to the vein lies the middle lobe bronchus. Usually the bronchus has to be divided in order to have optimal visualization of the middle lobe artery but at times the artery is seen slightly superior and posterior to the bronchus. Division of the bronchus facilitates division of the artery and provides the exposure needed to assess if there are other middle lobe arterial branches.

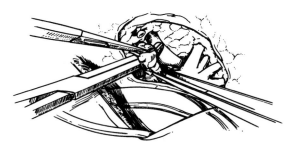

Figure 6–9. The middle lobe bronchus is encircled with a right-angle clamp and divided with a scalpel. It is important to identify the origin of the middle lobe bronchus to avoid damage to the bronchus intermedius. The bronchial stump is closed with interrupted absorbable sutures; alternatively, a stapler may be placed and the bronchus closed with staples. Note the relationship of the middle lobe artery to the bronchus.

After the bronchus is divided, the middle lobe arterial branch is easily seen and is circumferentially mobilized (Figure 6–10). The arterial branch or branches are ligated and divided. Once the bronchus, artery, and vein are divided, the minor fissure and the portion of the oblique fissure in contact with the middle lobe are divided with several firings of the linear stapler, and the lobe is removed.

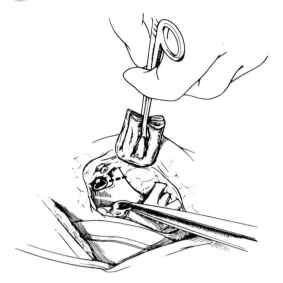

Figure 6–10. After the middle lobe bronchus is divided, the arterial branch (or branches) is easily visible and can be mobilized and divided (hatched line). Once the artery is divided, the minor fissure is divided with a linear stapler, as is the portion of the major fissure between the middle and lower lobes.

A mediastinal lymph node dissection is then completed in order to obtain the most accurate and complete staging information.

Despite the apparent simplicity of middle lobectomy as described, there are several potential trouble spots. The middle lobe bronchus comes off the bronchus intermedius at essentially a right angle and is quite fragile and susceptible to injury. The origin of the middle lobe bronchus is not easily seen from the anterior approach, and the bronchus intermedius may be damaged when the middle lobe bronchus is taken with a stapler. The middle lobe arterial supply may also present problems if there is more than one branch. Sometimes, the additional branch may be obscured and injured if its presence is not recognized. Care must also be taken when going around the middle lobe arterial branch from the anterior approach to avoid injuring the main pulmonary artery in the fissure.

Right Lower Lobectomy

The chest is entered through either a standard posterolateral thoracotomy incision (fifth intercostal space) or a vertical axillary muscle-sparing incision (fourth intercostal space). If disease is noted within the fissure or if the hilum is involved, it is best to obtain control of the proximal right main pulmonary artery.

The hilar pleura is incised anteriorly and superiorly with the lung retracted in a posterior direction, and the proximal pulmonary artery is encircled just lateral to the superior vena cava.

If the fissure is reasonably well developed, the pleura overlying the pulmonary artery is incised and the dissection is carried down on to the plane of the artery (Figure 6–11). The branch to the superior segment of the lower lobe is first identified, and the middle lobe arterial branch is most commonly found arising from the opposite aspect of the artery just across from the superior segmental origin. The dissection may be extended posteriorly along the superior aspect of the branch to the superior segment, which leads to the bifurcation of the upper lobe bronchus and bronchus intermedius.

With the lung retracted anteriorly, the pleura overlying this bifurcation posteriorly is incised, and a linear stapler may be inserted from just above the superior segmental arterial branch through the area of the bifurcation. This move is possible because there are no vascular structures present posterior to the origin of the superior segmental arterial branch. On the superior aspect of the artery, just opposite the superior

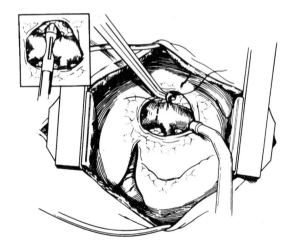

Figure 6–11. The pulmonary artery within the fissure has been identified and dissected. The position of the branch to the superior segment is such that it must be ligated and divided separately from the rest of the arterial supply to the lower lobe. The superior segmental branch is shown here being encircled by a right-angle clamp and the point of division of the basilar arterial trunk is marked (hatched line). Note the position of the superior segmental branch relative to the middle lobe artery. **Inset,** The basilar arterial trunk is shown being divided by the endoscopic vascular stapler, which both ligates and divides. The angle is usually ideal for placement of this stapler, which provides an extremely secure closure with three parallel rows of staples.

segment, the posterior segmental branch, the so-called recurrent branch, to the upper lobe arises and is easily visualized. Rarely, this branch to the upper lobe may arise from the superior segment branch to the lower lobe, and this possibility should be kept in mind. The posterior aspect of the major fissure is then divided and completed.

The relationship of the superior segmental branch to the middle lobe arterial branch determines whether the lower lobe artery may be divided as a complete trunk or whether the superior segmental branch and basilar trunk need to be taken separately. The superior segmental branch must be taken separately to avoid damage to the middle lobe arterial supply (see Figure 6–11).

Dividing the pulmonary artery reveals the bronchus, which lies just deep (medial) to the artery. With the artery retracted superiorly, the origin of the middle lobe bronchus may be visualized and the location for division of the lower lobe bronchus established (Figure 6–12).

The middle lobe artery lies superficial and superior to the middle lobe bronchus. Care must be taken to avoid compromising the origin of the middle lobe bronchus when the lower lobe bronchus is stapled or divided (see Figure 6–12). The bronchus may be closed either with a stapler or divided with a scalpel and closed with interrupted absorbable sutures.

With the lung retracted toward the apex of the chest the inferior pulmonary ligament is divided up to the level of the inferior pulmonary vein (Figure 6–13). An inferior pulmonary ligament lymph node (level 9) should be excised for staging purposes. The superior pulmonary vein is dissected free and encircled in preparation for division. A finger is passed around the vein after the appropriate dissection plane is entered, and the vein is divided between rows of staples placed by a vascular stapler (see Figure 6–13). Alternatively, the vein may be clamped, divided, and sutured with a running monofilament thread or doubly ligated before division. At the minimum, a tie and a suture ligature are placed to secure the vein. The anterior aspect of the major fissure is now easily completed with a firing of the linear stapler, which allows the lobe to be removed.

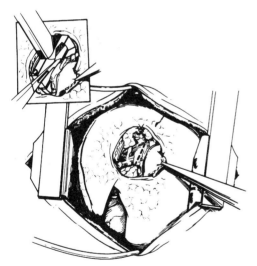

Figure 6–12. The stump of the lower lobe pulmonary artery is retracted superiorly to expose the lower lobe bronchus. The middle lobe bronchus that comes off the bronchus intermedius at a 90° angle must be identified and preserved. If a stapler is to be used, it must be placed in such an orientation as to avoid compromising the orifice of the middle lobe bronchus. The site of bronchial division is shown (hatched line). The bronchial division includes the bronchus to the superior segment as shown. Occasionally it is necessary to close and divide the superior segment bronchus separately. **Inset,** A stapler is placed across the lower lobe bronchus distal to the origin of the middle lobe bronchus. Often the stapler has to be oriented in an oblique fashion to include the superior segment bronchus and avoid the middle lobe.

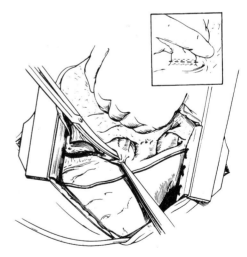

Figure 6–13. With the lung retracted superiorly, the inferior pulmonary ligament is incised up to the level of the inferior pulmonary vein. The vein is shown being dissected by incising the overlying pleura. The vein may then be encircled with a finger and divided between rows of vascular staples or clamped, divided, and sutured closed. **Inset,** The vein has been encircled and two rows of staples placed. The line of division is marked (hatched line). Often division of the vein precedes bronchial division, but there is no set order in which structures must be taken.

It is a common misconception that right lower lobectomy is difficult because it is necessary to identify the pulmonary artery within the fissure. If a difficult fissure is encountered, it is always best to obtain proximal control of the right main pulmonary artery as the initial maneuver. The artery may then be followed distally beyond the middle lobe branch that leads up to the fissure and facilitates dissection of the fissure, minimizing air leaks. Alternatively, the artery may be identified posteriorly from within the 'crotch' formed by the bronchus intermedius and the upper lobe bronchus, and the posterior aspect of the fissure completed. Once the artery is identified, further dissection within the fissure proceeds expeditiously. Rarely should it be necessary to dissect through the depths of the fissure to identify the artery.

Left-Sided Pulmonary Resections

Several features of the left chest make it unique. The aortic arch is a left-side structure and its position relative to the pulmonary artery and the left main bronchus is the major defining feature of resections on the left side. Access to the proximal left main bronchus and carina is limited because of the aortic arch. Thus, the left paratracheal area, a lymph-node-bearing area, is difficult to access at thoracotomy. There is no well defined area where a lymph node dissection is carried out as on the right side. Lymph nodes are dissected from the aortopulmonary window and the subcarinal space and, at times, from the paratracheal area.

Access to the most proximal aspect of the left main pulmonary artery may be gained by dividing the ligamentum arteriosum and then encircling the pulmonary artery. The left recurrent laryngeal nerve is highly vulnerable to injury because of its position in relation to the inferior surface of the aortic arch. This nerve originates from the vagus nerve as it crosses the arch and then 'recurs' around the ligamentum arteriosum. Any dissection in the aortopulmonary window places the left recurrent laryngeal nerve at risk of injury.

The left main bronchus also varies significantly from the right main bronchus. On the left there is a long segment of main stem bronchus before the bifurcation of the lobar bronchi; on the right, the right upper lobe bronchus originates within 2 cm of the carina. Sleeve resection of either the upper or lower lobe is certainly feasible, although left-sided sleeve resections account for only a minority of these resections in any series.

The lingular segment is analogous to the middle lobe in that it has a separate arterial and venous branch as well as a distinct bronchus. Lingular segmentectomy was one of the first segmental resections described, probably because of its well defined, discrete bronchovascular anatomy.

Contralateral mediastinal lymph node involvement is much more common with left-sided lesions, particularly lesions of the left lower lobe. For that reason, mediastinoscopy is particularly important when lesions of the left lower lobe are assessed.

Left Upper Lobectomy

The left upper lobectomy is perhaps the most technically challenging pulmonary resection because of the location of the pulmonary artery in relation to the aorta and the branching pattern of the left pulmonary artery. A number of potential pitfalls must be avoided in order to safely complete a left upper lobectomy.

Lymphatics from the left upper lobe commonly drain to lymph nodes in the aorto-pulmonary window (level 5) or para-aortic location (level 6), and these lymph nodes must be removed in order to obtain complete staging information. Despite the classification of these nodal locations as mediastinal (N2), involvement of these lymph nodes with tumor in the absence of other nodal disease is associated with a better prognosis than N2 disease in any other location. Survival with isolated involved level 5 or level 6 lymph nodes approximates that of patients who have only N1 lymph node involvement (approximately 40% at 5 years) as long as a complete resection can be performed.

Access to the superior mediastinum is difficult from the left side because of the location of the aortic arch in relation to the left main bronchus and tracheobronchial angle. For this reason, mediastinoscopy is extremely useful for left-sided lesions even without enlarged lymph nodes present on a CT scan, since it allows accurate sampling of the paratracheal area in a manner that is significantly simpler than trying to access this area during thoracotomy.

Left upper lobectomy is begun by incising the hilar pleura anteriorly and superiorly with the lobe retracted in a posterior direction. The pulmonary artery emerges from beneath the aortic arch and is located superior and posterolateral to the superior pulmonary vein. The apical segmental branch of the vein may cross the artery, partly obscuring the apical-posterior segmental trunk of the pulmonary artery and necessitating division of the venous branch first. The appropriate plane of dissection is entered on the pulmonary artery proximal to the take-off of the first branch, and careful circumferential dissection is carried out. The left main pulmonary artery is encircled with the index finger, and a blunt tipped clamp is passed toward the encircled finger to pass an umbilical tape around the vessel. A Rumel tourniquet is placed but not snared to allow the main pulmonary artery to be occluded if it should prove necessary. The superior pulmonary vein is dissected and encircled, care being taken to include the lingular branch. The vein may be doubly ligated or stapled with a vascular stapler and divided.

Once proximal control of the pulmonary artery is achieved, the branch is completely divided and the artery is repaired with 5–0 or 6–0 monofilament, nonabsorbable sutures. It is best to recognize that this arterial branch presents special problems and the recognition of this should lead to great caution when the left upper lobe is retracted, since avoiding problems with the pulmonary artery is far better and simpler than having to repair the artery, no matter how good you are at fixing problem situations.

Dissection of the artery continues distally, following the artery toward and into the fissure. The left main pulmonary artery resides in an epibronchial location relative to the left main bronchus (Figure 6–14). As the fissure is entered, the anterior segmental arterial branch to the upper lobe is encountered just proximal to and opposite the origin of the superior segmental branch to the lower lobe. Once the superior segmental branch is identified, the posterior portion of the fissure may be completed with a stapler. The anterior segmental branch is divided between silk ligatures (Figure 6–15) and the artery is followed further distally until the linear branches are encountered. There may be a single lingular trunk or two separate branches. The lingular branches are ligated and divided, and the anterior portion of the fissure is completed with a firing of the linear stapler (Figure 6–16). Alternatively, the fissure may be taken after the bronchus is divided, when it is all that remains holding the lobe in place.

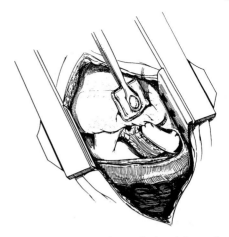

Figure 6–14. Relationship of the left main pulmonary artery to the left main bronchus seen from the posterior aspect. The main pulmonary artery lies in an epibronchial location. The inferior pulmonary vein is also visible from this posterior view.

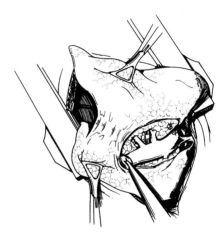

Figure 6–15. The anterior segmental branch of the pulmonary artery has been divided and the artery exposed in the fissure. Two lingular arterial branches are visible, as is the branch to the superior segment of the lower lobe.

Within the fissure, the artery is bluntly reflected inferiorly away from the underlying bronchus, which is located medially (or deep) (Figure 6–17). The bifurcation of the left main bronchus is visible at this point, and care should be taken to avoid damage to the lower lobe bronchus when the upper lobe bronchus is divided. The bronchus needs to be skeletonized and encircled before it is divided. Bronchial vessels should be either electrocoagulated or occluded with metal clips and divided, depending on their size. It should not be assumed that the stapler used to close the bronchus will occlude these vessels. Staplers used on the bronchus are not particularly

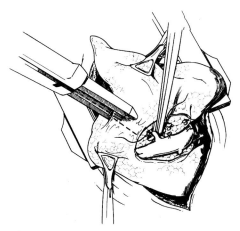

Figure 6–16. The anterior aspect of the fissure is taken with the linear stapler after the artery has been identified and dissected. A right-angled clamp is around a lingular arterial branch in preparation for ligation and division of the branch.

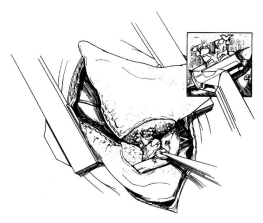

Figure 6–17. The pulmonary artery is retracted inferiorly to expose the origin of the left upper lobe bronchus. The point of division of the bronchus is shown (hatched line) just proximal to the bifurcation. The lingular bronchus and upper lobe proper are easily visible. **Inset,** The stapler is applied to the bronchus proximal to the lingula and upper lobe proper bifurcation. This is done from within the fissure.

the bronchus and sweeping any lymph nodes upward with the specimen. Incising the fibrous tissue on the plane of the bronchus at the level of the bifurcation also facilitates division of the anterior portion of the fissure. The thumb and first finger placed at the bifurcation may be used to thin out the parenchyma in this location so that the fissure can be divided by firing the linear stapler after the stapler is placed through the hole formed by the opposed thumb and forefinger. The upper lobe bronchus is stapled and divided as close as possible to the bifurcation (see Figure 6–17).

Alternatively, the bronchus may be divided with a scalpel (open technique) and closed with individual sutures of either a 3–0 or 4–0 monofilament or braided nonabsorbable material (Figure 6–18). The bronchus is divided in an open fashion – i.e. it is incised with a scalpel – in the presence of endobronchial disease that may be close to the bronchial margin, since the stapler, by virtue of its width, obscures what otherwise might be an adequate margin. The importance of a negative margin is obvious, and frozen-section examination of the bronchial margin should be obtained whenever an endobronchial lesion is present, if not routinely for all but small

hemostatic because of the size of the staples (3.5 mm or 4.8 mm). To avoid postoperative bleeding from a bronchial artery, these vessels should be identified and ligated before the bronchus is divided (or stapled).

Exposure of the left upper lobe bronchus is achieved from both the anterior aspect of the hilum and from within the fissure. Division of the superior pulmonary vein exposes the bronchus when the hilum is viewed from the anterior aspect. After division of the vein, there is a good opportunity to work on cleaning off

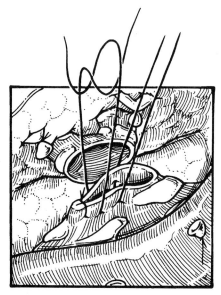

Figure 6–18. The bronchus has been divided with a scalpel and is being closed with sutures. The first suture should be placed at the midpoint of the closure, and all sutures should be placed before tying. The sutures should be evenly spaced and should be tied snugly but not so tight that they pull through the membranous bronchus, which is quite fragile. The bronchus is closed so that the membranous portion is apposed to the cartilaginous bronchus.

peripheral lung cancers. The bronchial stump is checked under saline to ensure that the closure is airtight.

The inferior pulmonary ligament is incised, freeing up the lower lobe, which it tethers, although the value of this maneuver is questionable. The purpose of incising the so-called inferior pulmonary ligament is to allow the lower lobe to more adequately fill the residual space after the upper lobe is removed. Lymph nodes in the para-aortic (level 6) and aorto-pulmonary window (level 5) locations are taken.

The subcarinal space is opened by incising the mediastinal pleura posteriorly and just inferior to the main bronchus. Small vagal branches going to the lung are divided between metal clips. The contents of the subcarinal space (level 7) are removed using blunt and sharp dissection along with the liberal use of metal clips.

The lymph nodes of the left paratracheal and tracheobronchial angles are most easily sampled at mediastinoscopy, but if exposure of these nodal locations is required, it is obtained by dissecting inferior to the aortic arch heading medially. The pulmonary artery must be retracted inferiorly to permit this dissection, which is facilitated by dividing the ligamentum arteriosum (Figure 6–19). On the left side there is no well-defined packet of superior mediastinal lymph nodes that yield to a nice clean dissection. The nodes must be removed individually. Great care must be taken to avoid the left recurrent laryngeal nerve, which 'recurs' around the ligamentum arteriosum. If the patient is hoarse in the postoperative period, the vocal cords should be examined with a laryngoscope to ensure that the left vocal cord is moving. If the left vocal cord is paralyzed, the patient's ability to cough and clear secretions in the postoperative period is markedly impaired, and aspiration with subsequent pneumonia becomes a significant risk.

Left Lower Lobectomy

Carcinomas of the left lower lobe involve contralateral mediastinal lymph nodes more commonly than lesions in any other lobe because of the almost constant occurrence of lymphatics that cross the midline. For left lung lesions, mediastinoscopy is the definitive invasive procedure for sampling right paratracheal lymph nodes but also provides access to the left paratracheal (level 2) and tracheobronchial

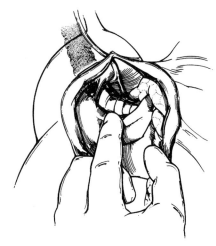

Figure 6–19. Exposure of the tracheobronchial angle is difficult from the left side because of the relationship of the left main bronchus to the aortic arch. To gain access to the tracheobronchial angle, the pulmonary artery must be retracted inferiorly. The ligamentum arteriosum is shown intact, but access to the left tracheobronchial angle is facilitated by dividing the ligamentum. The vagus nerve and the left recurrent laryngeal nerve are nicely demonstrated, showing how vulnerable the recurrent nerve is to injury during dissection in the aortopulmonary window.

angle (level 4) lymph nodes. The left-sided lymph nodes are actually easier to access with the mediastinoscope than at thoracotomy because of the location of the aortic arch relative to the left main bronchus.

The chest is entered through either a standard posterolateral thoracotomy incision (fifth intercostal space) or a muscle-sparing vertical axillary incision (fourth intercostal space). Even for lower lobectomy, there is no advantage to being in a lower intercostal (sixth) space, since the position of the hilar structures remains constant, although it seems intuitive that, if the fifth space is used for upper lobectomy, the sixth must be appropriate for lower lobectomy. The pleural space is thoroughly explored to rule out visceral or parietal pleural spread of tumor, assess lymph node involvement, assess nodal disease within the fissure, and establish whether left lower lobectomy is the procedure of choice.

It is safest, especially for a less experienced surgeon, to begin the dissection with the upper lobe retracted posteriorly to allow access to the proximal pulmonary artery, which is exposed by incising the pleura anteriorly and superiorly and dissecting down onto the artery. The appropriate plane is entered, the artery is encircled with a finger, an umbilical tape is passed, and a Rumel tourniquet is placed but not cinched down. This establishes proximal control if needed, which is a maneuver that is much easier to carry out at this point than at a time of sudden hemorrhage if the pulmonary artery or one of its branches is entered inadvertently.

If the fissure is complete – that is, if the pulmonary artery is visible from within the fissure – dissection may begin in the fissure by incising the pleura overlying the pulmonary artery to enter the appropriate plane on the vessel (Figure 6–20). Once this plane is reached, dissection may proceed in both an anterior and posterior direction along the artery. The superior segmental branch to the lower lobe is identified, usually just opposite the lingular branch of the artery to the upper lobe. This branch often needs to be divided separately depending on its location relative to the lingular branch (see Figure 6–20). At times the basilar segmental trunk of the artery may be divided along with the superior segmental branch, but this is dependent on the superior segment branch coming off distal (i.e., inferior) to the takeoff of the lingular branch. The artery to the lower lobe may be taken with a vascular stapler or doubly ligated. A linear endoscopic vascular stapler is ideally suited for ligation and division of the basilar arterial trunk.

Once the superior segmental branch of the artery is identified, the posterior aspect of the fissure may be completed by incising the pleura overlying the pulmonary artery posteriorly just before the artery enters the lung parenchyma. There are no branches coming off the inferior aspect of the artery posterior to the superior segment branch, and a finger may be inserted along the artery between this branch and the posterior aspect of the lung. This allows for placement of a linear stapler and completion of the fissure. Rarely should it be necessary to directly cut into lung parenchyma overlying the artery in order to complete a fissure. Likewise, the anterior aspect of the fissure may be completed with the linear stapler once the artery has been identified.

The inferior pulmonary ligament, a fibrofatty band tethering the lower lobe medially, is incised with electrocautery and divided up to the level of the inferior pulmonary vein (Figure 6–21). The vein may be visualized from either the anterior or posterior aspect of the hilum and is encircled with a finger or right-angled clamp once the plane of dissection is entered. The vein is then ligated and divided with a vascular stapler or clamped and sutured (see Figure 6–21).

By retracting the proximal pulmonary artery stump superiorly, the bronchus to the lower

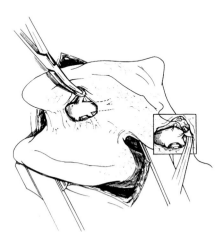

Figure 6–20. View of the left pulmonary artery in the fissure, showing the branch to the superior segment to the lower lobe being exposed. Note the position of this branch relative to the anterior segmental branch (upper lobe) and lingular branch. Often the superior segment branch needs to be taken separately, but may, at times, be taken in combination with the basilar trunk. **Inset,** The superior segment branch has been ligated and divided and the basilar trunk is being ligated.

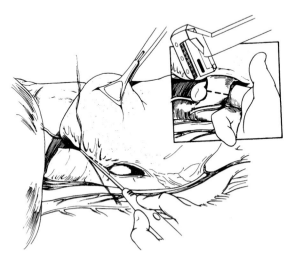

Figure 6–21. The inferior pulmonary ligament, a fibrofatty band tethering the lower lobe, is being incised with electrocautery as the lower lobe is elevated upward. The ligament is incised up to the level of the inferior pulmonary vein. **Inset,** Once the inferior vein is dissected free, it is encircled with a finger or clamp. A vascular stapler may be used to ligate the vein; alternatively, the vein may be doubly ligated or clamped, divided, and closed with sutures.

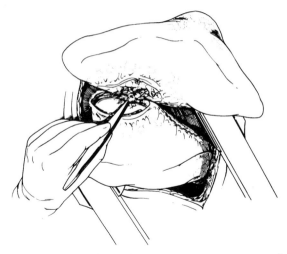

Figure 6–22. The pulmonary artery is retracted superiorly to reveal the lower lobe bronchus. The line of division (hatched line) is just proximal to the bifurcation between the superior segment bronchus and the basilar segmental bronchus. The line of division needs to be slightly oblique to encompass the origin of both of these. Most commonly the bronchus is closed with a stapler but it may also be cut and sutured closed.

lobe is identified (Figure 6–22). The bifurcation of the left main bronchus will be seen with this maneuver, confirming its identity. Care must be taken to include the superior segmental bronchus with the division of the lower lobe bronchus. This may require division of the bronchus in a slightly oblique orientation, but this should be done as close as possible to the bifurcation. Identification of the lower lobe bronchus is also facilitated after division of the inferior pulmonary vein because the bronchus is just posterior and superior to the vein. This identification may be helpful when there is lymph node involvement or tumor within the fissure, making it difficult to approach the bronchus from that aspect.

A lymph node dissection is performed by taking the contents of the aortopulmonary window (level 5), the para-aortic location (level 6), and the subcarinal space (level 7). The subcarinal space is entered by retracting the lung anteriorly and incising the pleura just inferior to the left main bronchus posteriorly. Several vagal branches are encountered going to the lung. These need to be clipped and divided. The contents of the subcarinal space are removed with the aid of metal clips placed on the small bronchial vessels. An inferior pulmonary ligament lymph node (level 9) is also taken. This is most often encountered as the inferior pulmonary ligament is incised and is usually found near the inferior pulmonary vein. These are the nodal levels not sampled by mediastinoscopy and their excision completes the staging evaluation.

Pneumonectomy

Rarely is it possible even for a well trained and experienced surgeon to know in advance that a pneumonectomy will be required if he or she is thinking about conserving lung parenchyma. Recognizing that pneumonectomy is associated with a significantly higher mortality than lobectomy, it is best to look at pneumonectomy as a procedure of last resort, when it is impossible to do any other procedure. We tend to look at any resection as an opportunity to conserve lung tissue as long as it is not at the expense of an adequate cancer operation. This mandates recognizing when a bronchoplastic procedure or sleeve resection is appropriate, as well as when an arterioplasty or partial resection of the pulmonary artery is required in order to avoid pneumonectomy. Pneumonectomy is an easier operation to perform than lobectomy because it requires only mobilization of hilar structures and is certainly technically less demanding than a bronchoplastic procedure.

It is illustrative to look at the situations in which pneumonectomy may be required. Very proximal involvement of the pulmonary artery, especially on the left side, usually mandates pneumonectomy, especially if it is difficult to encircle the artery proximally. To better assess the proximal extent of involvement of the left pulmonary artery, it is often necessary to divide the ligamentum arteriosum, which is a move that frees up a considerable portion of the proximal left main pulmonary artery. Occasionally, a sleeve resection or partial resection of the pulmonary artery is possible in order to avoid pneumonectomy if the artery can be controlled proximally and if there is a trunk of distal pulmonary artery that remains intact. Involvement of the main stem bronchus with tumor rarely, by itself, mandates pneumonectomy if the surgeon is familiar with bronchoplastic procedures. The situation becomes more difficult if the minor carina on the left (bifurcation of the main stem bronchus) is extensively involved and precludes salvaging the 'uninvolved' bronchus for reattachment. Tumor or lymph node involvement that encases the pulmonary artery in the fissure often makes lobectomy difficult and may require pneumonectomy, but it is best to proceed with an extensive dissection proximal and distal to the involved area to ensure that lobectomy is not possible before making the decision. A 'difficult' or incomplete fissure without tumor involvement should not be an indication for pneumonectomy. Involvement of the confluence of the pulmonary veins is another situation in which pneumonectomy may be required, since it is usually necessary to take a cuff of left atrium in order to complete this resection.

Lesions that mandate right pneumonectomy again are mainly those that involve the most proximal portion of the pulmonary artery or larger lesions that arise within the center of the lung and involve all three lobes. With the length of the right main pulmonary artery, it is often possible to have significant involvement of the pulmonary artery yet still be able to get proximal enough to place a clamp and resect a portion of the artery and obviate having to perform pneumonectomy. A significant length of the right pulmonary artery may be mobilized posterior to the superior vena cava. Because of the short length of the right main bronchus proximal to the right upper lobe takeoff, there is a tendency on the part of many surgeons to think that pneumonectomy is required when there is tumor in the main bronchus. Resection of the right main bronchus including the upper lobe allows the bronchus intermedius to be anastomosed to the origin of the right main bronchus, thus obtaining effectively the same bronchial margin but conserving lung tissue.

Relative contraindications to pneumonectomy include baseline pulmonary function that would leave inadequate pulmonary reserve after resection, inability to remove all disease, and advanced age. Low preoperative diffusing capacity as well as pulmonary hypertension may also contradict pneumonectomy. A quantitative ventilation-perfusion lung scan should be performed to assess relative blood flow to each lung if the forced expiratory volume in 1 second (FEV$_1$) is less than 2 L. As a guideline, the calculated FEV$_1$ remaining after pneumonectomy should be at least 800 mL, but this may vary depending on the size of the patient. It is not surprising to find that even patients with seemingly borderline lung function may be candidates for pneumonectomy because of relatively little perfusion going to the lung proposed for resection. In a sense, some of these patients are already 'auto-pneumonectomized.'

Lung conservation should always be kept in mind at the start of any pulmonary resection, and it is only rarely that a resection should be begun when a pneumonectomy will have to be performed. Most commonly, the decision to remove an entire lung is made intraoperatively after thorough exploration of the chest and assessment of the extent of the lesion. Subjecting a patient to the increased morbidity and mortality that accompany pneumonectomy if the resection will not be 'curative' – i.e. with total removal of all disease – rarely proves worthwhile if one looks at survival benefit. Assessing the extent of the lesion often goes as far as beginning the resection as if lobectomy or sleeve lobectomy is possible and only converting to pneumonectomy when it is impossible to complete a lesser resection.

Right Pneumonectomy

The chest is entered through either a standard posterolateral thoracotomy (fifth intercostal space) or a vertical axillary muscle-sparing incision (fourth intercostal space). The lung is retracted posteriorly by the surgeon to expose the anterior hilum where the pleura is incised, carrying this superiorly over the bronchus and inferiorly to the level of the inferior pulmonary vein (Figure 6–23). The inferior pulmonary ligament is incised up to the level of the inferior vein, and the vein is encircled. The right main pulmonary artery is identified, as is the superior pulmonary vein. The artery is followed proximally to where it lies posterior to the vena cava. After the appropriate dissection plane is entered, the proximal pulmonary artery is encircled with the finger.

Depending on the location of the tumor, or of proximal lymph node involvement, it may not be possible to isolate the proximal pulmonary artery without entering the pericardium. Opening the pericardium also allows for a more complete exploration to assess resectability if the lesion is quite proximal and there is a concern about involvement of the pulmonary venous confluence. The pericardium should be opened anterior to the phrenic nerve, if possible, and the opening extended along the length of the hilum. A finger may be inserted to assess the depth of invasion of the tumor into the pericardium and whether there is enough proximal pulmonary artery to allow it to be encircled. The superior and inferior pulmonary veins are also identified, and an assessment is made whether these vessels may be encircled, since sometimes a shelf of tumor

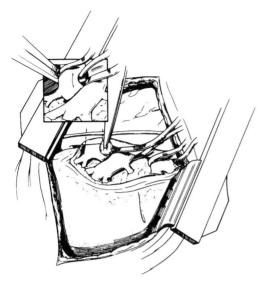

Figure 6–23. View of the right hilum from the right side of the operating table. The hilar pleura has been incised and dissection has begun on the pulmonary artery and veins. The superior and inferior veins are encircled with tapes. Note that the artery courses posterior to the vena cava; an additional length of the artery can be obtained by retracting the vena cava medially. The phrenic nerve courses along the superior vena cava as shown. **Inset,** The right main pulmonary artery is encircled with a tape to establish proximal control. This is a prudent move at the start of any pulmonary resection. The artery courses posterior to the superior pulmonary vein and may be injured if care is not taken when encircling the vein.

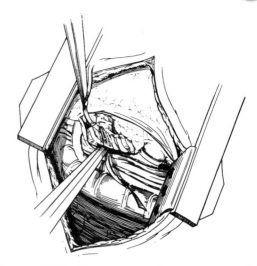

Figure 6–24. The azygos vein crosses the right main bronchus just proximal to the origin of the right upper lobe bronchus. This is a constant anatomic finding. The vein may be taken if necessary to expose the bronchus. The view in this drawing is from the posterior aspect of the hilum. The right main bronchus may be encircled from this approach.

is found posterior to the veins that is not readily apparent. Entering the pericardium is often the key move in assessing resectability of a central lesion.

If the resection is possible outside the pericardium, the superior pulmonary vein is dissected and encircled. Care must be taken to avoid injury to the continuation of the pulmonary artery as it courses medial to the superior pulmonary vein. The plane between these two vessels must be entered in order to separate them (see Figure 6–25).

Once the vessels are encircled, the proximal main stem bronchus is dissected. Depending on the location of the tumor, division of the azygos vein may facilitate this dissection as the vein traverses the bronchus just proximal to the takeoff of the right upper lobe (Figure 6–24). This is a consistent landmark. The dissection around the bronchus is carried out with the lung retracted anteriorly. Once the artery has been dissected, it is easy to encircle the bronchus after the pleura overlying the subcarinal space has been incised. Either a finger or

blunt right-angled clamp is passed around the right main bronchus as close to the origin of the bronchus as possible. From the right side this is relatively easy, since the carina is so easy to mobilize from this side. There should be no difficulty encountered in encircling the right main bronchus at its origin.

The location of the tumor dictates to some extent the order in which the vascular structures are divided. With proximal involvement of the artery, it is often easier to divide the veins first, followed by the bronchus, leaving the artery until last when the exposure is at a maximum. The main pulmonary artery and the superior and inferior pulmonary veins are divided between rows of staples placed with a vascular stapler (Figure 6–25). Alternatively, a vessel may be divided between clamps and closed with a running, monofilament, nonabsorbable suture. It is not adequate to place only a tie on the main pulmonary artery or on the veins; proximal vessels should at least be doubly ligated with a suture ligature if a stapler is not used or the vessels are not sutured. Occasionally, dividing the bronchus first provides significantly better exposure, which allows for easier division of vascular structures. The bronchus may be safely closed with a stapler or sewn with interrupted sutures of absorbable material. A pedicle of pleura or intercostal muscle is placed to buttress the pneumonectomy stump closure, although

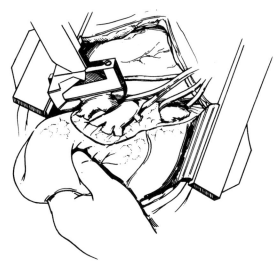

Figure 6–25. The vascular stapler is applied to the right main pulmonary artery. The artery is divided between rows of vascular staples. Alternatively, the artery may be clamped, divided, and sutured closed. The superior and inferior veins may also be divided between rows of vascular staples. Simple ligation of any of these structures is inadequate. At the least, a ligature should be placed, followed by a suture ligature. It makes no difference in what order the vascular structures are divided. If it is easier to take the veins first, that should be done. There is nothing magical or advantageous to dividing the artery first.

there is little experimental evidence to support the contention that this decreases the already small incidence of pneumonectomy stump breakdowns.

Mediastinal lymph node dissection should be carried out in the standard fashion, removing the contents of the superior mediastinum and subcarinal space. If an intrapericardial pneumonectomy has been performed, it is mandatory that either the pericardial edges are reapproximated or, if pericardium has been excised as part of the resection, prosthetic material is used to close the pericardium at the completion of the resection. This is necessary to prevent the heart from migrating out of the pericardium, as it is no longer kept in place by the lung on that side. The closure should not be constricting, and the prosthetic material should be fenestrated to allow drainage and prevent even a minimal amount of tamponade.

Left Pneumonectomy

A standard posterolateral thoracotomy or muscle-sparing incision is performed and the chest entered through the fourth (muscle-sparing) or

fifth intercostal space. A thorough exploration is carried out to assess the extent of tumor involvement and resectability. Extensive direct mediastinal invasion usually precludes resection, and this type of involvement cannot be accurately evaluated by any preoperative imaging studies.

If there is extensive tumor encasing the hilum, further exploration is required, and the pericardium should be incised along the length of the hilum to permit a finger to be inserted (Figure 6–26). This allows the extent of involvement of the atrium and the confluence of the pulmonary veins as well as proximal involvement of the pulmonary artery to be assessed. The pericardial incision should be made anterior to the phrenic nerve (on the lung side of the nerve), if possible. Damage to the nerve should be avoided and the nerve sacrificed only if resection is possible and the nerve is involved by tumor.

Extensive proximal (medial) invasion of the atrium often precludes resection, since the amount of atrium that may be safely and prudently resected is limited. How extensive is too extensive is difficult both to judge and to convey, but the feasibility of resection is borderline once involvement of the venous confluence is recognized. It is important to assess

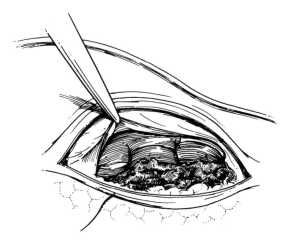

Figure 6–26. View from the left side of the table of the left pulmonary hilum. The pericardium has been opened to assess the extent of invasion of this hilar mass and determine the feasibility of resection. It must be possible to encircle the artery and both veins, and there has to be enough room to place a clamp. The confluence of the veins should be closely examined to make sure the veins may be encircled. Division of the ligamentum arteriosum might be required in order to gain enough additional length on the artery to place a clamp so that resection can proceed.

involvement of the posterior hilum as well, and to ensure resectability it must be possible to pass a finger around the hilum. Often a shelf of tumor extending further medially is encountered when the posterior hilum is palpated, and this precludes safe resection.

The proximal extent of involvement of the pulmonary artery must also be ascertained via intrapericardial exploration. Division of the ligamentum arteriosum allows for a complete assessment of the entire length of the left main pulmonary artery and may be necessary in order to complete a resection.

Once it has been established that the lesion is resectable and that pneumonectomy is required, the hilar structures must be mobilized. If an intrapericardial assessment has been necessary, the pulmonary artery is encircled within the pericardium, as are the superior and inferior pulmonary veins. If the procedure is feasible, the hilar pleura is incised anteriorly and superiorly, with the lung retracted posteriorly (Figure 6–27). The left main pulmonary artery is encircled either with a blunt-tipped clamp or preferably with a finger. The superior pulmonary vein is also encircled, and the inferior pulmonary ligament is divided, allowing the inferior pulmonary vein to be encircled.

The order in which the hilar structures are divided varies depending on the location of the tumor. Occasionally, it may even be preferable to divide the left main bronchus before any of the vascular structures are divided. The main pulmonary artery is divided between two rows of vascular staples. Alternatively, a vascular clamp is placed on the proximal pulmonary artery and the artery is divided and closed with a running monofilament suture. The superior pulmonary vein is also divided between rows of vascular staples or may be clamped and sewn, as described above (Figure 6–28). The inferior pulmonary vein may be approached from either the anterior or posterior aspect of the hilum, stapled or clamped, and divided. The bronchus is approached from the posterior aspect of the hilum, with the lung retracted anteriorly and divided as close as possible to the carina (Figure 6–29). Dissection of the proximal left main bronchus is difficult because of the location of the aortic arch, but a long bronchial stump should be avoided.

In contrast to the situation on the right side, the carina is not easily visible from the left and cannot be mobilized, thus making the approach to the proximal left main bronchus more difficult. The bronchus is retracted laterally, being pulled upward toward the incision to facilitate the dissection and the placement of the stapler on the proximal bronchus. Alternatively, the bronchus may be incised and closed with interrupted sutures (see Figure 6–29). A flap of parietal pleura is sewn to the bronchial stump using fine silk sutures to reinforce the closure of the pneumonectomy stump (Figure 6–30). This flap is usually based superiorly and takes the pleura overlying the descending thoracic aorta for approximately 5 cm.

If the pericardium has been opened, it must be closed to prevent herniation of the heart

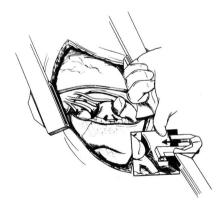

Figure 6–27. Tapes have been placed around the superior and inferior pulmonary veins and a finger is being placed around the left main pulmonary artery. Placing a finger around the artery to ensure that the plane is free is preferable to blind placement of a clamp and possibly damaging the back side of the artery. **Inset,** A vascular stapler is used to ligate the artery and the vessel is divided between rows of vascular staples.

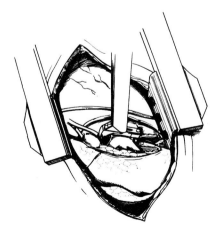

Figure 6–28. The superior pulmonary vein is divided between rows of vascular staples. The artery has been divided and the cut ends are visible.

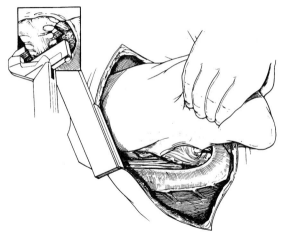

Figure 6–29. View of the left hilum from the posterior aspect showing the relationship of the left main bronchus to the aorta. The bronchus is dissected as far proximally as feasible so that the division occurs as close to the carina as possible. It is disadvantageous to leave a long bronchial stump that is relatively ischemic. Because of the aortic arch, the mobilization of the carina from the left side is not possible, but the left main bronchus may be traced back almost to its origin. **Inset,** Once the bronchus has been dissected proximally and skeletonized, it is closed with a firing of the stapler and divided. Here the stapler is being placed around the bronchus.

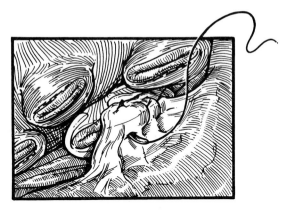

Figure 6–30. A flap of pleura is sewn to the left main bronchial stump for additional protection. The stumps of the vessels are easily seen. The incidence of stump breakdown is low, and there is no definitive evidence that placing a flap on a bronchial stump lowers the incidence; however, there is something intuitively attractive about reinforcing a bronchial stump that spurs us on.

into the pneumonectomy space. This is important for either a right or left pneumonectomy. If the pericardium only has been incised, a few sutures may be all that is required to close the defect, but constriction of the heart must be avoided. If a piece of pericardium has been excised, a patch of prosthetic material should be used to close the defect. The prosthetic patch, with fenestrations, should be loosely sewn into place to prevent even minimal tamponade.

A chest tube is placed into the pneumonectomy space to allow the position of the mediastinum to equilibrate and to monitor bleeding into the space. The tube is removed within 24 hours. Alternatively, to 'set' the mediastinum, air may be withdrawn from the pleural space after closure until negative pressure is obtained and the use of a tube is avoided. A moderate amount of subcutaneous emphysema is to be expected during the early postoperative course, as the space fills with fluid, displacing the air from the pneumonectomy space into the subcutaneous tissue.

Postoperative Considerations

After the chest tube is removed, it is common to note subcutaneous emphysema of the chest and neck. This occurs when the air that remains in the pleural space is displaced as the space fills with fluid. The presence of a moderate amount of subcutaneous air in the early postoperative period does not indicate a bronchial stump leak but is a normal and expected sequelae to pneumonectomy. An excessive and increasing amount of subcutaneous air, however, may be indicative of a small leak from the bronchial stump, and the patient may have to be re-explored to assess this possibility. This is strictly a technical error and must be avoided by checking the bronchial stump closure at the time of the initial resection. This is potentially a devastating complication, which should be preventable. A bronchial stump leak early in the postoperative course may be repaired primarily, but the space must be considered infected. Tube drainage for several days may prevent late infection, but there should be a high index of suspicion for a late postpneumonectomy empyema.

Pulmonary edema is perhaps the most dreaded early complication after pneumonectomy, most commonly right pneumonectomy. This may present any time from 24 to 96 hours after pneumonectomy, with the patient showing some increased work of breathing and mild hypoxemia. Chest radiographs may look perfectly clear, or a very fine reticular pattern may be seen. Usually within 24 hours after these initial findings the patient requires mechanical ventilation, and there is very little that can be done other than to support the patient's hemodynamics. If deemed necessary, and it often is of significant help in these situations, a pulmonary artery catheter may be placed despite the pulmonary artery stump. The catheter should be floated with the balloon inflated, which is standard procedure.

It is not necessary to ventilate these patients with a double-lumen endobronchial tube, but peak airway pressures should be kept as low as possible (<40 cm H_2O), and the ventilation mode of choice is pressure-controlled ventilation. Most of these patients benefit from sedation and paralysis to more effectively oxygenate them, but some may be supported, for a time, with a pressure support mode and either continuous positive airway pressure or a low setting of intermittent mandatory ventilation. There is no absolute contraindication to positive end-expiratory pressure, which should be used to keep the inspired oxygen concentration as low as possible, preferably below 60%. Long periods of high inspired oxygen concentrations should be avoided if possible. Continuous inhaled nitric oxide has been used as an adjunct in these patients with varying degrees of efficacy. It remains to be determined how useful nitric oxide may be in these situations.

Sometimes the oxygenation improves, but most commonly these patients continue to deteriorate and ultimately die. Mortality from this complication is more than 50% and probably closer to 75%; the figure has not improved over the past few years. There is no known cause for this syndrome, if we can call it that, which appears to be associated with an increase in vascular permeability. Steroids, even if given early, seem ineffective in attenuating the development of the problem. Intraoperative fluid administration should be minimal if pneumonectomy is even being contemplated. Postoperative fluid replacement should be milliliter for milliliter, with correction for insensitive losses to maintain an acceptable urine output (15 mL/hr).

Early in the postoperative period patients may be somewhat more dyspneic than expected, but this usually resolves over a short period of time as the pain of the operation lessens, making splinting with breathing less prominent. Patients should also be informed that over time they will develop some degree of scoliosis away from the side of the resection – that is, the spine moves toward the side of the pneumonectomy. This is one of the compensatory mechanisms, along with a shift of the mediastinum and elevation of the ipsilateral hemidiaphragm, that serve to decrease the size of the space.

The pneumonectomy space fills at a variable rate. Often the space may be filled within 7–10 days, but it is not uncommon to see patients return to the office for the first postoperative visit 3 weeks after discharge with an incompletely filled space. Space infections, however, often are not obvious or easy to diagnose. One needs to be wary if the patient is failing to thrive after several weeks. These patients complain of not feeling quite right, of no appetite with continued weight loss, and often of low-grade fevers. These infections may be quite insidious, and the only way to identify them in a timely fashion is to maintain a high index of suspicion.

When a question exists, fluid should be withdrawn from the space after appropriate sterile precautions are taken. A Gram's stain and culture of the fluid should be obtained. If the fluid is infected, the space must be drained. It is not adequate to simply place a patient with a postpneumonectomy space infection on antibiotics, even if there is no overt evidence of a bronchial stump breakdown. Tube drainage is not feasible in these patients over the long term, and an open window thoracostomy (Clagett) should be made. The window should be large and in the most dependent location possible. This procedure is the only one that effects complete drainage of the space whether or not there is an air leak, but often there is some hesitation on the part of the surgeon to carry out this necessary procedure because of the presumed disfigurement. Ultimately, the window may be closed as the second stage of the Clagett procedure or muscle flaps rotated into the space for closure, so it is not necessarily permanent. Anything less than complete drainage of the space is usually doomed to failure, if not early on then sometimes years later.

The 30-day mortality from pulmonary resections is approximately 4%. Lobectomies and lesser resections have a mortality of 1–2%, whereas pneumonectomy still carries a mortality of 6–7%. The mortality rate is directly proportional to increased age, associated diseases, and the extent of resection. Respiratory complications, not surprisingly, are the most common cause of postoperative mortality in patients undergoing pulmonary resection. Cardiac complications also account for a significant percentage of mortality, whereas technical problems such as hemorrhage, bronchopleural fistula, and empyema account for a small but significant percentage of complications leading to death.

Approximately 30% of patients undergoing pulmonary resection will sustain a postoperative complication, of which approximately two-thirds are minor and the other one-third nonfatal major complications. The most common complication is supraventricular arrhythmia, which occurs in up to 20% of patients, depending on how closely patients are monitored. Most of these respond to simple pharmacologic manipulation and rarely are hemodynamically significant at onset. With appropriate treatment the rhythm reverts to sinus rhythm quickly and patients may be taken off the antiarrhythmic drugs, usually after 1 month. Other minor complications include postoperative air leaks lasting more than 7 days and atelectasis. Major nonfatal events most commonly are respiratory-related, with patients developing significant infiltrates and pneumonitis. A small percentage of patients require reintubation in the postoperative period for respiratory failure that is usually related to the development of an infiltrate.

There are no definitive predictors for postoperative pulmonary complications, although significant risk factors for major complications include age above 60 years, FEV_1 of less than 2 L, weight loss of more than 10%, associated systemic disease, and extent of disease. Pulmonary complications can be minimized with meticulous attention to postoperative respiratory maneuvers, including chest physiotherapy and preoperative teaching.

Other complications of pulmonary resection include wound infections and disturbances in mental status, especially in older patients. Notwithstanding our best efforts to avoid them, complications do occur. If recognized early, many can be treated without sequelae. Meticulous attention to detail in all phases of management – preoperative, intraoperative, and postoperative – goes a long way toward keeping problems to a minimum.

Key Readings

Conlan AA, Kopec SE. Indications for pneumonectomy. Pneumonectomy for benign disease. *Chest Surg Clin North Am* 1999;9:311–326. *Discusses the decision to perform a pneumonectomy.*

Dewey TM, Mack MJ. Lung cancer. Surgical approaches and incisions. *Chest Surg Clin North Am* 2000;10:803–820. *Review of alternative approaches to enter the thoracic cavity.*

Selected Readings

Kittle CF. The history of lobectomy and segmentectomy including sleeve resection. *Chest Surg Clin North Am* 2000;10:105–130, ix.

Roviaro G, Varoli F, Vergani C, Maciocco M. Techniques of pneumonectomy. Video-assisted thoracic surgery pneumonectomy. *Chest Surg Clin North Am* 1999;9:419–46, xi–xii.

Tronc F, Gregoire J, Rouleau J, Deslauriers J. Techniques of pneumonectomy. Completion pneumonectomy. *Chest Surg Clin North Am* 1999;9:393–405, xi.

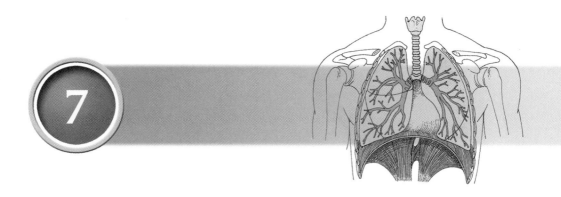

7

Congenital Lung Diseases

Congenital Lung Diseases: Key Points

- Describe the process of developing emphysema in the infant and the appropriate management
- Know the management of pulmonary cystic disease and congenital cystic adenomatoid malformation in the neonate
- Describe the differences between an intralobar and extralobar pulmonary sequestration

Pulmonary Embryology

A brief understanding of the morphogenesis of the trachea, bronchi, and lungs is necessary to understand congenital lesions (Table 7–1). Lung growth and development begins at approximately 3 weeks of gestation and proceeds until about 8 years of age. At 3 weeks of gestational age, the respiratory diverticulum (tracheobronchial groove) forms as a ventral epithelial evagination of the foregut. The groove begins to elongate in a caudal direction and soon becomes separated from the foregut by formation of an esophagotracheal septum.

By 4 weeks the separation is nearly complete and the respiratory diverticulum begins to form a left and right lung bud. These first branches form lung buds that correspond to the lobar bronchi, three on the right and two on the left. The lung bud continues to grow caudally and laterally and undergoes 20 generations of airway subdivisions.

As the lung buds grow caudally and laterally, they grow into a second primordium, which is a mass of splanchnic mesoderm. As the lung buds branch and extend, they carry this mass of mesodermal tissue along with them (Figure 7–1).

The lung buds and the associated splanchnic mesoderm undergo a reciprocal inductive interaction that is essential for normal pulmonary development. The epithelium lining the entire

147

TABLE 7–1 • *Normal Embryologic Development of the Lower Respiratory Tract*

Age	Embryologic Development
Embryonic period	
22 days	Median pharyngeal groove appears on foregut
24–26 days	Lung bud appears and soon bifurcates
5–6 weeks	Lung sac acquires lobar buds
7th week	Mesoderm forms bronchial muscle Pulmonary capillary plexus develops Truncus arteriosus separates into aorta and main pulmonary artery Pulmonary plexus and the sixth pharyngeal arches fuse
8th week	Distinct lobar architecture
Pseudoglandular period	
8–16 weeks	The bronchial divisions are established and proliferate rapidly
Canalicular period	
4–6 months	Respiratory bronchioles and alveoli develop; mature alveolar cells appear
Terminal sac period	
6 months to birth	Alveolar walls become progressively thinner as alveoli mature

Adapted from Luck SR, Reynolds M, Rafensperger JG. Congenital bronchopulmonary malformations. *Curr Probl Surg* 1986;23:245.

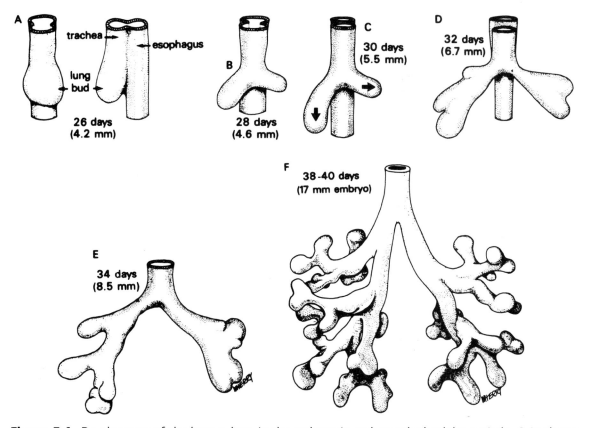

Figure 7–1. Development of the human lung in the embryonic and pseudoglandular periods. **A** is shown from the side; all others are shown from the front only. (From Fraser RG, Pare JAP, Pare PD, *et al. Diagnosis of diseases of the chest*, 3rd ed. Philadelphia: WB Saunders, 1988.)

BOX 7-1 CHARACTERISTICS OF SURFACTANT

Composition
- Phospholipids (80–85%) – lecithin is most abundant agent
- Protein (5–10%) – apoproteins A, B, C
- Neutral lipids (10%)

Source
- Secreted by type II granular pneumocytes

respiratory system forms from the respiratory diverticulum and is of endodermal origin. The splanchnic mesoderm forms the connective tissue, cartilage, smooth muscle cells, and blood vessels surrounding the epithelium.

During the histological development, the lungs pass through three developmental stages. The glandular stage extends from the branching of the respiratory diverticulum to the fourth month of development. During this time, the lung buds proliferate and branch into the surrounding splanchnic mesenchyme. During the canalicular stage between the fourth and sixth months of fetal life, the airways become lined by a cuboidal epithelium and the parenchyma of the lung becomes highly vascularized. Finally, during the saccular stage, which extends until term, the epithelium that lines the lung bud branches becomes thinner and thinner, while the blood vessels proliferate and become intimately associated with the alveolar epithelium.

Between the sixth and seventh months, the alveolar epithelium begins to differentiate into two types of alveolar cell: squamous type I cells and surfactant-secretory type II cells. Type II cells process intracellular inclusion bodies, which represent a storage form of the pulmonary surfactant (Box 7-1). Pulmonary surfactant is composed of phospholipid protein complexes. Lecithin is the most abundant phospholipid in surfactant. Once an adequate number of type II cells have formed, a fetus is viable in the extrauterine environment. The secretion of surfactant is a clinically useful indication of fetal lung maturity.

Congenital Lobar Emphysema

Congenital lobar emphysema is responsible for 50% of the congenital malformations of the lung. Pathophysiologically, congenital lobar emphysema is caused by overexpansion of the air spaces of a segment or lobe of the lung. The left upper lobe is most often involved. In contrast to adult emphysema, there is no damage to the lung parenchyma. The mechanism of action involves a ball-valve obstruction of a lobar or segmental bronchus. This results in distal air trapping with hyperinflation, which compounds bronchial obstruction (Figure 7-2). Several conditions have been shown to cause obstruction in congenital lobar emphysema. Bronchial obstruction due to mucous plugs, inflammation, stenosis, atresia, or bronchial wall abnormalities trap air after inspiration. Bronchial obstruction occasionally is also caused by extrinsic compression due to pulmonary artery sling, aneurysmal dilation, and congenital heart abnormalities (Table 7-2).

Patients can have a full range of symptoms. Some infants have mild symptoms that do not progress and have a stable overexpanded lobe without mass effect on other pulmonary tissue. Other infants will develop tachypnea, dyspnea, wheezing, and cyanosis within several days of birth, severe enough to require endotracheal intubation and urgent surgical intervention. In general, 80% of affected patients present within the first 6 months of life. Patients with this disorder who are older than 1 year at presentation are less frequently seen, and rarer still are those who present as adults. In the newborn, there is usually a history of tachypnea, chest retraction, and wheezing from birth. An upper respiratory infection may complicate the condition and precipitate severe respiratory distress. Later symptoms can include failure to thrive, psychomotor retardation and thoracic malformation.

Chest radiographs will demonstrate radiolucency of the involved lobe with mediastinal shift to the opposite side (Figure 7-3). Because of air trapping, the mediastinal shift can increase on expiration. Occasionally, the emphysematous segment herniates into the opposite side anterior to the heart and great vessels. Chest radiography is usually sufficient to make the diagnosis, although other studies may prove useful. A computed tomography (CT) scan of the chest may show a bronchial obstruction caused by the overinflated lung, mediastinal masses, bronchogenic cysts, and pulmonary artery slings (Figure 7-4). Ventilation/perfusion scans can reveal unventilated pulmonary segments and provide confirmatory data in patients suspected

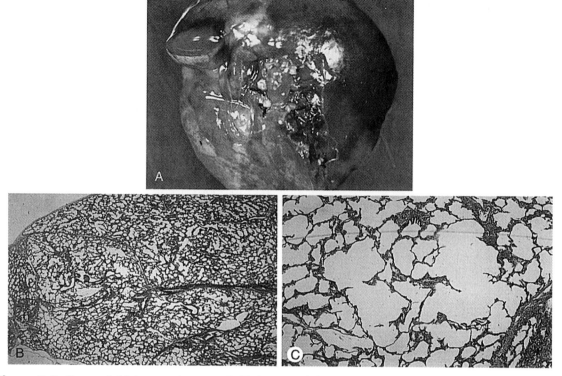

Figure 7–2. Congenital lobar emphysema. **A,** Right upper lobectomy specimen resected at 3 weeks of age. Note the turgid appearance of the lung parenchyma. **B,** Overdistended alveoli (hematoxylin and eosin, original magnification ×10). **C,** Interalveolar septa show focal rupture. No fibrosis is present (hematoxylin and eosin, original magnification ×20). (From Schwartz DS, Reyes-Mugica M, Keller MS. Imaging of surgical diseases of the newborn chest. Intrapleural mass lesions. *Radiol Clin North Am* 1999;37:1067–1078.)

TABLE 7–2 • *Causes of Bronchial Obstruction*		
Intrinsic		Bronchomalacia
		Bronchial atresia
		Bronchial stenosis
		Bronchial granulations
		Mucosal folds
		Mucous plugs
		Inflammatory exudates
Extrinsic	Cardiac	Patent ductus arteriosus
		Pulmonary artery sling
		Pulmonary stenosis
		Aneurysmal dilation
		Tetralogy of Fallot
	Non-cardiac	Bronchogenic cyst
		Esophageal duplication cyst
		Mediastinal adenopathy
		Accessory diaphragm

of having congenital lobar emphysema on chest radiographs. Diagnostic bronchoscopy should be performed when there is a question of bronchial compression by vascular structures.

Surgical intervention is required for life-threatening progressive pulmonary insufficiency from compression of adjacent normal lung. Surgical excision of the involved lobe should be done immediately in a critically ill patient. In most patients, lobectomy results in complete cure. At operation, the chest is opened as soon as possible after induction of anesthesia. Positive end-expiratory pressure ventilation (PEEP) causes further overinflation of the involved lobe and increases the risk of cardiovascular compromise due to this phenomenon of 'auto-PEEP.' Repair of any heart defects or vascular abnormalities should be given precedence, although a lobectomy may still be required. The mortality rate associated with surgical correction is 10–30%. The prognosis

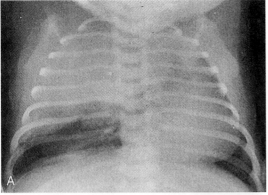

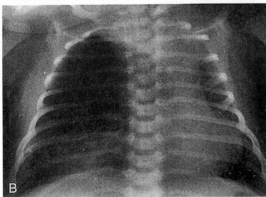

Figure 7–3. Congenital lobar emphysema. **A,** Newborn presented with respiratory distress and a homogeneous mass in the right upper hemithorax with mediastinal shift. Congenital lobar emphysema should be considered, despite the absence of obvious emphysema, because on early radiographs the lesion can be filled with lung fluid. **B,** After 36 hours the fetal lung fluid has cleared and the true emphysematous nature of the mass is revealed. This lesion was surgically resected. (From Rencken I, Patton WL, Brasch RC. Airway obstruction in pediatric patients. From croup to BOOP. *Radiol Clin North Am* 1998;36:175–187.)

depends on the presence of associated anomalies.

Congenital Pulmonary Cysts

Congenital pulmonary cystic lesions occur as a result of entrapment of part of the developing lung bud. These occur early in the fetal development, a time when completion of the terminal bronchioles and development of the alveoli is occurring. No specific cause has been determined. Most hypotheses regarding the development of pulmonary cysts suggests a process of pouching out of the primitive lung bud and then an abortive pinching off of the

segment from the foregut. It is unusual for pulmonary cysts to be associated with other congenital abnormalities.

Grossly, cystic lung lesions are usually unilobar. The lower lobes are involved more often than the upper lobes. In general, pulmonary cysts are singular and multilobular. They are usually larger than 1 cm in diameter. The location within the chest is more peripheral than central. Unlike bronchogenic cysts, communication between the cyst and tracheobronchial tree is always present.

Pathologically, the cystic wall structure depends on the site of origin of the cyst and determines its composition. Proximal cysts typically are composed of bronchial glands, smooth muscle, cartilage, and columnar epithelium. Distal cysts have alveolus-like histology. Most are air-filled, although in up to 25% of cases they can be fluid-filled. Because they originate from the foregut, cysts may be lined with ciliated columnar (respiratory) or squamous epithelium. Both linings have mucous bronchial glands, which causes the cyst to fill under pressure. This causes pressure on surrounding structures, particularly the membranous trachea or bronchi, and may lead to severe respiratory obstruction.

Clinically, these cysts usually produce symptoms early in life such as respiratory distress, infection with fever, cough, and sepsis. Respiratory distress is secondary to expansion of the cyst. Air can enter the cyst through the pores of Kohn but often is entrapped due to a ball-and-valve mechanism. As the cyst expands, there is compression of the ipsilateral lung and diaphragm, along with a shift of the mediastinum to the contralateral side. This shift results in atelectasis of the normal contralateral lung. This combination of expansion of the cyst and loss of normal lung tissue leads to worsening respiratory distress (Figure 7–5). Later in life, recurrent infection of the cyst is the primary mode of presentation. Poor ventilation allows the cyst to easily become infected and, because of the poor drainage, reinfection is a common occurrence.

Radiographically, a cystic lesion that communicates with the airways and contains secretions or pus has an air–fluid level on a decubitus or upright chest radiograph. The surrounding lung parenchyma may have a pneumonia.

Surgery is the definitive therapy for a congenital pulmonary cyst. Surgery in infancy is indicated for respiratory distress due to expansion or infection. If the cyst does not

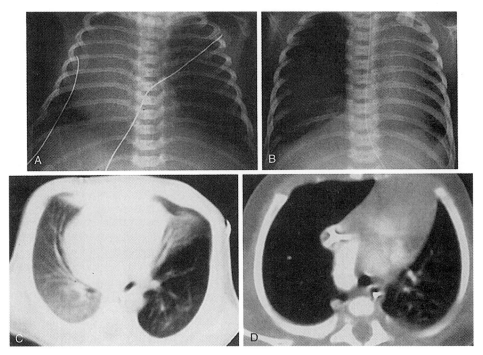

Figure 7–4. Two cases of lobar emphysema. **A**, Conventional radiograph of the chest of a neonate with respiratory distress shows overdistention of the left upper lobe, with atelectasis of the left lower lobe and a mediastinal shift to the right. **B**, Chest radiograph of an asymptomatic infant shows hyperinflation of the right upper lobe, with mediastinal shift to the left. There is atelectasis of the right middle and lower lobes. **C**, Unenhanced computed tomography (CT) of the chest of the patient in **A** shows a hyperlucent left upper lobe, with attenuation of the vessels out towards the lung periphery, collapse of the adjacent left lower lobe, and mediastinal shift to the right. **D**, Contrast-enhanced CT of the chest of the patient in **B** shows emphysematous changes in the right upper lobe, with mediastinal shift to the left. Note the incidental right aortic arch. (From Schwartz DS, Reyes-Mugica M, Keller MS. Imaging of surgical diseases of the newborn chest. Intrapleural mass lesions. *Radiol Clin North Am* 1999;37:1067–1078.)

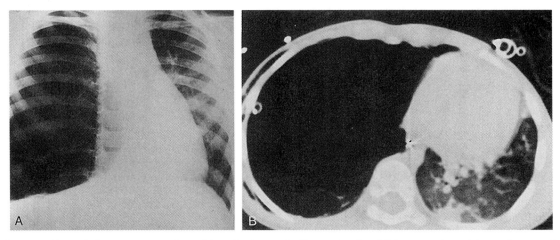

Figure 7–5. A, Pulmonary parenchymal 'tension' cyst. Radiograph of a child presenting with respiratory distress demonstrates the hyperlucent cyst on the right, producing ipsilateral and contralateral mass effect. **B**, Computed tomography scan at the lung bases demonstrates the large, air-filled cyst with internal septa and accompanying mediastinal shift. (From Hernanz-Schulman M. Cysts and cystlike lesion of the lung. *Radiol Clin North Am* 1993;31:631–649.)

spontaneously resolve after 1 year, lobectomy may be necessary, although preliminary work with cystectomy is promising. For an infected cyst, lobectomy is usually necessary. Infants occasionally can have rupture of cysts causing tension pneumothorax. Patients will rapidly deteriorate into respiratory stridor and cyanosis.

Congenital cystic adenomatoid malformation (CCAM) is a unilateral hamartomatous lesion that is symptomatic within the first few days of life. The cause of this overgrowth is undetermined but it probably occurs in the first 35 days of gestation.

Pathophysiologically, CCAM develops from excessive overgrowth of bronchioles beyond a segment of atretic bronchus. The exact cause of the bronchial atresia is multifactorial: a possible mechanism includes vascular interruption by the proximal bronchial segment. The blood supply is via the pulmonary artery with drainage via the pulmonary vein into the left atrium. These lesions have intracystic communications and, unlike bronchogenic cysts, a connection to the tracheobronchial tree. The vascular supply is from the bronchial circulation.

Pathologically, CCAM forms a large rubbery mass that can enlarge rapidly by air-trapping in the cystic areas (Figure 7–6). Unlike lobar emphysema, most CCAMs are observed in the lower lobes. An adenomatoid increase of terminal respiratory bronchiole-like structures lined by ciliated columnar epithelium occurs. Interspersed cysts may resemble immature alveoli. Connective tissue stroma contains disorganized elastic tissue and smooth muscle.

Cystic adenomatoid malformations are classified into three types (Box 7–2). Type I occurs as multiple cysts larger than 2 cm or as a single, large, dominant cyst surrounded by smaller cysts within a single pulmonary lobe. It is lined with ciliated columnar epithelium and mucus-secreting cells are present. Type I malformations

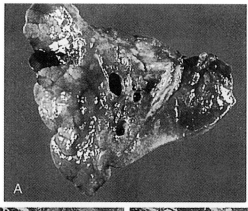

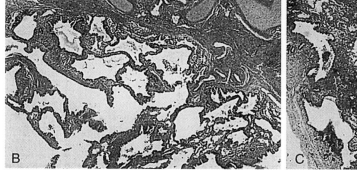
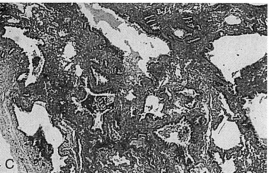

Figure 7–6. Congenital cystic adenomatoid malformation of the lung, Type II. **A,** Right lower lobectomy specimen resected at 4 days of age. There are several cysts ranging from 0.5 to 1.5 cm in diameter. **B,** Photomicrograph shows several cysts resembling bronchioles (hematoxylin and eosin, original magnification ×20). **C,** A trichrome stain reveals some interstitial fibrosis and alveolar duct-like structures between the cysts. (From Schwartz DS, Reyes-Mugica M, Keller MS. Imaging of surgical diseases of the newborn chest. Intrapleural mass lesions. *Radiol Clin North Am* 1999;37:1067–1078.)

BOX 7–2 CLASSIFICATION OF CONGENITAL CYSTIC ADENOMATOID MALFORMATIONS

- Type I (50%) – typically a single large cyst surrounded by smaller cysts within a single pulmonary lobe
- Type II (40%) – small (<1 cm), evenly spaced cysts
- Type III (<10%) – bulky cysts composed of several tiny cysts (<0.5 cm)

are the most common form, accounting for up to 50% of cases. Type II malformations account for 40–45% of cases. They are multiple, evenly spaced cysts, generally less than 1 cm in diameter. The cellular lining is usually cuboidal to columnar. The malformation appears as dilated terminal bronchioles when observed on histologic sections. Type III malformations are rare and include firm, bulky cysts composed of numerous tiny cysts, each less than 0.5 cm (Figure 7–7).

Most infants demonstrate respiratory distress at birth or before 1 month of age. Ultrasound is instrumental in diagnosing CCAM in a fetus as early as the 20th week of gestation. A predominantly solid lung mass is associated with fetal anasarca, ascites, and maternal polyhydramnios. A combined solid–cystic lesion presents with respiratory distress in the newborn. Older infants and adults have the primary cystic lesion. Plain chest radiographs are the most important initial diagnostic study. The findings observed on plain chest radiographs include single or multiple large cysts, multiple smaller cysts of uniform size, and solid-appearing masses.

Masses are typically intrapulmonary and contain scattered radiolucent areas. Some cysts within the malformation may contain air–fluid levels. CT scans are used to preoperatively assess cystic lesions, although ultrasound is arguably equally efficacious. Chest CT can delineate the nature of the cyst. Multiple cysts that are not seen on a posteroanterior chest film can be easily seen on a CT scan (Figures 7–8, 7–9).

Congenital cystic adenomatoid malformation can be a life threatening emergency. The presence or evolution of hydrops in association with isolated CCAM before lung maturity should prompt consideration of fetal surgery (Figure 7–10) Lobectomy is usually performed, although pneumonectomy is occasionally carried out. In the older child or adult, surgical resection is required to remove the source of recurrent pneumonia. Prognosis and likelihood of survival depends on the presence of hydrops, degree of hypoplasia of the remaining lung, histologic subtype, and prompt diagnosis.

Pulmonary Sequestration

Pulmonary sequestration refers to a segment or a lobe of lung tissue that has no bronchial communication with the tracheobronchial tree. The arterial blood supply is from a systemic source, usually coming directly from the aorta (Figure 7–11). The vessel often comes off the abdominal aorta, passes through the diaphragm, and supplies the lobar sequestration. The venous return is usually through pulmonary veins. Pulmonary sequestration can be either intralobar or extralobar (Table 7–3).

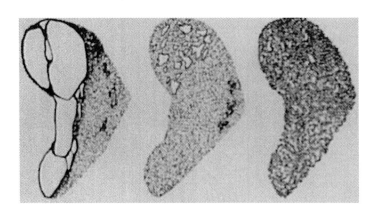

Figure 7–7. The three types of congenital cyst adenomatoid malformation of the lung. **A,** Type 1 lesions have large cysts of variable sizes. **B,** Type 2 lesions have smaller cysts. **C,** Type 3 lesions appear solid because of reflections from numerous adenomatoid structures along with scattered, thin-walled structures similar to bronchioles. (From Stocker JT, Madewell JE, Drake RM. Congenital cyst adenomatoid malformation of the lung. *Hum Pathol* 1977;8:155.)

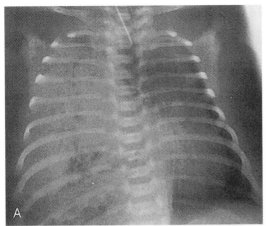

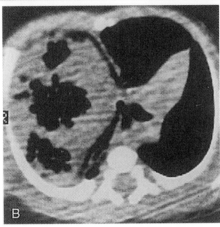

Figure 7–8. Congenital cystic adenomatoid malformation. Newborn presented with increasing respiratory distress. **A,** Frontal chest radiograph shows a complex mass in the right hemithorax and shift of heart and mediastinum to the left. It is difficult to define the nature and complete extent of the mass lesion. **B,** Computed tomography scan localizes the lesion to the right middle lobe and characterizes the mass as a type 1 malformation. The lucent area between the mass and the heart is an uninvolved, but displaced, right upper lobe. (From Rencken I, Patton WL, Brasch RC. Airway obstruction in pediatric patients. From croup to BOOP. *Radiol Clin North Am* 1998;36:175-187.)

An intralobar sequestration is situated within the normal lung parenchyma while an extralobar sequestration is independent of the normal lung and has its own visceral pleural investment. Extralobar sequestration is believed to occur later in gestation than intralobar sequestration. It forms in the more distal part of the developing lung bud and remains extrapulmonary in location. It is usually attached to the mediastinum through a pedicle and most commonly occurs at the lung base. It is

commonly associated with diaphragmatic hernia.

The majority of sequestrations are intralobar. Intralobar lesions may contain air spaces but have no normal communication with the tracheobronchial tree. Communication with lung parenchyma can lead to chronic infections in the sequestered lobe. Children and young adults with recurrent left lower lobe pneumonia should be suspected of having an intralobar sequestration (Figure 7–12). Air–fluid levels suggest communication to the tracheobronchial tree, probably caused by erosion and fistulization. Most cases of intrapulmonary sequestration are asymptomatic and present in late adolescence.

Extralobar sequestration occurs in the left chest 90% of the time, usually in the posterior costophrenic angle. There is a 4:1 male:female predominance. Most cases of extralobar sequestration present in the first year of life. Extralobar sequestrations are associated with congenital malformation in up to 50% of cases.

In most infants with extralobar sequestration, the lesion is found in an incidental radiograph of the chest (Figure 7–13). Repeated infection may develop if the sequestration communicates with the foregut and failure of separation during the third/fourth week of embryogenesis. Extralobar sequestrations have the consistency of liver and do not contain air spaces (Figure 7–14).

Diagnosis in the newborn can be made with chest radiographs, CT and color flow Doppler ultrasound. In the case of extralobar sequestration, a plain radiograph demonstrates the lung as a mass, usually between the lower lobe and the diaphragm. This is due to the firm consistency of the lung resulting from the lack of connection of the lung tissue to the bronchial tree. Intralobar sequestrations may resemble a mass. Sometimes intralobar lesions contain air secondary to abnormal communication with the tracheobronchial tree. Aortography with a demonstration of the abnormal systemic feeding vessel to the sequestration can be used as a confirmatory procedure (Figure 7–15). Doppler ultrasound can demonstrate the anomalous aortic branches without the morbidity of aortography. CT scans and magnetic resonance angiography (MRA) allow visualization of the arterial inflow and give information similar to that provided by contrast aortography (Figure 7–16).

Treatment consists of a segmental resection or lobectomy depending on the degree of inflammation and infection. Most important

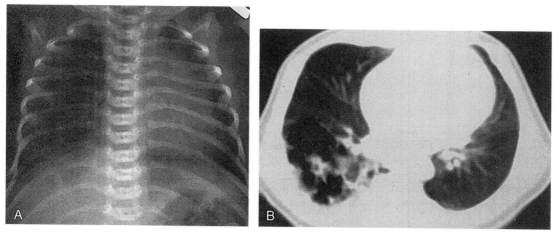

Figure 7–9. Congenital cystic adenomatoid. **A**, Asymptomatic neonate demonstrates an ill-defined, aerated mass at the right lung base in the cardiophrenic sulcus. There is no effect on the mediastinum. **B**, Unenhanced computed tomography shows right lower lobe cysts of variable sizes. The remaining lung parenchyma is normal. (From Schwartz DS, Reyes-Mugica M, Keller MS. Imaging of surgical diseases of the newborn chest. Intrapleural mass lesions. *Radiol Clin North Am* 1999;37:1067–1078.)

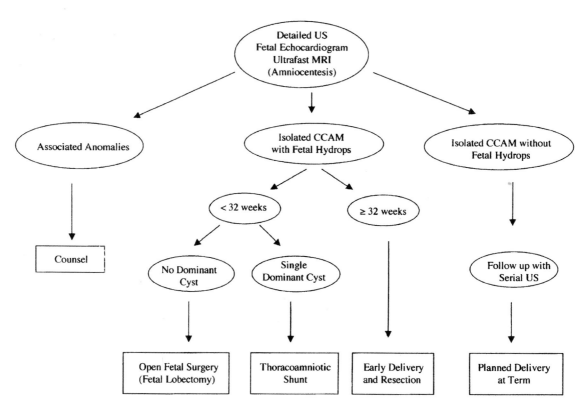

Figure 7–10. Algorithm for the fetus with a prenatally diagnosed congenital cystic adenomatoid malformation (CCAM). (From Kitano Y, Flake AW, Crombleholme TM, *et al*. Open fetal surgery for life-threatening fetal malformations. *Semin Perinatol* 1999;23:448–461.)

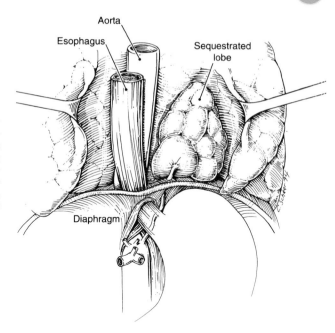

Figure 7–11. An illustration of a left posterior pulmonary sequestration showing the systemic arterial supply arising from below the diaphragm. Major hemorrhage can result from a failure to recognize this anomaly and inadvertent division of these vessels during resection. (From Pearson FG, Cooper JD, Deslauriers J, *et al. Thoracic surgery*, 2nd ed. New York: Churchill Livingstone, 2002:511.)

TABLE 7–3 • *Common Distinguishing Features of Pulmonary Sequestrations*

Feature	Extralobar	Intralobar
Sequestered bronchopulmonary tissue		
Location	Found above, below, or within diaphragm	Usually posterior basilar segments of lower lobe
Laterality	Left side: 90%	Often right side: 40%
Pleural covering	Separate from rest of lung by definition	No pleural separation from adjacent lung, by definition
Age at diagnosis	<1 year: 60%	>20 years: 50%
Neonatal presentation	Often	Never
Gender distribution	M:F 4:1	M = F
Foregut communication present	Occasionally	Rarely
Associated anomalies	Frequent: 15–40%	Uncommon
Caliber of anomalous artery	Usually small	Usually large
Venous drainage	Azygous, hemizygous or portal vein	Usually pulmonary vein
Complications	Rarely infected	Frequent infections

Data from Carter R. Pulmonary sequestration. *Ann Thorac Surg* 1969;7:68; Hutchin P. Congenital cystic disease of the lung. *Rev Surg* 1971;28:79; Panicek DM, *et al*. The continuum of pulmonary developmental anomalies. *Radiographics* 1987;7:747; Sade RM, *et al*. The spectrum of pulmonary sequestration. *Ann Thorac Surg* 1974;18:644.

is to identify the arterial and venous supply to the sequestration prior to removal (Figure 7–17). Serious hemorrhage may occur if complete vascular control is not obtained. Resections can usually be performed without major morbidity and is curative. Intralobar lesions almost always require lobectomy. Extralobar sequestrations that are invested with a separate layer of visceral pleura are simply resected.

Bronchial Atresia

Congenital bronchial atresia is a rare disorder characterized by a bronchocele due to a blindly ending segmental or lobar bronchus with hyperinflation of the obstructing lung segment. The most frequent location is the left upper lobe, followed by the left lower and right upper lobes. The pathophysiology is suspected

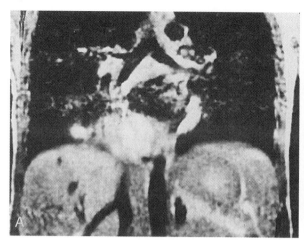
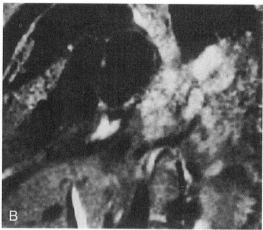

Figure 7–12. Intralobar sequestration – 8-year-old girl with a history of multiple episodes of pneumonia at right base. **A,** Coronal magnetic resonance image with T1-weighted spin-echo sequence demonstrates the anterior origin of the feeding artery from the aorta. There is high signal intensity emanating from the highly proteinaceous fluid within the sequestered parenchymal cysts. **B,** Oblique magnetic resonance image, obtained by outlining the course of the vessel on axial images and determining the appropriate angle of section, demonstrates the oblique, cephalad course of the vessel as it enters the sequestration. (From Hernanz-Schulman M. Cysts and cystlike lesion of the lung. *Radiol Clin North Am* 1993;31:631–649.)

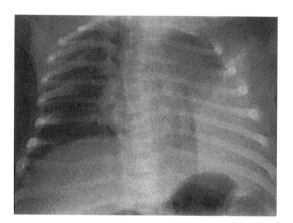

Figure 7–13. Pulmonary sequestration. Chest radiograph of an asymptomatic neonate demonstrates a solid mass at the left chest base. There is no mediastinal shift. (From Schwartz DS, Reyes-Mugica M, Keller MS. Imaging of surgical diseases of the newborn chest. Intrapleural mass lesions. *Radiol Clin North Am* 1999;37:1067–1078.)

mal bronchial structures leads to emphysematous lung changes. Patients usually present in young adulthood, although neonates and infants can present in respiratory distress. There is significant risk of pulmonary infection. Chest radiography typically demonstrates a hilar mass with radiating solid channels surrounded by hyperaerated lung. Indications for surgical resection include prevention of pulmonary sepsis. The natural history of these lesions usually involves degeneration into pulmonary infection; therefore, resection should always be performed.

Unilateral Lung Atresia

Unilateral pulmonary atresia is a rare occurrence resulting in an average life expectancy of 6 years for right-sided agenesis and 16 years for left-sided agenesis. The majority of infants have other associated congenital abnormalities that are responsible for their early mortality. Without associated defects, patients have a normal life expectancy. Pathophysiologically, there is no pulmonary tissue or ipsilateral pulmonary artery. The degree of mediastinal shift and total loss of tissue determines ventilatory ability. A large diaphragmatic hernia can interfere with normal alveolar development. A newborn with unilateral pulmonary agenesis

to be due to vascular insult during the fourth or sixth week of gestation during lung budding. Initially, the portion of lung adjacent to the atretic bronchus is filled with fluid. The fluid is reabsorbed and replaced by air from adjacent lung tissue. Retained secretions result in a mucocele. Compression of adjacent nor-

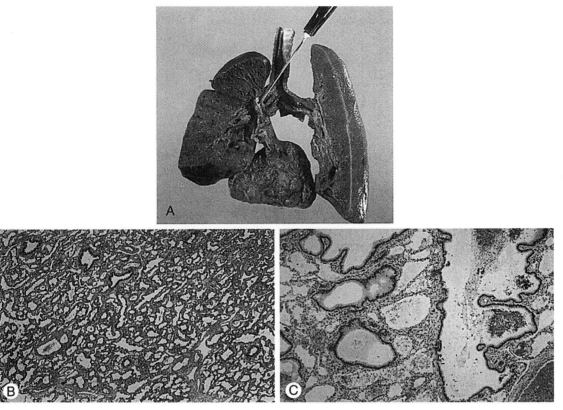

Figure 7–14. Extralobar pulmonary sequestration. **A,** Coronal section of both lungs shows an extralobar sequestration attached to the right lung. The pedicle of attachment contained the systemic vessel; there was no airway connection to the tracheobronchial tree. **B,** Photomicrograph of an extralobar pulmonary sequestration shows immature lung morphology (hematoxylin and eosin, original magnification ×10). **C,** Photomicrograph of an extralobar pulmonary sequestration shows hamartomatous dilated airways reminiscent of congenital cystic adenomatoid malformation type II (hematoxylin and eosin, original magnification ×20). (From Schwartz DS, Reyes-Mugica M, Keller MS. Imaging of surgical diseases of the newborn chest. Intrapleural mass lesions. *Radiol Clin North Am* 1999;37:1067–1078.)

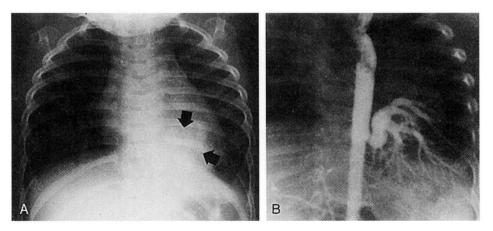

Figure 7–15. Pulmonary sequestration. **A,** Chest radiograph of a child with recurrent pneumonia. The film shows a focal radiodensity in the left retrocardiac region (arrows). **B,** Aortogram demonstrates a large aberrant arterial vessel arising from the descending aorta supplying the lesion. (From Kravitz RM. Congenital malformations of the lung. *Pediatr Clin North Am* 1994;41:453–472.)

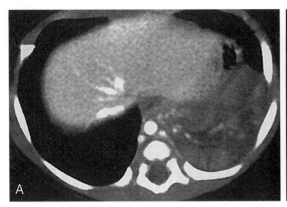 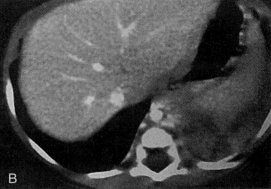

Figure 7–16. Extralobar pulmonary sequestration. Contrast-enhanced computed tomography scans of the chest (same infant as in Figure 7–13). show a solid soft tissue mass at the left lung base, with patchy parenchymal enhancement. An aberrant arterial supply arising from the aorta to the soft tissue mass is identified, which was diagnosed as an extralobar pulmonary sequestration. (From Schwartz DS, Reyes-Mugica M, Keller MS. Imaging of surgical diseases of the newborn chest. Intrapleural mass lesions. *Radiol Clin North Am* 1999;37:1067–1078.)

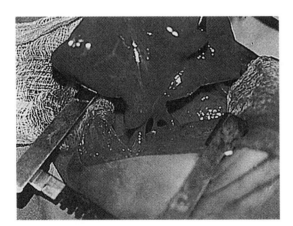 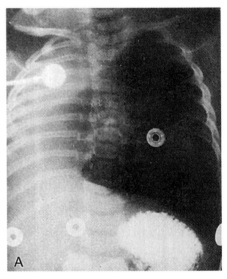

Figure 7–17. Extralobar pulmonary sequestration. Surgical excision of the left lung base with demonstration of the systemic arterial connection. (From Schwartz DS, Reyes-Mugica M, Keller MS. Imaging of surgical diseases of the newborn chest. Intrapleural mass lesions. *Radiol Clin North Am* 1999;37:1067–1078.)

Figure 7–18. Agenesis of the right lung. **A**, Anteroposterior chest radiograph shows an opaque, small-volume right hemithorax and a large-volume left lung that herniates across the midline.

may be asymptomatic or have tachypnea, dyspnea, and cyanosis. Older infants may present with wheezing that suggests asthma. On physical examination, the trachea and mediastinal structures are shifted to the involved side. The overall shape of the chest is normal. Chest radiographs will reveal a free pleural cavity with mediastinal shift and diaphragmatic variation (Figure 7–18). There is no surgical intervention, although many of the patients go to the operating room for associated cardiac abnormalities.

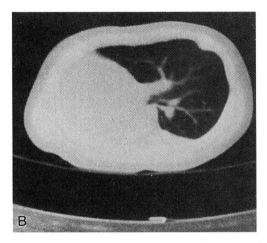

Figure 7–18. Continued. **B,** Computed tomography scan shows that the left lung vasculature is normal or slightly increased; the opacity in the right side is largely composed of displaced mediastinal and cardiac structures. No aerated lung is seen in the right hemithorax. (From Kravitz RM. Congenital malformations of the lung. *Pediatr Clin North Am* 1994; 41:453–472.)

Key Readings

Bush A. Congenital lung disease: a plea for clear thinking and clear nomenclature. *Pediatr Pulmonol* 2001;32:328–337. *Attempt to clear some of the misnomers and problems with labeling congenital anomalies.*

Devine PC, Malone FD. Noncardiac thoracic anomalies. *Clin Perinatol* 2000;27:865–899. *Comprehensive review of congenital thoracic anomalies.*

Selected Readings

Morin L, Crombleholme TM, D'Alton ME. Prenatal diagnosis and management of fetal thoracic lesions. *Semin Perinatol* 1994;18:228–253.

Nuchtern JG, Harberg FJ. Congenital lung cysts. *Semin Pediatr Surg* 1994;3:233–243.

Ouzidane L, Benjelloun A, el Hajjam M, *et al.* Segmental bronchial atresia – a case report and a literature review. *Eur J Pediatr Surg* 1999;9:49–52.

Plattner V, Haustein B, Llanas B, *et al.* Extra-lobar pulmonary sequestration with prenatal diagnosis. A report of 5 cases and review of the literature. *Eur J Pediatr Surg* 1995;5:235–237.

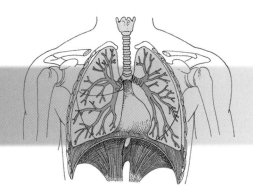

8

Bronchogenic Cancer

EPIDEMIOLOGY   STAGING

ETIOLOGY/RISK FACTORS   MANAGEMENT

PATHOGENESIS   SURGICAL MANAGEMENT

PATHOLOGY   PREVENTION

DIAGNOSIS

Bronchogenic Cancer: Key Points

- Understand the major trends in lung cancer epidemiology in the past 50 years
- Know the role of smoking in lung cancer and the other less common environmental exposures
- Describe the pathogenesis of lung cancer based on several current models of oncogenesis
- Know the essential differences between the two major classifications of bronchogenic carcinoma
- Develop an algorithm for management of the asymptomatic versus symptomatic thoracic patient
- Know the controversial features of the TNM staging system for non-small-cell lung cancer
- Develop an outline for management of non-small-cell lung cancer and small-cell lung cancer

Lung cancer is the leading cause of cancer death in both men and women in the USA. Smoking is the major risk factor for development of lung cancer. More than 99% of malignant lung tumors arise from the respiratory epithelium and are termed bronchogenic carcinoma. Bronchogenic carcinoma is divided into two subgroups: small-cell lung cancer (SCLC) and non-small-cell lung cancer (NSCLC). NSCLC includes adenocarcinoma, squamous-cell carcinoma, and large-cell carcinoma. A correct tissue diagnosis is critical because SCLC has a high response rate to chemotherapy and radiation and is rarely treated by surgery alone. Conversely, NSCLC can be cured by surgery in certain stages and is not curable by chemotherapy alone. The overall 5-year survival rate for lung cancer remains 15%.

Epidemiology

Lung cancer is the second most common cancer in the USA and, although it accounts for 15% of all cancers, it is the most lethal, accounting for approximately one-fourth of all cancer deaths. The deaths attributed to lung cancer in 2000 were approximately 160 000, exceeding the combined total deaths of breast, prostate, and colorectal cancer patients (Figures 8–1, 8–2). In terms of both cancer deaths and years of life lost, the effect of lung cancer is greater than that of breast, prostate, colon, and rectal cancer combined.

Lung cancer is the most common cause of cancer death in women (78 000 in 2000) and the second most common cause of cancer death in men. Historically, lung cancer was diagnosed predominantly in men but, with the increase in smoking among women, the estimated male-to-female lung cancer prevalence ratio escalated to 1.2:1. Among men, the mortality rate for lung cancer has declined significantly as a result of decreased cigarette smoking over the last 30 years. However, smoking cessation in women has lagged behind smoking cessation in men and the incidence of lung cancer in women continues to climb. Since 1987, more women have died of lung cancer than breast cancer, which traditionally has been the major cause of death (Figure 8–3). African-American men have the highest incidence of lung cancer but racial differences are confounded by differences in socioeconomic status and smoking behavior (Figure 8–4).

Etiology/Risk Factors

Cigarette smoking is the most important risk factor in the development of lung cancer. Smokers have a 10–25-fold increase in lung cancer incidence compared to nonsmokers. The relationship between cigarette smoking and lung cancer was not widely appreciated until the early 1950s (Figure 8–5). Since then it has become apparent that cigarette smoking accounts for the majority (>85%) of lung cancer cases seen in the USA and the rest of the world. The risk of lung cancer developing in an active smoker is difficult to estimate but appears to be related to the number of cigarettes smoked, the duration of smoking in years, the age at initiation of smoking, the depth of smoke inhalation, and the tar and nicotine content of the cigarettes smoked. The American Cancer Society estimates that approximately 175 000 cancer deaths are attributed to tobacco use and an additional

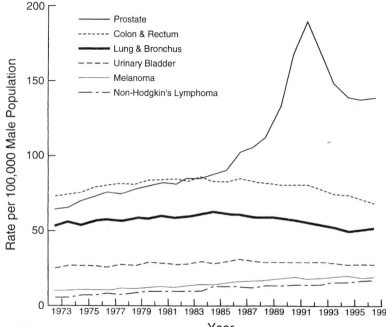

Figure 8–1. Age-adjusted cancer incidence rates for men by site, 1973–1997. Rates are per 100 000 and age-adjusted to the 1970 standard population. Because of changes in the international classification of diseases (ICD) coding, numerator information has changed over time. Rates for cancers of the liver, lung and bronchus, and colon and rectum are affected by these coding changes. (From Greenlee RT, Hill-Hampton MB, Murray T, *et al.* Cancer Statistics, 2001. *CA Cancer J Clin* 2001; 51:15–36.)

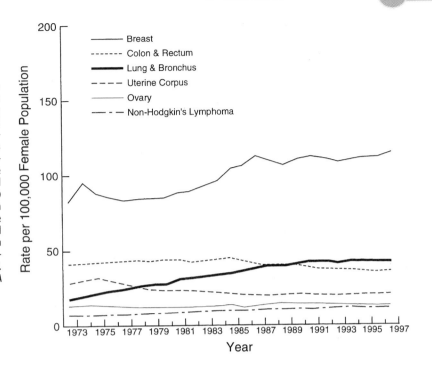

Figure 8–2. Age-adjusted cancer incidence rates for women by site, 1973–1997. Rates are per 100 000 and age-adjusted to the 1970 standard population. Uterus cancer death rates are for uterine cervix and uterine corpus combined. Because of changes in the international classification of diseases (ICD) coding, numerator information has changed over time. These coding changes affect lung and bronchus and colon and rectum figures. (From Greenlee RT, Hill-Hampton MB, Murray T, *et al.* Cancer Statistics, 2001. *CA Cancer J Clin* 2001;51:15–36.)

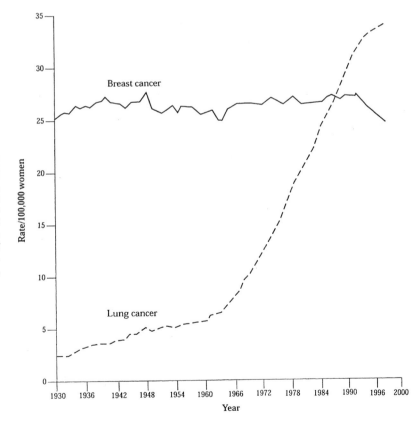

Figure 8–3. Age-adjusted death rates for lung cancer and breast cancer among women, USA, 1930–1997. Death rates are adjusted to 1970 population. (From US Department of Health and Human Services. *Women and Smoking. A Report of the Surgeon General.* Washington, DC: USDHHS, 2001:193–109.)

19 000 cancer deaths per year are related to excessive alcohol use (in combination with tobacco use). SCLC has the strongest association with smoking.

Cigarette smoke contains a number of active carcinogens and procarcinogens, and the pattern of mutations seen in oncogenes and tumor suppressor genes isolated from smokers with

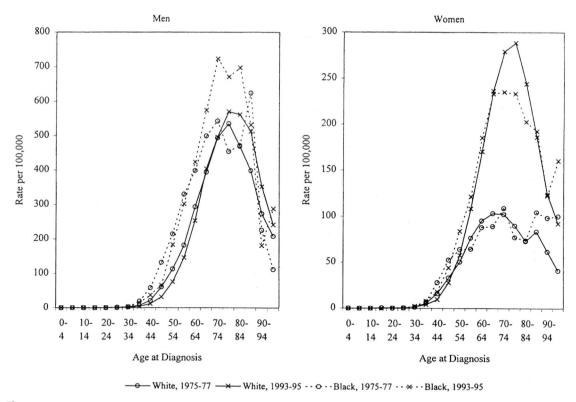

Figure 8–4. Age-specific lung cancer incidence rates by gender, race, and age at diagnosis. (From Merrill RM. Measuring the projected public health impact of lung cancer through lifetime and age-conditional risk estimates. *Ann Epidemiol* 2000;10:88–96.)

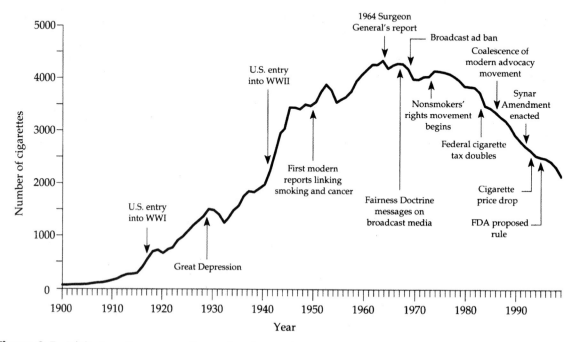

Figure 8–5. Adult cigarette consumption and major smoking and health events per capita, USA, 1900–1999. (From US Department of Health and Human Services. *Reducing tobacco use: A report of the US Surgeon General.* Centers for Disease Control and Prevention, Office on Smoking and Health, 2000, p 33.)

lung cancer is that expected from the mechanism of action of the major cigarette smoke carcinogens. The carcinogenic substances in cigarette smoke are only partially understood. More than 40 carcinogens have been identified in cigarette smoke. Some of these include polycyclic aromatic hydrocarbons, nickel, vinyl chloride, aldehydes, catechols, peroxides, and nitrosamines. The use of filter-tipped, low-tar, and low-nicotine cigarettes may lower exposure to some of these agents and thus lower lung cancer rates; however, smokers have been found to increase their nicotine (and thus carcinogen) intake by increasing either the number of cigarettes smoked or the depth of inhalation when using these cigarettes.

Smoking cessation causes a gradual drop in lung cancer risk, but not a complete normalization of risk, over a number of years. Once smoking is discontinued, there is a progressive decline in lung cancer risk such that after 10–15 years of abstinence the risk of cancer developing approaches that of a lifelong nonsmoker (Figure 8–6).

An area now receiving greater examination is the potential carcinogenic effect of secondhand or passive smoke exposure in nonsmokers. Secondhand smoke contains significant amounts of carcinogens, which may be inhaled and absorbed into the blood of nonsmokers. The majority of studies have shown a significantly increased risk of lung cancer from secondhand smoke exposure, with a relative risk in the range of 1.3. This is approximately 10–15-fold less than the risk of lung cancer in active smokers.

A number of studies have demonstrated increased risk for lung cancer in the spouses of smokers. The tobacco smoke exposure of a smoker's child is greater than that of a spouse. Exposure to 25 smoker-years in childhood approximately doubles the risk of lung cancer in a nonsmoker.

Inhalation of asbestos fibers may cause both pulmonary and pleural malignancies, including bronchogenic carcinoma and pleural mesothelioma. All four lung cancer cell types occur with asbestos exposure, although adenocarcinoma may occur with greater frequency in the lower lobes and periphery. The relative risk of lung cancer in a nonsmoking asbestos worker is approximately fivefold. The lag between the time of first exposure to asbestos and the development of lung cancer ranges from 20 to 30 years. A rough dose–response relationship exists between cumulative asbestos exposure and the development of lung cancer (Table 8–1).

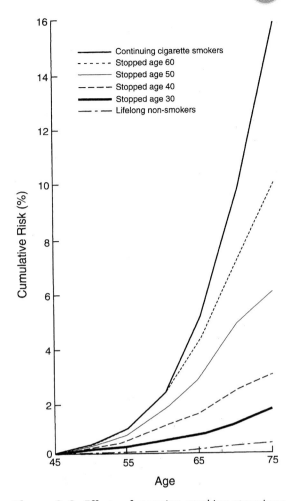

Figure 8–6. Effects of stopping smoking at various ages on the cumulative risk for death from lung cancer up to age 75; death rates for men in the UK in 1990. Nonsmoker risks are taken from a US prospective study of mortality. (From Peto R, Darby S, Deo H, *et al.* Smoking, smoking cessation, and lung cancer in the UK since 1950: combination of national statistics with two case-control studies. *Br Med J* 2000; 321:323–329.)

It has been estimated that, in the USA, as many as 30 000 lung cancer deaths may be attributable to radon exposure each year. The mining of radioactive ores was the first occupation to be linked to the development of lung cancer. The association between ionizing radiation and lung cancer was made in classic studies of uranium miners exposed to radon daughters. Radon daughters are radon decay products with alpha-, beta-, and delta-particle emission. The alpha particles are believed to deliver significant radiation to bronchial epithelium following inhalation of the particles attached to aerosols. Exposure of respiratory epithelium to radioisotope emission

TABLE 8–1 • *The Association between Cumulative Asbestosis Mortality Rate and Cumulative Excess Lung Cancer Mortality Rate in One Study**

Cohort Category	No. in Cohort	Asbestosis Death Rate/1000	Excess Lung CancerDeath Rate/1000
Male factory workers			
Light/moderate exposure <2 years	884	0	8.48
Light/moderate exposure >2 years	554	3.61	19.49
Severe exposure <2 years	936	2.14	25.00
Severe exposure >2 years	512	17.58	103.71
Laggers (men)	1369	4.38	19.94
Female factory workers	694	7.20	46.11
Total	4949	4.85	31.14

* Newhouse *et al.*, 1985.
From Weiss W. Asbestosis: a marker for the increased risk of lung cancer among workers exposed to asbestos. *Chest* 1999;115:543.

results in carcinogenic changes. Studies on miners have demonstrated that nonsmokers with a significant exposure to radon daughters have a 15-fold increased risk of lung cancer. Other miners in areas of significant subterranean radioactivity can also be exposed. As with asbestos and smoking, the risks of ionizing radiation exposure and smoking are synergistic.

The presence of chronic obstructive pulmonary disease (COPD), defined as either airflow obstruction on pulmonary function testing or symptoms of chronic bronchitis, increases the risk of lung cancer several-fold. COPD is a risk factor by itself and is not just a reflection of the number of cigarettes smoked.

Epidemiologic studies demonstrate increased risk for lung cancer in individuals with a diet low in fruit and vegetables. The effect of dietary intervention by increasing fruit and vegetable intake on risk for lung cancer has not been determined. Other factors linked to an increased risk of lung cancer include vitamin A and E deficiency.

Other well documented but less potent pulmonary carcinogens include chromium, nickel, mustard gas, vinyl chloride, arsenic, isopropyl oil, hydrocarbons, and chloromethyl ether (Table 8–2). Many if not all of these materials are additive or synergistic with cigarette smoke in the induction of bronchogenic carcinoma. Other known occupational lung carcinogens include chloromethyl ethers, coke oven emissions, iron and steel founding, beryllium, cadmium, and silica.

Pathogenesis

The occurrence of lung cancer is consistent with mendelian inheritance of a major autosomal gene governing susceptibility. Major categories of genes that potentially determine susceptibility to lung cancer include proto-oncogenes, tumor suppressor genes, genes encoding enzymes that metabolize procarcinogens to active carcinogens (such as the p450 enzymes), and genes that detoxify carcinogens (such as glutathione-*S*-transferase) (Table 8–3). Although relatives with germ line mutations in either *p53* or the retinoblastoma tumor suppressor genes have higher incidences of lung cancer, these abnormalities do not appear to be a common mechanism in the general population. Combinations of susceptibility genes appear to increase lung cancer risk significantly.

The respiratory epithelium develops as an outpouching from the endoderm of the primitive foregut. All respiratory epithelial cells differentiate from the primitive respiratory epithelium. Animal studies demonstrate that, in the airway epithelium, both the secretory and basal cells can dedifferentiate and subsequently redifferentiate into the various epithelial subtypes. In the alveolar epithelium, the type II cell is the proliferative stem cell. All histologic subtypes of bronchogenic carcinoma are believed to be derived from the respiratory epithelium. The different histologic subtypes are a reflection of the differentiation pathway taken by a particular tumor.

TABLE 8–2 • *Environmental Agents Linked to Lung Carcinogenesis*

Established Risk Factors	Possible Risk Factors
Arsenic	Acrylonitrile
Asbestos	Beryllium
BCME and CMME	Cadmium
Environmental tobacco smoke	Coal combustion products
Mustard gas	Cooking oil vapors
Nickel	Diesel exhaust
PAHs	Dietary cholesterol
Radon	Dietary fat
Tobacco smoke	Urban air pollution
Vinyl chloride	
Established Protective Agents	**Possible Protective Agents**
Dietary fruits and vegetables	Dietary beta-carotene
	Dietary vitamin C

BCME, bis(chloromethyl) ether; CMME, chloromethyl methyl ether; PAHs, polycyclic aromatic hydrocarbons.
From Roth JA, Ruckdeschel JC, Weisenburger TH. *Thoracic oncology*, 2nd ed. Philadelphia: WB Saunders, 1995:16.

The development of bronchogenic carcinoma follows a multistep carcinogenesis process with the successive accumulation of mutations in a number of genes involved in regulating growth (Figure 8–7). DNA damage occurs after exposure to carcinogens. These substances may act as initiators and promoters of carcinogenesis, with the resulting development of genetic changes characteristic of a malignant cell. A progression of histologic changes occurs:

1. Proliferation of basal cells
2. Development of atypical nuclei with prominent nucleoli
3. Stratification
4. Development of squamous metaplasia
5. Carcinoma *in situ*
6. Invasive carcinoma.

Premalignant lesions have been described and widely accepted only for squamous-cell carcinoma. Microdissection of bronchial epithelium has allowed the identification of genetic lesions, including chromosome 3p deletion, chromosome 9p deletion, and *p53* gene mutations in premalignant lesions. The usual order of occurrence and prognostic import of these genetic alterations is not yet known. Increased cellular proliferation is also necessary for carcinogenesis. It is likely that growth factors, derived from inflammatory cells, epithelial cells, and neuroendocrine cells, may be elevated in tobacco smokers and play a role in pathogenesis of lung cancer.

During the process of lung neoplasia, a number of biologic events occur that are believed to play a crucial role in the malignant process. Proto-oncogenes, a class of genes that encode proteins involved in normal cell growth processes, may be activated or altered to oncogenes through gene mutations, deletions, insertions, abnormal regulation, or rearrangement. Several oncogenes have been found to be consistently associated with lung cancer. These include the *myc* family (c-*myc*, N-*myc*, L-*myc*) in small-cell carcinoma (SCLC) and *ras* genes (H-*ras*, K-*ras*, N-*ras*) and c-*erb*B-2 in non-small-cell lung cancer (NSCLC). The presence of *myc* gene amplification in SCLC appears to be associated with more aggressive subtype. The *ras* gene family encodes a 21 kDa guanosine triphosphate (GTP)-binding protein (p21) that has been found to have point mutations (usually codon 12) or p21 overexpression in lung cancer (Figure 8–8). Other oncogenes reported to be expressed abnormally include *erb-B*, *myb*, *fes*, *kit*, *jun*, *fos*, *raf*, and *fms* (Table 8–4).

Another molecular mechanism involved in the development of human tumors is the loss of function of tumor suppressor genes. Loss of activity of these genes may allow for uncontrolled proliferation of cells. There are two well-described tumor suppressor genes – *p53* and the retinoblastoma gene (*Rb*) – both of which have been reported to be abnormal in lung cancer. Inactivation of

TABLE 8–3 • *Major Molecular Alterations in Lung Cancer*

	Small Cell Lung Cancer	Non-small Cell Lung Cancer
Tumor suppressor genes		
p53 abnormalities		
Mutation with 17p13 LOH	75–100	≈50
Abnormal p53 expression (IHC)	40–70	40–60
p16–cyclin D1–CDK4–RB pathway lesions		
p16 mutation or DNA methylation with 9p21 LOH	<1	10–40
Absent p16 expression (IRC²)	0–10	30–70
Absent Rb expression with 13q14 LOH	≈90	15–30
APC (5q21 LOH) DNA methylation	26	46
Chromosome 3p LOH (several sites)	100	90
RAR-β 3p24 (DNA methylation)	76	40
RASSF1A 3p21.3 (DNA methylation)	90	30–40
FHIT 3p14.2 (DNA methylation and deletion)	64	≈50
CDH13 (HCAD) (DNA methylation)	20	45
Proto-oncogenes and growth stimulation		
Putative autocrine loops	GRP/GRP receptor SCF/Kit	HGF/Met NDF/Erb-B
ras mutation	<1	15–20
myc amplification*	15–30	5–10
Other molecular changes		
bcl-2 expression	75–95	10–35
Telomerase activity	≈100	80–85
Microsatellite instability	≈35	≈22
Promoter hypermethylation	Marker-dependent	Marker-dependent

*Overexpression without amplification is observed in other cases. SCLC amplifications include *myc*, N-*myc*, and L-*myc*.

Erb-B, epidermal growth factor receptor; GRP, gastrin-releasing peptide; HGF, hepatocyte growth factor; IHC, immunohistochemistry; Met, metastasis oncogene; NDF, new differentiation factor; NSCLC, non-small-cell lung cancer; SCF, stem cell factor; SCLC, small-cell lung cancer.

From Fong KM, Minna JD. Molecular biology of lung cancer: clinical implications. *Clin Chest Med* 2002;23:85.

the *Rb* gene occurs in almost all cases of SCLC and approximately one third of cases of NSCLC (Figure 8–9). In NSCLC, loss of *Rb* protein expression has been reported to be an independent prognostic marker for decreased survival. Abnormalities of *p53* expression occur in up to 100% of SCLC and 75% of NSCLC (Figure 8–10).

The finding of these changes in early tumor specimens suggests that this gene may play a role in the early stages of lung carcinogenesis. Alterations in *p53* may correlate with more aggressive tumors with a poorer prognosis. If both *p53* and *Rb* mutations are present, survival expectation is only 12 months compared with 46 months in patients with normal expression of these proteins. These mutations can lead to loss of tumor-suppressor function,

cellular proliferation, and inhibition of apoptosis. Several other tumor-suppressor genes have been identified, including the c-*raf*-1 proto-oncogene, the protein-tyrosine phosphatase-gamma gene, the *FHIT* (fragile histidine triad) gene, the beta-retinoic acid receptor gene, and the von Hippel–Lindau gene.

Genetic deletions are a fairly common occurrence in lung cancer. The exact relationship between the deletion of certain genes and tumor cell growth is not well defined but may be related to either the loss of tumor suppressor genes or the activation of growth-promoting oncogenes through gene rearrangement and abnormal control of oncogene expression. A particularly frequent genetic loss is the short arm of chromosome 3 in SCLC. Other

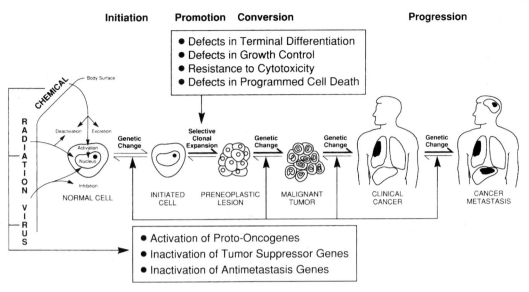

Figure 8–7. Multistep carcinogenesis. Carcinogenesis is a multistage process characterized by the accumulation of alterations to cellular proto-oncogenes and tumor-suppressor genes. The current model describes four conceptual steps: (1) tumor initiation, (2) tumor progression, (3) malignant conversion, and (4) tumor progression. (From Roth JA, Ruckdeschel JC, Weisenburger TH. *Thoracic Oncology*, 2nd ed. Philadelphia: WB Saunders, 1995.)

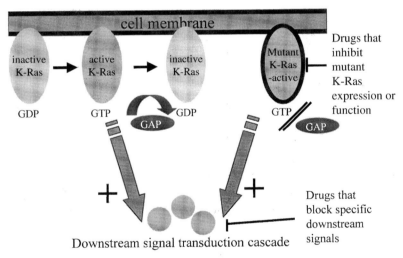

Figure 8–8. Mutant K-Ras pathway. Ras is active when bound to guanosine triphosphate (GTP) and inactive when bound to guanosine diphosphate (GDP). The intrinsic GTPase activity of Ras is stimulated by GAP, resulting in inactive Ras. Oncogenic Ras mutations inhibit GTPase activity, causing it to remain permanently activated with ensuing positive signaling to downstream molecules. Drugs that could interfere with the localization of mutant K-Ras in the membrane (and thus inactivate it) or interfere with its expression such as antisense compounds, or with components of the downstream signaling cascade, such as mitogen-stimulated extracellular regulated kinase (MEK) inhibitors, all have therapeutic potential. (From Fong KM, Minna JD. Molecular biology of lung cancer: clinical implications. *Clin Chest Med* 2002;23:91.)

genetic deletions have been detected in chromosomes 5, 9, 11, 13, and 17.

A number of growth factors have been reported to be secreted by tumor cells or neighboring stromal cells and to have a positive influence on tumor cell growth. The most widely studied is bombesin, a neuropeptide that appears to play an autocrine growth role in SCLC cells in vitro. Other neuropeptides such as bradykinin, neurotensin,

TABLE 8–4 • *Examples of Oncogenes and Tumor Suppressor Genes Found to be Altered in Lung Cancer*

SCLC	NSCLC
Oncogenes	
c-myc	K-ras*
L-myc	N-ras
N-myc	H-ras
c-raf	c-myc
c-myb	c-raf
c-erb-B1 (EGF-R)	c-fur*
c-fms	c-fes
c-rif	c-erb-B1 (EGF-R)*
	c-erb-B2 (Her2, neu)
	c-sis
	bcl-1
Tumor-Suppressor Genes	
p53*	p53*
RB*	RB

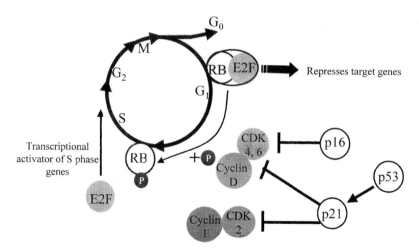

Figure 8–9. The p16–cyclin D1–CDK4-RB pathway. The product of the retinoblastoma tumor suppressor gene (RB) binds to the E2F transcription factor during the resting (G0/G1) phase of the cell cycle. When complexed to RB, E2F cannot activate the genes needed to initiate the S phase. Moreover, the RB–E2F complex also represses the transcription of other target genes. RB is phosphorylated at the end of G1 by cyclin/cyclin-dependent kinase (CDK) complexes – e.g., cyclin D/CDK4, 6 – and dephosphorylated at the end of mitosis (M). Phosphorylation of RB releases E2F, which initiates the S phase, overcoming the block to the cell cycle. In quiescent cells, RB is unphosphorylated, cyclin D levels are low, and CDK inhibitors – e.g., p16, p21, and p27 – inhibit the cyclin/CDK complexes. In lung cancers, acquired loss of RB function allows continued cell cycling. This pathway can be turned on by mutations inactivating RB, inactivating p16, overexpression of cyclin D1, or overexpression of CDK4. Mutations inactivating p53 function also can impinge on this pathway. p21 abnormalities have not been reported. Drugs that replace RB or p16 function or that would inhibit cyclin D1 or CDK4 would represent new therapeutics. In small-cell lung cancer the abnormality is usually in RB and in non-small-cell lung cancer the abnormality is usually in p16. (From Fong KM, Minna JD. Molecular biology of lung cancer: clinical implications. *Clin Chest Med* 2002;23:87.)

endothelin, and vasopressin may also have a mitogenic effect on small-cell carcinoma. Growth factors reported to be involved in lung cancer cell growth through autocrine or paracrine mechanisms include insulin-like growth factor type 1, transforming growth factor a, transferrin, and possibly the colony-stimulating factors.

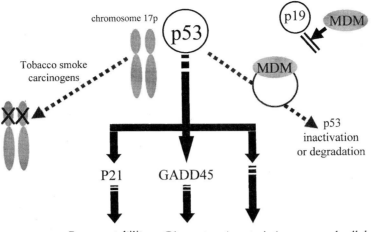

Figure 8–10. The *p53* tumor suppressor gene pathway. *p53* is situated on the short arm of chromosome 17. It helps maintain genomic stability, inhibits the cell cycle at G1, and causes apoptosis if DNA is damaged beyond repair. These functions are lost because of mutation in *p53* in 90% of small-cell lung cancers (SCLCs) and more than 50% of non-small-cell lung cancer (NSCLCs). *p53* activity is antagonized by *MDM2* (which thus functions as an oncogene), with the two forming a negative feedback loop. *MDM2* is not frequently abnormal in lung cancers. In addition, *p19* alternate reading frame (ARF) is an alternatively spliced transcript from the same chromosome 9p21 locus that gives rise to p16. It antagonizes *MDM2*, thus functioning as a tumor suppressor. *p19*ARF mutations are apparently not common in lung cancer. *p53* is inactivated by damage to both alleles, often by allelic loss and somatic missense mutations. Tumor suppressor genes also can be inactivated by promoter hypermethylation but this is apparently not common for *p53*. Gene therapy with wild-type *p53* replacement is clinically successful in some NSCLCs. (From Fong KM, Minna JD. Molecular biology of lung cancer: clinical implications. *Clin Chest Med* 2002;23:86.)

Pathology

In general, there is a slight preponderance of lung cancer developing in the right lung because the right lung has approximately 55% of the lung parenchyma. Also, lung cancer more frequently occurs in the upper lobes than in the lower lobes. The blood supply to these tumors, which arise from the bronchial epithelium, is from the bronchial arteries.

The clinical behavior of bronchogenic carcinoma will vary depending on the cell type. The World Health Organization (WHO) histologic classification of lung cancer, which is widely accepted, falls into two general groups: non-small-cell lung cancer (NSCLC) and small-cell lung cancer (SCLC) (Table 8–5). This classification has important implications for prognosis and treatment.

Among NSCLC histologies, subtypes include epidermoid (including squamous), adenocarcinoma (including bronchioloalveolar), large cell (including giant cell and clear cell), and combinations of these histologies such as adenosquamous. The adenocarcinoma histologic subtype has proportionally increased in frequency over the past decade; at present, it accounts for approximately 35% of NSCLC cases. Slower growth kinetics are seen with adenocarcinoma and large-cell carcinoma which tend to spread systemically relatively early in their course. In contrast, squamous-cell carcinoma invades locally before systemic spread, so these patients often have symptoms resulting from local tumor invasion.

The small-cell subtype is distinguished by the presence of neurosecretory granules visualized by electron microscopy and other clinicopathologic features. These tumors have a relatively rapid growth rate, a tendency to metastasize, and are highly responsive to chemotherapy. Small-cell carcinoma is the most aggressive of lung tumors, with a rapid doubling time and early mediastinal and extrathoracic spread.

In the case of mixed tumors, biologic behavior is thought to depend on the predominant cell type; however, tumors with any significant degree of small-cell characteristics are believed to behave in a more aggressive fashion.

Non-Small-Cell Lung Cancer

Squamous-cell carcinoma accounts for a third of all lung cancers. Until recently, this was the most common lung cancer cell type but, in most centers, squamous-cell subtypes have

TABLE 8–5 • 1999 WHO/IASLC Histologic Classification of Lung and Pleural Tumors

1. Epithelial Tumors

1.1 Benign

   1.1.1 Papillomas

     1.1.1.1 Squamous cell papilloma

       1.1.1.1.1 Exophytic

       1.1.1.1.2 Inverted

     1.1.1.2 Glandular papilloma

     1.1.1.3 Mixed squamous cell and glandular papilloma

   1.1.2 Adenomas

     1.1.2.1 Alveolar adenoma

     1.1.2.2 Papillary adenoma

     1.1.2.3 Adenomas of salivary gland type

       1.1.2.3.1 Mucous gland adenoma

       1.1.2.3.2 Pleomorphic adenoma

       1.1.2.3.3 Other

     1.1.2.4 Mucinous cystadenoma

     1.1.2.5 Others

1.2 Preinvasive Lesions

   1.2.1 Squamous dysplasia/carcinoma *in situ*

   1.2.2 Atypical adenomatous hyperplasia

   1.2.3 Diffuse idiopathic pulmonary neuroendocrine cell hyperplasia

1.3 Invasive Malignant

   1.3.1 Squamous-cell carcinoma

     Variants:

     1.3.1.1 Papillary

     1.3.1.2 Clear-cell

     1.3.1.3 Small-cell

     1.3.1.4 Basaloid

   1.3.2 Small-cell carcinoma

     Variant:

     1.3.2.1 Combined small-cell carcinoma

   1.3.3 Adenocarcinoma

     1.3.3.1 Acinar

     1.3.3.2 Papillary

     1.3.3.3 Bronchioloalveolar carcinoma

       1.3.3.3.1 Nonmucinous

       1.3.3.3.2 Mucinous

       1.3.3.3.3 Mixed mucinous and nonmucinous or indeterminate

     1.3.3.4 Solid adenocarcinoma with mucin formation

     1.3.3.5 Mixed

     1.3.3.6 Variants:

       1.3.3.6.1 Well-differentiated fetal adeno-carcinoma

       1.3.3.6.2 Mucinous ('colloid')

       1.3.3.6.3 Mucinous cysta-denocarcinoma

       1.3.3.6.4 Signet-ring

       1.3.3.6.5 Clear-cell

   1.3.4 Large-cell carcinoma

     Variants:

     1.3.4.1 Large-cell neuroendocrine carcinoma

       1.3.4.1.1 Combined large-cell neuroendocrine carcinoma

     1.3.4.2 Basaloid carcinoma

     1.3.4.3 Lymphoepithelioma-like carcinoma

     1.3.4.4 Clear-cell carcinoma

     1.3.4.5 Large-cell carcinoma with rhabdoid phenotype

   1.3.5 Adenosquamous carcinoma

   1.3.6 Carcinomas with pleomorphic, sarcomatoid, or sarcomatous elements

     1.3.6.1 Carcinomas with spindle and/or giant cells

       1.3.6.1.1 Pleomorphic carcinoma

       1.3.6.1.2 Spindle-cell carcinoma

       1.3.6.1.3 Giant-cell carcinoma

     1.3.6.2 Carcinosarcoma

     1.3.6.3 Blastoma (pulmonary blastoma)

     1.3.6.4 Others

   1.3.7 Carcinoid tumor

     1.3.7.1 Typical carcinoid

     1.3.7.2 Atypical carcinoid

   1.3.8 Carcinomas of salivary gland type

     1.3.8.1 Mucoepidermoid carcinoma

     1.3.8.2 Adenoid cystic carcinoma

     1.3.8.3 Others

   1.3.9 Unclassified carcinoma

2. Soft Tissue Tumors

2.1 Localized fibrous tumor

2.2 Epithelioid hemangioendothelioma

2.3 Pleuropulmonary blastoma

2.4 Chondroma

2.5 Calcifying fibrous pseudotumor of the pleura

2.6 Congenital peribronchial myofibroblastic tumor

IASLC, International Association for the Study of Lung Cancer; WHO, World Health Organization. From Pearson FG, Cooper JD, Deslauriers J, *et al. Thoracic surgery,* 2nd ed. New York: Churchill Livingstone, 2002:799.

diminished and adenocarcinoma has become the most prevalent cell type. Squamous-cell carcinoma tends to originate in the central airways. Squamous-cell carcinoma arises from areas of chronically damaged bronchial epithelium in a progressive fashion from metaplasia to dysplasia and to neoplasia. The origin of squamous-cell carcinoma from damaged bronchial epithelium explains the occasional occurrence of positive sputum cytology in the absence of chest radiographic abnormalities. Squamous-cell carcinoma is the cell type most prone to cavitation. Histologically, squamous-cell carcinomas are characterized by keratinization with 'pearl' formation (i.e. flattened cells surrounding central cores of keratin). Squamous carcinomas are also characterized by predominant desmosomes that can be visualized on histologic sections as intercellular bridges (Figure 8–11).

Large-cell carcinoma, often referred to as large-cell undifferentiated carcinoma, accounts for 15–20% of tumors but this diagnosis may be overestimated, since tumors without clear differentiation are often placed in this category. Large-cell carcinoma is a group of carcinomas undifferentiated at the light microscopic level.

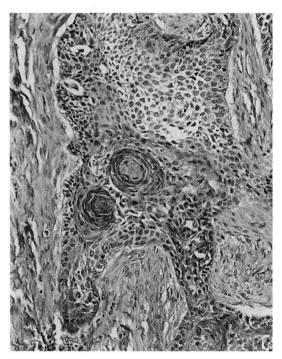

Figure 8–11. Squamous-cell carcinoma, well differentiated. These tumor cells have abundant eosinophilic keratinized cytoplasm and form nests and keratin pearls characteristic of squamous differentiation. (Hematoxylin and eosin, original magnification ×160.) (From Travis WD. Pathology of lung cancer. *Clin Chest Med* 2002;23:69.)

They exhibit neuroendocrine or glandular differentiation markers when studied by immunohistochemistry or electron microscopy (Figure 8–12). The location and behavior of large-cell carcinoma tend to be similar to adenocarcinoma, although certain large-cell variants such as giant-cell tumors may be extremely aggressive. Most of these tumors are large peripheral lesions unrelated to bronchi except for contiguous growth. Two rare subtypes of large-cell carcinomas are the giant-cell carcinomas, associated with peripheral leukocytosis, and clear-cell carcinomas, which resemble renal-cell carcinomas.

Adenocarcinoma is the most common histologic type and accounts for approximately 45% of all lung cancers. The increasing prevalence of this tumor is due to more frequent occurrence in women and changing environmental exposure. Most of these tumors (75%) are peripherally located. Adenocarcinomas tend to metastasize earlier than squamous-cell carcinomas. Because of the frequent peripheral origin of this type of carcinoma, sputum cytology is seldom positive even when the disease is detected early by chest radiography. Histologically, ade-

nocarcinoma comes from mucus-producing bronchial epithelial cells. These cuboidal to columnar cells have abundant vacuolated cytoplasm with evidence of gland formation. Half of adenocarcinomas exhibit markers for type II or Clara cells, such as mRNA for the surfactant proteins A, B, and C. The hallmark of adenocarcinomas is the tendency to form glands (Figure 8–13). Special stains demonstrate that the tumor cells contain mucins.

Bronchioloalveolar carcinoma, a subcategory of adenocarcinoma, arises in the periphery from terminal bronchioloalveolar regions and tends to spread in along pre-existing alveolar septa (Figure 8–14). Bronchioloalveolar carcinoma of the lung is more indolent than adenocarcinoma. It has the best prognosis of any kind of lung cancer because it is highly differentiated. These tumors can appear as interstitial infiltrates on chest radiographs and can be confused with infectious pneumonitis. The diagnostic confusion is compounded by the predominant manifestation of this tumor type in nonsmokers. Bronchioloalveolar carcinoma may require resection to confirm the diagnosis but the lobar type rarely is cured by opera-

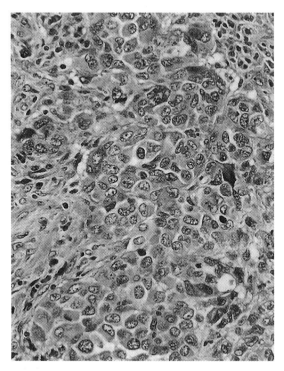

Figure 8–12. Large-cell carcinoma. This tumor consists of sheets and nests of large cells with abundant cytoplasm and vesicular nuclei with prominent nucleoli. (Hematoxylin and eosin, original magnification ×640). (From Travis WD. Pathology of lung cancer. *Clin Chest Med* 2002;23:74.)

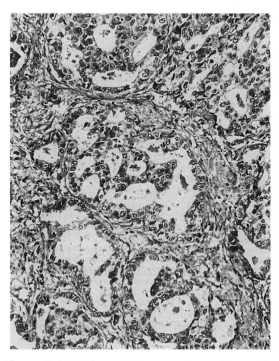

Figure 8–13. Adenocarcinoma, acinar subtype. The malignant epithelial cells form glands or acini. (Hematoxylin and eosin, original magnification ×320.) (From Travis WD. Pathology of lung cancer. *Clin Chest Med* 2002;23:69.)

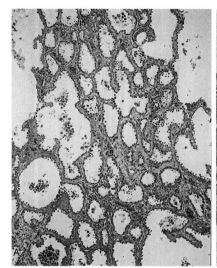
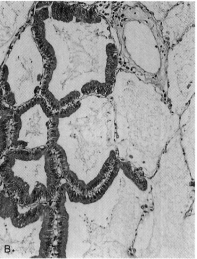

Figure 8–14. Adenocarcinoma, bronchioloalveolar subtype. **A,** Nonmucinous bronchioloalveolar carcinoma. This tumor consists of uniform cuboidal cells proliferating along the alveolar septa. The alveolar architecture is preserved. The tumor contrasts with the normal alveolar walls. **B,** Mucinous bronchioloalveolar carcinoma. The tumor consists of tall columnar cells with abundant apical cytoplasmic mucin growing along alveolar walls. (Hematoxylin and eosin, original magnification ×160.) (From Travis WD. Pathology of lung cancer. *Clin Chest Med* 2002;23:70.)

tion. These lesions are usually multicentric in origin and recurrence in the lung is common. The nodular type of bronchioloalveolar carcinoma is treated like any other type of adenocarcinoma and has an excellent prognosis. Of note, bronchioloalveolar carcinoma is particularly resistant to chemotherapy.

Small-Cell Lung Cancer

Small-cell carcinoma represents 20–25% of primary lung malignancies. Approximately 80% of small-cell tumors originate centrally and are found in airway submucosa. These tumors spread rapidly to regional hilar and mediastinal lymph nodes without involving the respiratory tract directly. They also expand against the bronchus, causing extrinsic compression. They tend to undergo central necrosis and cavitation. The disease is characterized by a very aggressive tendency to metastasize. It spreads very early to mediastinal lymph nodes and distant sites, especially bone marrow and brain.

This tumor, once thought to originate from neural ectoderm, may actually develop from a pulmonary stem cell with secondary differentiation into a cell type with neural characteristics (Table 8–6). Microscopically small-cell tumors appear as sheets or clusters of cells with dark nuclei and very little cytoplasm. This 'oatlike' appearance under the microscope explains the term 'oat-cell carcinoma' for this disease. The nuclear chromatin is finely distributed, and nucleoli are inconspicuous. Keratinization, stratification, and intercellular bridge formation are exhibited.

Diagnosis

Patients typically present either in the early stages with an asymptomatic mass or in the late stages with symptoms from the mass. It is important to delineate management of the two. Once a decision is made to investigate, a firm diagnosis should be obtained. Usually, diagnosis requires a tissue biopsy.

Management of Solitary Pulmonary Nodule

High-risk individuals (i.e. smokers with COPD) often receive frequent chest radiographs for a variety of indications. A significant number of lung cancers are initially detected as asymptomatic radiographic abnormalities, many as a solitary pulmonary nodule, defined as an asymptomatic mass within the lung parenchyma that is less than 3 cm in size and is circumscribed. Overall, 33% of these masses are malignant; 50% are malignant if the patient is older than 50 years.

The investigation of patients with a newly discovered solitary pulmonary nodules should begin with the review of previous chest radiographs (Figure 8–15). Lesions that are new or

TABLE 8–6 • *Light Microscopic Features for Distinguishing Small-Cell Carcinoma and Large Cell Neuroendocrine Carcinoma*

Histologic Feature	Small cell Carcinoma	Large Cell Neuroendocrine Carcinoma
Cell size	Smaller (less than diameter of three lymphocytes)	Larger
Nuclear cytoplasmic ratio	Higher	Lower
Nuclear chromatin	Finely granular, uniform	Coarsely granular or vesicular Less uniform
Nucleoli	Absent or faint	Often (not always) present May be prominent or faint
Nuclear molding	Characteristic	Less prominent
Fusiform shape	Common	Uncommon
Polygonal shape with ample pink cytoplasm	Uncharacteristic	Characteristic
Nuclear smear	Frequent	Uncommon
Basophilic staining of vessels and stroma	Occasional	Rare

From Travis WD, Linnoila RI, Tsokos MG, *et al.* Neuroendocrine tumors of the lung with proposed criteria for large-cell neuroendocrine carcinoma. An ultrastructural, immunohistological, and flow cytometric study of 35 cases. *Am J Surg Pathol* 1991;15:529–553.

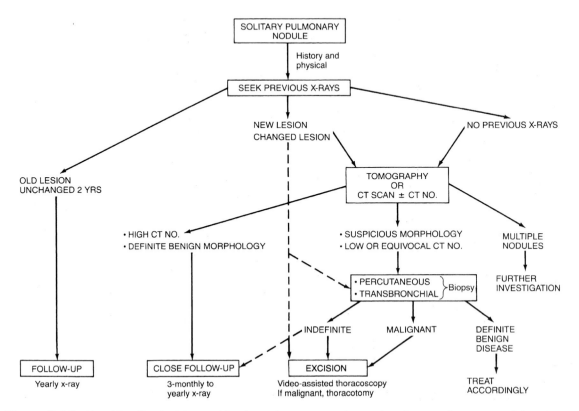

Figure 8–15. Algorithm for decision-making in patients presenting with solitary pulmonary nodules. (From Roth JA, Ruckdeschel JC, Weisenburger TH. *Thoracic oncology*, 2nd ed. Philadelphia: WB Saunders, 1995:126.)

increasing in size should be treated as pulmonary malignancies. In general, a patient with a single mass should undergo resection for definitive diagnosis and treatment. A subset of patients, however, may be managed conservatively:

- Patients with a mass unchanged for more than 2 years (documented upon serial radiographic examinations)
- Patients with benign patterns of calcification such as a hamartoma
- Patients with masses clearly caused by an inflammatory process such as tuberculosis. If the mass represents active tuberculosis or other infectious process, the lesion may disappear after therapy.
- Patients with prohibitive operative risk
- Patients in whom small-cell carcinoma is suspected.

Fine-needle aspiration should be performed when trying to identify a reason not to operate or if small-cell carcinoma is expected. If the fine-needle aspiration is positive, resection of the nodule is recommended; if the result is nondiagnostic, definitive treatment or other diagnostic maneuvers should be carried out. Sputum cytology is frequently nondiagnostic in this situation, whereas the sensitivity of transthoracic fine-needle aspiration approaches 100%.

A wedge resection may not always be possible, particularly if the mass is located centrally within the lobe. A lobectomy may be necessary for a diagnosis (and treatment) in the patient who is physiologically fit to undergo a lobectomy. If a cancer diagnosis is obtained, a mediastinal lymph node dissection should be performed as part of the definitive procedure. A pneumonectomy should not be performed for a presumed cancer until the diagnosis is confirmed at time of operation.

Symptomatic Presentation of Cancer Patient

Patients with lung cancer are usually 50–70 years of age; lung cancer is rarely seen in patients younger than 30 years. Lung cancer is clinically silent for most of its course. The presence of symptoms is associated with later-stage disease and prognosis is worse than with a carcinoma that presents as an asymptomatic radiographic abnormality.

Patients have bronchopulmonary symptoms such as cough (75%), dyspnea (60%), chest pain (50%), and hemoptysis (30%) (Table 8–7).

TABLE 8–7 • Presenting Signs and Symptoms of Patients with Lung Cancer

Finding	Percentage
Cough	74
Weight loss	68
Dyspnea	58
Chest pain	49
Sputum production	45
Hemoptysis	29
Malaise	26
Bone pain	25
Lymphadenopathy	23
Hepatomegaly	21
Fever	21
Clubbing	20
Neuromyopathy	10
Superior vena cava syndrome	4
Dizziness	4
Hoarseness	3
Asymptomatic	12

Modified from Hyde L, Hyde CI. Clinical manifestations of lung cancer. *Chest* 1974;65:229–306 and Cromartie RS, Parker EF, May JE, *et al.* Carcinoma of the lung: a clinical review. *Ann Thorac Surg* 1980;30:30–35.

Fever, wheezing, or stridor may also occasionally be present. Other symptoms may include hoarseness, superior vena cava syndrome, chest wall pain, Horner syndrome, dysphagia, pleural effusion, or phrenic nerve paralysis. Nonspecific symptoms such as anorexia, malaise, fatigue, and weight loss may occur in up to 70% of patients.

Because the pulmonary parenchyma does not contain nerve endings, many lung cancers grow to a large size before they cause local symptoms of hemoptysis, a change in sputum production, dyspnea, obstruction, or pain (Table 8–8). Obstruction of a main stem bronchus or lobar bronchus may impair mucus passage. With this partial obstruction and bacterial overgrowth, pneumonia may develop. Frequently, patients are seen by their local physician with clinical evidence of pneumonia of several days' onset. The pneumonia may be treated intermittently with antibiotics for a period of several weeks. If the clinical picture does not clear, a chest x-ray is obtained, which identifies the lung cancer.

Either a new cough or a change in the nature of a chronic cough is the most common presenting symptom of bronchogenic carcinoma.

TABLE 8–8 • *Signs and Symptoms Due to Primary Tumor*

Symptoms from Endobronchial and Central Tumor Growth	Symptoms from Peripheral Tumor Growth
Cough	Sharp pain (pleura, chest wall)
Obstruction dyspnea	Restrictive dyspnea
Segmental atelectasis	Effusion: serous or bloody fluid
Segmental emphysema	Cough
Pneumonic (fever, productive cough)	Lung abscess from tumor cavitation
Dull chest pain	
Wheeze or stridor	

This symptom in a smoker should always cause concern. Cough productive of copious thin secretions, often with a salty flavor, has been described as classically occurring in bronchiolo-alveolar carcinoma, but it occurs in only a minority of cases. Hemoptysis, either gross or minor, commonly occurs when mucosal lesions ulcerate. Although the most common cause of hemoptysis is bronchitis, this sign should always lead to further investigation.

Tumors that obstruct major airways can produce wheezing, and unilateral wheezing suggests a localized obstruction. Airway obstruction can result in atelectasis or post-obstructive pneumonia. Bronchogenic carcinomas are often associated with cavitation and lung abscess formation, due either to airway obstruction with postobstructive pneumonia or to necrosis of a large tumor mass. Clinical signs particularly indicative of malignancy-associated lung abscess include chronicity of symptoms, lack of high fever, and lack of leukocytosis.

Local invasion can produce chest pain, dyspnea from pleural effusion, and symptoms referable to nerves, heart, and great vessels. Pleural effusions occur in approximately 10–20% of patients at the time of diagnosis and are most frequently a sign that the tumor is not operable. Invasion of the pericardium can lead to cardiac tamponade as well as to arrhythmias.

A number of syndromes have been described associated with locally invasive disease. The superior vena cava syndrome is due to obstruction of the superior vena cava either by tumor or by associated thrombosis. Although this syndrome is no longer considered a medical emergency, it should be treated promptly following establishment of a tissue diagnosis.

Horner syndrome results from involvement of the superior cervical ganglion and is characterized by unilateral facial anhidrosis, pto-

sis, and miosis. Hoarseness can occur from invasion of the recurrent laryngeal nerve, either by tumor directly extending into the mediastinum or by adjacent malignant lymph nodes. The symptom of hoarseness is important because recurrent nerve involvement, usually the left, most commonly is associated with unresectability.

The Pancoast syndrome occurs in tumors involving the apex and superior sulcus of the lung and results from local invasion into the brachial plexus as well as the cervical sympathetic chain. Clinical manifestations are dominated by shoulder and arm pain and may include Horner syndrome. The tumor may not be readily apparent on plain radiographs, and computed tomographic (CT) scanning or magnetic resonance imaging (MRI) may be necessary for diagnosis. Delay in diagnosis is common in these individuals, who may be treated for their musculoskeletal symptoms for long periods before any chest imaging is obtained.

Other poor prognostic indicators include esophageal obstruction and vertebral body invasion. Distant extrathoracic tumor effects may be due to direct tumor infiltration and metastasis, commonly involving lymph nodes, the central nervous system, liver, bone and bone marrow, the adrenal gland, and other areas of the lung. Bone and central nervous system involvement frequently causes symptoms, whereas liver and adrenal involvement may be asymptomatic at diagnosis. The frequent involvement of the bone marrow (up to 50%) in small-cell carcinoma may occur without hematologic abnormalities. Each of the bronchogenic carcinoma cell types may involve any of these organs, although it is much more common for the more rapidly spreading small-cell carcinoma to have metastasized at the time of initial presentation.

In addition, lung cancer has the potential to spread to almost any organ in the body at some point in the clinical course.

Paraneoplastic syndromes occur in 10% of patients with bronchogenic carcinoma and occasionally are the presenting symptom. Paraneoplastic manifestations can be divided into systemic, endocrine, neurologic, cutaneous, hematologic, and renal categories (Table 8–9). Systemic manifestations are often nonspecific and can include weight loss, anorexia, and fever. The endocrine and neurologic manifestations of bronchogenic carcinoma are more specific (Table 8–10).

Digital clubbing is seen in a variety of pulmonary conditions but occurs most commonly in association with bronchogenic carcinoma. Clubbing is due to subungual thickening that involves the fingernails, resulting in loss of the normal angle between the fingernail and nail bed. In addition, the fingernails are easily compressed against the nail bed and have a spongy feel. Hypertrophic pulmonary osteoarthropathy is often associated with clubbing and commonly presents with exquisite tenderness over the long bones. Hypercoagulable states can result from bronchogenic carcinoma. Invasion of the bone marrow rarely can produce anemia or leukocytosis with a leukoerythroblastic reaction.

Endocrine abnormalities are relatively common in lung cancer. Hypercalcemia is most commonly associated with squamous-cell carcinoma and may occur directly through bone invasion or indirectly through the effect of a parathyroid-hormone-related peptide on bone. Small-cell carcinoma may be associated with the syndrome of inappropriate antidiuretic hormone release (SIADH) and Cushing syndrome. Elevations in adrenocorticotropic hormone (ACTH) levels may be found in 30–50% of cases of small-cell carcinoma. Cushing syndrome, as manifested by muscle weakness, hypokalemia, metabolic alkalosis, diabetes, and other signs and symptoms such as hirsutism, truncal obesity, facial swelling, and bruising, only occurs in 1–5% of patients.

An interesting neuromuscular disorder in lung cancer is the association between small-cell carcinoma and the Eaton–Lambert myasthenic syndrome. This syndrome is characterized by proximal muscle weakness, decreased or absent deep tendon reflexes, paresthesias, and autonomic dysfunction. The diagnosis may be made by electromyography, showing a decreased action potential that improves following maximal voluntary contraction or repetitive nerve stimulation. Diagnosis is made by detecting antibodies that react with calcium channel components extracted from small-cell carcinoma. Therapy consists of treatment of the underlying malignancy, increasing acetylcholine release through the use of 3,4-diaminopyridine, cholinesterase inhibitors, and immunomodulation by plasmapheresis or plasma exchange, corticosteroids, azathioprine, and immunoglobulin.

Laboratory Evaluation

In addition to a complete blood count, an electrolyte panel, liver function tests, and a serum calcium assay, a number of serum tumor markers have been described in lung cancer. These are substances produced by the tumor or by host cells in response to the tumor and may be useful in staging, prognostication, and clinical follow-up of patients. Because these factors may be produced by normal cell types, they are less useful in diagnosis. The tumor markers most often used include carcinoembryonic antigen (CEA), creatine kinase BB (CK-BB), and neuron-specific enolase (NSE). Other substances that hold promise but require further study include bombesin/gastrin-releasing peptide (GRP), tissue polypeptide antigen (TPA), and CA-125.

The clinical role for serum tumor markers in lung cancer remains to be defined. If elevated at diagnosis, markers may be helpful in the clinical evaluation of patients. NSE and CEA are the markers used most frequently in lung cancer. In the majority of patients with small-cell carcinoma, NSE levels are elevated and may be useful in staging, prognosis and follow-up.

Imaging Evaluation

A radiologic evaluation is an integral part of the diagnosis and treatment of lung cancer. In NSCLC patients without clinical evidence of metastasis, a chest radiograph and a CT scan of the chest and upper abdomen (with cuts through the adrenal gland) are performed. Pretreatment bone scan and MRI scan of the brain are performed in the presence of any organ-specific or nonspecific symptoms. In patients with limited stage SCLC, MRI scans of the brain and radionuclide bone scans are typically obtained because of the frequency of bony and intracranial metastases. The standard chest

TABLE 8–9 • *Paraneoplastic Syndromes in Lung Cancer Patients*

Endocrine

Hypercalcemia (ectopic parathyroid hormone)

Cushing syndrome

SIADH

Carcinoid syndrome

Gynecomastia

Hypercalcitonemia

Elevated growth hormone

Elevated prolactin, follicle-stimulating hormone, luteinizing hormone

Hypoglycemia

Hyperthyroidism

Neurologic

Encephalopathy

Subacute cerebellar degeneration

Progressive multifocal leukoencephalopathy

Peripheral neuropathy

Polymyositis

Autonomic neuropathy

Eaton–Lambert syndrome

Optic neuritis

Skeletal

Clubbing

Pulmonary hypertrophic osteoarthropathy

Hematologic

Anemia

Leukemoid reactions

Thrombocytosis

Thrombocytopenia

Eosinophilia

Pure red cell aplasia

Leukoerythroblastosis

Disseminated intravascular coagulation

Cutaneous

Hyperkeratosis

Dermatomyositis

Acanthosis nigricans

Hyperpigmentation

Erythema gyratum repens

Hypertrichosis lanuginosa acquisita

Other

Nephrotic syndrome

Hypouricemia

Secretion of vasoactive intestinal peptide with diarrhea

Hyperamylasemia

Anorexia–cachexia

SIADH, syndrome of inappropriate antidiuretic hormone secretion.

TABLE 8–10 • *Paraneoplastic Syndromes of the Nervous System Associated with Lung Cancer*

Syndrome	Clinical Features
Subacute cerebellar degeneration	Subacute, progressive bilateral, symmetric cerebellar failure often with dementia, dysarthria, cerebrospinal fluid (CSF) lymphocytosis, and elevated protein. Some reports of improvements with removal of primary tumor
Dementia	Variable presentation, acute to slowly progressive. Often associated with abnormalities in other areas of the neuraxis. Electroencephalogram shows slowing. CSF pleocytosis sometimes seen
Limbic encephalitis	Dementia with degenerative changes in the hippocampus and amygdaloid nuclei. Often associated with inflammatory and degenerative lesions in other areas of the neuraxis. May or may not improve with removal of primary tumor (Ophelia syndrome)
Optic neuritis	Decrease in visual acuity, papilledema; unilateral or bilateral. Rare
Subacute necrotic myelopathy	Rapidly ascending motor and sensory paralysis to thoracic level. Elevated CSF protein. Severe tissue destruction of gray and white matter
Sensory neuropathy	Subacute onset of sensory loss including deep tendon reflexes, with normal strength and normal motor conduction velocity. Elevated CSF protein. Uncommon. Also called dorsal root ganglionitis
Sensorimotor peripheral neuropathy	Distal weakness and wasting, areflexia, distal sensory loss. Elevated CSF protein. Quite common. Recovery rare even with removal of primary tumor
Autonomic and gastrointestinal neuropathy	Orthostatic hypotension, neurogenic bladder, intestinal pseudo-obstruction. Many cases of Ogilvie syndrome (colonic pseudo-obstruction) may be paraneoplastic
Dermatomyositis and polymyositis	Progressive muscle weakness developing gradually over weeks to months (proximal to distal). Usually not disabling. Elevated muscle enzymes and sedimentation rate. Stringent association in older males
Myasthenic syndrome (Eaton–Lambert syndrome)	Weakness and fatigability of proximal muscles, especially pelvic girdle and thigh. Dryness of mouth, dysphagia, dysarthria, and peripheral paresthesias common. Electromyelograms show a facilitated response in active muscles. Poor response to edrophonium chloride. Should respond to therapy of primary tumor. Guanidine may also be useful

Modified from Bunn PA, Minna JD. Paraneoplastic syndromes. In: DeVita VT, Hellman S, Rosenberg SA, eds. *Cancer: principles and practice of oncology,* 4th ed. Philadelphia: JB Lippincott, 1993.

x-ray and CT scan of the chest and upper abdomen (to include the adrenals) are the most frequent diagnostic imaging studies performed in patients with lung cancer.

Computed tomography chest scan and MRI can identify the location of the primary tumor with respect to the other mediastinal structures; however, it is difficult to determine whether lung cancer has invaded specific structures or simply abuts adjacent structures. Often this distinction may only be made at the time of surgical exploration.

Chest X-ray

The chest x-ray provides information regarding the size, shape, density, and location of the tumor in relation to the mediastinal structures. The chest x-ray is performed to evaluate the location of the mass, the presence or absence of thoracic lymphadenopathy, pleural effusion, pericardial effusion, pulmonary infiltrates, pneumonia, or consolidation. Changes in the contour of the mediastinum secondary to lymphadenopathy, and metastasis to ribs or other bone structure may be visualized. Clues to the histology may also be provided. In general, squamous carcinomas have a tendency to be large and central in location, adenocarcinoma tends to be more peripheral in its initial presentation, and a small-cell carcinoma tends to present as a central lesion associated with bulky mediastinal adenopathy. Specific attention should be paid to whether the mass has cavitation or not and its relationship to the thoracic structures and mediastinum, and whether it is limited or diffuse in appearance. Also sought is the presence or absence of segmental or lobar collapse or consolidation, hilar and mediastinal enlargement, or evidence of intrathoracic metastasis or extrapulmonary intrathoracic extension.

Most asymptomatic lung cancers are detected on chest radiographs. Although it is possible to visualize lesions as small as 3 mm, in practice, lesions smaller than 5–6 mm in diameter are rarely noticed. The radiographic appearance of a lesion cannot reliably distinguish between a benign and a malignant process. Radiographic appearances characteristic of malignant lesions include lobulation, shaggy margins, and poorly defined margins but the radiographic appearance on plain chest radiograph may be misleading.

The majority of squamous-cell carcinomas occur centrally. They may cause partial or complete obstruction of airways, with radiographic changes of atelectasis, postobstructive pneumonia (usually with volume loss and lack of air bronchograms), lung abscess, bronchiectasis, and mucoid impaction (Figure 8–16). Peripheral squamous-cell carcinomas are particularly liable to cavitate and resemble a lung abscess. Cavitation is less common in adenocarcinoma and large-cell carcinoma and rare in small-cell carcinoma.

Small-cell carcinoma also occurs centrally, usually associated with hilar and mediastinal adenopathy due to rapid lymphatic spread (Figure 8–17). Although the primary lesion does not tend to obstruct, occasionally the metastatic adenopathy will cause external compression of airways. Small-cell carcinoma may also occur peripherally but this is extremely uncommon and a peripheral 'small-cell' tumor must be differentiated from other neuroendocrine lesions, in particular carcinoid tumor.

Adenocarcinomas are most frequently peripheral lesions. About half of these tumors present less than 4 cm in diameter. Pleural involvement may occur in approximately 20%

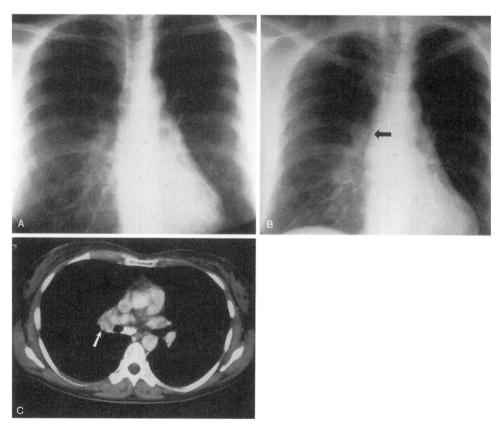

Figure 8–16. Primary squamous-cell carcinoma, seen as a hilar mass. **A,** On a baseline chest radiograph, the hila are normal. **B,** Six months after *A* was taken, an abnormal convexity in the superior right hilum (arrow) has developed. **C,** CT confirms the right hilar mass (arrow), which was due to squamous-cell carcinoma. (From Roth JA, Ruckdeschel JC, Weisenburger TH. *Thoracic oncology*, 2nd ed. Philadelphia: WB Saunders, 1995:69.)

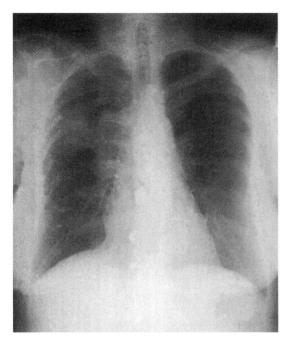

Figure 8–17. Chest radiograph from a patient with limited-stage small-cell lung cancer who presents with a right hilar lesion and mediastinal adenopathy. (From Johnson BE. Management of small cell lung cancer. *Clin Chest Med* 2002;23:226.)

of cases. Radiographic signs suggestive of malignancy include a lobular contour, shaggy or ill-defined margins, and eccentric calcification if the tumor develops in a scar or granuloma. Bronchioloalveolar carcinoma may occur either

as a solitary nodule or as a diffuse infiltrate. These two distinct types of bronchioloalveolar carcinoma have distinct behaviors, with the nodular type often being quite indolent and slow growing. The lobar type rarely if ever is cured by operation and commonly recurs early (Figure 8–18).

Large-cell carcinomas are more frequently peripheral than central. They tend to be sharply defined lobulated masses that occasionally cavitate and are not associated with scars.

When an abnormality is visualized on a chest radiograph, it is extremely helpful to obtain old chest radiographs, if available. The stability of the lesion over time can be very helpful in suggesting either a benign or malignant diagnosis. Doubling times of less than 6 weeks or more than 18 months strongly suggest a benign diagnosis. Another sign of benign disease is the presence of heavy calcification within a lesion, particularly when present in a concentric, solid, or popcorn pattern. It must be kept in mind, however, that carcinomas can arise adjacent to calcified granulomas; therefore, if a lesion that contains a significant amount of calcium enlarges over time, it should be considered to be malignant.

Computed Tomography

More recently, low-resolution CT of the chest has revealed small nodules undetectable on routine chest x-ray. Some of these subcentimeter

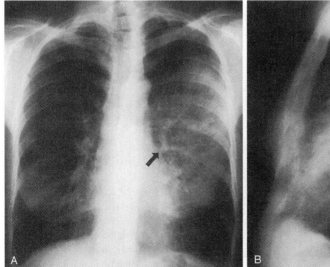
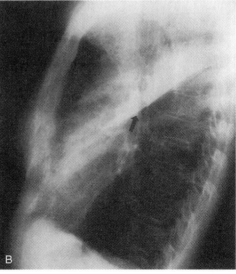

Figure 8–18. Bronchoalveolar-cell carcinoma presenting as an alveolar infiltrate. **A,** The posteroanterior chest film shows diffuse air-space (alveolar) infiltrate in the left upper lobe (arrow). **B,** The lateral chest film shows the tumor/consolidation to be delimited posteriorly by the major fissure (arrow). (From Roth JA, Ruckdeschel JC, Weisenburger TH. *Thoracic oncology*, 2nd ed. Philadelphia: WB Saunders, 1995:75.)

nodules (approximately 10%) prove to be lung cancers (Figure 8–19). CT of the chest provides more detail than chest x-ray regarding the surface characteristics of the tumor, relationships of the tumor to the mediastinum and mediastinal structures, and metastasis to lung, bone, liver, and adrenals. Enlargement of the mediastinal lymph nodes can be identified if present (Figure 8–20). Although CT cannot accurately or consistently predict invasion, it can identify size of mediastinal lymph nodes. CT of the chest has a 65% specificity and an 80% sensitivity for identifying mediastinal lymphadenopathy. When lymph nodes are greater than 1.5 cm in diameter, CT is approximately 85% specific in identifying metastasis to mediastinal lymph nodes.

A high-quality CT evaluation of the chest and upper abdomen to include the adrenal glands is mandatory in the patient with a lung lesion. This examination evaluates the presence or absence of enlarged (>1 cm) mediastinal lymph nodes, and evaluates the liver, adrenals, and kidneys for metastasis.

Computed tomographic scanning of the thorax is now frequently undertaken in patients with suspicious nodules. In many cases, dense or diffuse calcification (suggesting a high likelihood that the lesion is a granuloma) or fat (suggesting a hamartoma) can be detected. CT scans also reliably detect enlarged lymph nodes, although biopsy is required to determine whether the lymphadenopathy is due to metastatic tumor.

Magnetic Resonance Imaging

Magnetic resonance imaging is frequently used to complement CT in evaluating the

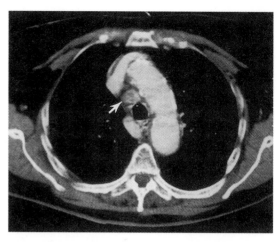

Figure 8–20. Enlarged benign mediastinal lymph node. CT at the level of the aortic arch shows a pretracheal node measuring 15 mm in diameter (arrow). This node was enlarged owing to healed granulomatous disease. (From Roth JA, Ruckdeschel JC, Weisenburger TH. *Thoracic oncology*, 2nd ed. Philadelphia: WB Saunders, 1995:82.)

location of tumors within the chest. Specifically, MRI is helpful for evaluating apical lung lesions where the coronal reconstruction may help to identify proximity to the brachiocephalic vessels and the brachial plexus and the spine (Figures 8–21, 8–22). MRI studies are particularly useful to detect vertebral, spinal cord, and mediastinal invasion in selected patients.

Positron-Emission Tomography

Positron-emission tomographic (PET) scanning can often reliably discriminate between benign and malignant parenchymal nodules in most circumstances. PET determines the presence or absence of cancer based on the different metabolism manifest by cancer cells compared with normal cells. Cancer cells metabolize glucose more rapidly than normal cells. The 18-fluorodeoxyglucose ([18]FDG) given intravenously as a substrate is taken up by both normal and malignant tissue. Phosphorylated FDG is trapped within malignant cells and can be imaged with PET. Various nuclear scanning devices can scan the patient to determine whether there are areas of increased uptake. These areas of increased uptake are commonly associated with malignancy and may identify areas of unsuspected metastatic disease (Figure 8–23). PET coupled with CT yields increased sensitivity and specificity in determining the

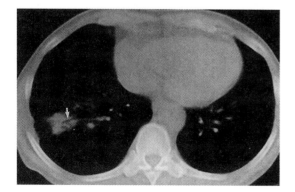

Figure 8–19. Bronchioalveolar carcinoma solitary nodule. Solitary nodule with an air bronchogram (arrow). (From McLoud TC. *Thoracic radiology: the requisites*. St Louis: Mosby Yearbook, 1998.)

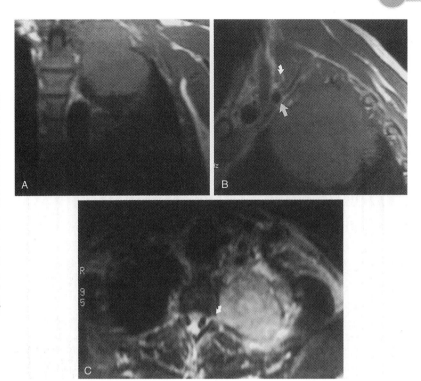

Figure 8–21. Magnetic resonance image of superior sulcus carcinoma. **A**, T1-weighted coronal scan demonstrates a large mass in the apex of the left lung extending into the chest wall and base of the neck. **B**, Sagittal T1-weighted scan shows that the subclavian artery (straight arrow) and brachial plexus (curved arrow) are not involved by the tumor. **C**, T2-weighted axial scan shows widening of the intervertebral foramen with tumor extension at the T2 level (arrow). (From McLoud TC. Imaging techniques for diagnosis and staging of lung cancer. *Clin Chest Med* 2002;23:132.)

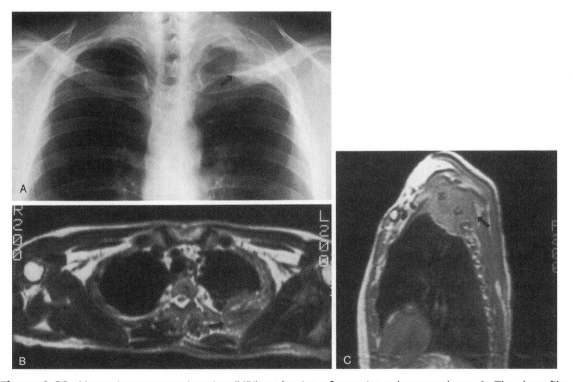

Figure 8–22. Magnetic resonance imaging (MRI) evaluation of superior sulcus neoplasm. **A**, The chest film shows a superior sulcus mass (arrow) and apical pleural thickening. No rib destruction or extrapleural mass is seen. **B**, The axial MRI demonstrates the tumor mass extending into the posterior chest wall (arrow). **C**, The sagittal MRI shows extension of tumor into the posterior chest wall (arrow) and encasement of the ribs. (From Roth JA, Ruckdeschel JC, Weisenburger TH. *Thoracic oncology*, 2nd ed. Philadelphia: WB Saunders, 1995:71.)

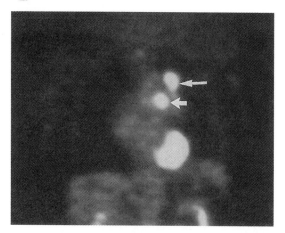

Figure 8–23. 18-fluorodeoxyglucose positron-emission tomography (FDG-PET) scan in a patient with a left upper lobe cancer. Hypermetabolic focus in the left upper lobe corresponds to the primary tumor (long arrow). There is also uptake in the left-sided mediastinal nodes (short arrow), proved by biopsy. (From McLoud TC. Imaging techniques for diagnosis and staging of lung cancer. *Clin Chest Med* 2002;23:134.)

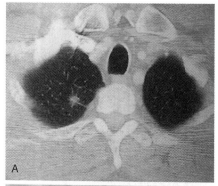

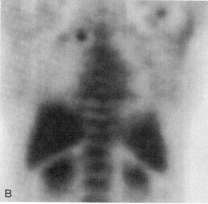

Figure 8–24. Adenocarcinoma. 18-fluorodeoxyglucose positron-emission tomography (FDG-PET). **A,** CT scan demonstrates a small spiculated lesion in the right upper lobe. **B,** PET scan shows marked uptake in the lesion. (From McLoud TC. Imaging techniques for diagnosis and staging of lung cancer. *Clin Chest Med* 2002;23:128.)

stage of patients with lung cancer before treatment interventions are instituted (Figure 8–24). The sensitivity and specificity of PET with FDG for detecting nonmalignant lesions ranges from 94% to 97% for benign lesions and from 80% to 100% for malignant lesions. Active inflammation may yield false-positive results and carcinoid tumors as well as bronchioloalveolar tumors take up the radiolabeled glucose poorly, leading to false-negative scans.

Obtaining Tissue Diagnosis

The definitive diagnosis of lung cancer requires histopathologic or cytologic confirmation. Tissue may be obtained through several procedures. Invasive procedures that may be included in the evaluation of patients with lung lesion include bronchoscopy, transthoracic needle aspiration/biopsy, mediastinoscopy, or thoracoscopy. Surgical or pathologic staging (pTNM) provides the most accurate staging of the TNM status of the tumor. Invasive staging identifies those patients most likely to benefit from resection and those patients with metastases to mediastinal lymph nodes for prospective clinical studies (protocols) or for definitive chemotherapy and radiation therapy.

Sputum cytology is positive in more than 50% of cases, especially in centrally located tumors. Sputum cytology, as demonstrated in the lung cancer screening trials, is helpful in diagnosing central squamous-cell carcinomas. However, the results are highly variable and interpretation may be difficult because of poor samples, purulence, malignant cell degeneration, poor sample preparation, and inexperienced cytologists. Thus negative sputum cytologic findings in a suspicious setting should not be the basis for ending the evaluation. Needle biopsy of suspicious pulmonary masses under either fluoroscopic or CT guidance is highly accurate, with a sensitivity of 90–95% (Figure 8–25). Fine-needle aspiration is not always needed in the patient with good physiologic reserve who is otherwise an appropriate candidate for surgery. If the patient does have suspicious lymph nodes in the cervical or supraclavicular area, fine-needle aspiration or biopsy will provide the confirmation of metastatic involvement. Otherwise, an excisional lymph node biopsy could be performed to obtain tissue for further evaluation.

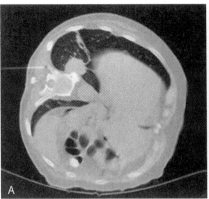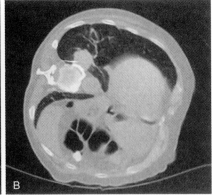

Figure 8–25. Computed-tomography-guided transthoracic needle biopsy. **A,** The needle is traversing the soft tissue, avoiding as much lung parenchyma as possible. **B,** The needle tip is seen within the mass. (From Mazzone P, Jain P, Arroliga AC, Matthay RA. Bronchoscopy and needle biopsy techniques for diagnosis and staging of lung cancer. *Clin Chest Med* 2002;23:151.)

Involvement of a cervical or supraclavicular lymph node indicates N3 disease and precludes surgical resection.

Flexible fiberoptic bronchoscopy to visualize all the central, lobar, segmental, and subsegmental airways can be performed on awake patients with local sedation. For endoscopically visible endobronchial lesions, bronchoscopy is diagnostic in over 90% of cases (Figure 8–26). The sensitivity of fiberoptic bronchoscopy for peripheral lesions is lower than for directly visualized airway lesions, with a sensitivity dependent on the size and location of the lesion. Peripheral nodules can also be biopsied with fluoroscopic guidance. Bronchoscopy may also be diagnostic in peripheral carcinomas, particularly those greater than 4 cm in size. The diagnostic yield falls to 25% or less in lesions smaller than 2 cm and bronchoscopy as a separate procedure is not indicated for these lesions. Bronchoscopy may also be useful in the localization of occult carcinomas (i.e. sputum-cytology-positive, chest-radiograph-negative lesions). Most of these lesions will be located in the proximal bronchi. Serious complications of bronchoscopy are minimal. These include hemorrhage, pneumothorax, laryngospasm, and hypoxemia.

Bronchoscopy is recommended before any planned pulmonary resection if the sputum is positive with a negative chest x-ray or if atelectasis or an infiltrate fails to clear with medical management. The surgeon always performs a bronchoscopy before resection to independently assess the endobronchial anatomy, exclude secondary endobronchial primary tumors, and ensure that all known cancer will be encompassed by the planned pulmonary resection. More centrally located lung cancers are more likely to be biopsy-positive by bronchoscopy, whereas smaller and more peripheral lung cancers are more likely to be 'negative' on bronchoscopy.

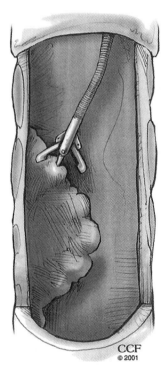

Figure 8–26. Use of spear forceps for biopsy of lesions located on lateral wall of trachea or bronchus. (Mazzone P, Jain P, Arroliga AC, Matthay RA. Bronchoscopy and needle biopsy techniques for diagnosis and staging of lung cancer. *Clin Chest Med* 2002;23:139.)

Transbronchial biopsy may be performed with a special 21-gauge needle through the flexible bronchoscope. This technique may be used to sample mediastinal lymph nodes or other masses adjacent to the larger bronchi.

Cervical mediastinoscopy with sampling of lymph nodes is also highly accurate in selected patients with lymphadenopathy. A mediastinoscopy or anterior mediastinotomy (Chamberlain procedure) should be part of the evaluation in all patients with clinically suspicious lymph nodes based on size as evaluated by CT scan. The information obtained from staging (pathologic staging) of suspicious mediastinal lymph nodes determines the definitive management. Enlarged lymph nodes (>1.5 cm) are more likely to be involved with metastases from lung cancer than nodes less than 1.5 cm in size. Other causes of mediastinal lymphadenopathy include mediastinal inflammation, peripheral pulmonary obstruction, atelectasis, consolidation, bronchitis, pneumonitis, or pneumonia, or some patients may have normally enlarged lymph nodes.

The decision to perform mediastinoscopy varies according to the individual surgeon's preference. Some surgeons routinely perform mediastinoscopy on all patients with presumed lung cancer while the majority of surgeons choose to perform the procedure on the basis of the size of the lymph nodes imaged by the CT scan. Sensitivity and specificity will vary according to the site of the mediastinal lymph nodes, with those larger than 2 cm approximately 95–100%.

Mediastinoscopy can evaluate lymph nodes of both the right and left side (Figure 8–27). Aortopulmonary window (level 5) or anterior mediastinal nodes (level 6) can be evaluated using a left parasternal incision (Chamberlain procedure) or via an extended cervical mediastinoscopy. Video-assisted thoracic surgery (VATS) techniques can evaluate enlarged level 5 or 6 lymph nodes, and enlarged level 8 or 9 or low level 7 lymphadenopathy. Complications of mediastinoscopy are infrequent but include massive hemorrhage, injury to the trachea or bronchi, esophageal injury, pneumothorax, and esophageal injury.

Staging

After performing a thorough history and physical examination, with particular attention to signs and symptoms consistent with individ-

ual organ involvement, laboratory data are obtained, including liver function tests, alkaline phosphatase, and calcium. Any abnormalities require follow-up with appropriate radionuclide and CT scans (Figure 8–28).

Since the majority of lung cancers metastasize to the liver, central nervous system, bone, and adrenal glands, extrathoracic staging procedures focus on the detection of tumor in these sites. Imaging techniques frequently used in tumor detection include CT scans of the central nervous system, liver, and adrenal glands. In NSCLC, the frequency of extrathoracic metastases is low enough to make routine scanning of these organ sites in asymptomatic patients unnecessary and potentially misleading.

Occasionally, intracranial metastases may be discovered in asymptomatic patients, particularly those with adenocarcinoma. Whether this justifies routine head MRI scanning is undetermined. Adrenal glands are usually included when doing chest CT scans. The finding of an adrenal mass on CT scan necessitates further evaluation, most commonly an MRI scan and possibly needle biopsy. Likewise, liver lesions seen on CT scan also require MRI scanning for further evaluation. PET scan also may be useful in these situations where the burden is to prove metastatic disease so as to avoid a needless surgical procedure.

After tissue diagnosis of lung cancer, staging determines the extent of local and distant disease. Accurate staging is crucial in the selection of correct therapy and determination of prognosis (Figure 8–29). The most widely accepted system of staging for NSCLC is the TNM anatomic classification (Table 8–11, Box 8–1).

Stage I and II tumors are completely contained within the lung and may be completely resected with surgery. Stage IV disease includes metastatic disease and is not typically treated by surgery, except in those patients requiring surgical palliation. 'Resectable' stage IIIA and IIIB tumors are locally advanced tumors with metastasis to the ipsilateral mediastinal structures or involving mediastinal structures. These tumors, because of their advanced nature, may be mechanically removed with surgery; however, surgery does not control the micrometastases.

Small-cell carcinoma is not generally included in the TNM classification because the majority of these tumors are systemic at the time of diagnosis. The staging system used for SCLC is the two-stage system devised by the Veterans Administration Lung Cancer Study Group, in which disease is classified as either 'limited' or

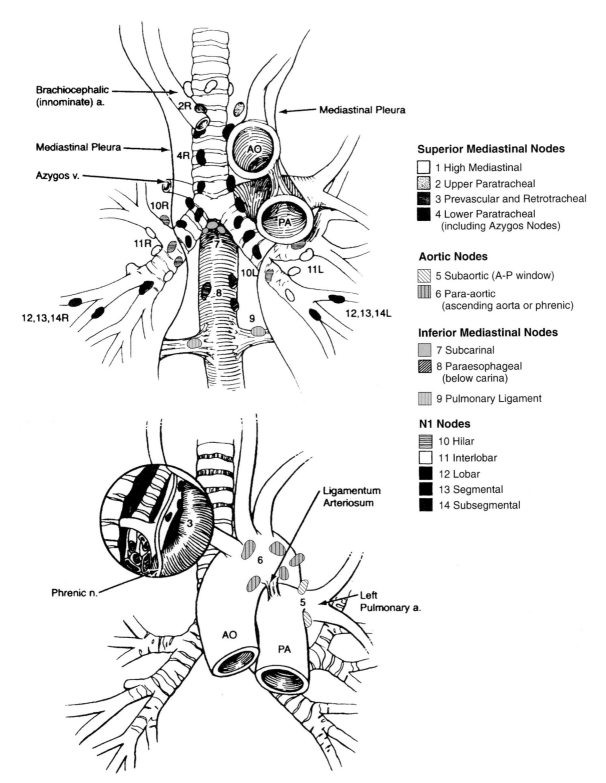

Figure 8–27. Regional lymph node stations for lung cancer staging. (From Mountain CF, Dresler CM. Regional lymph node classification for lung cancer staging. *Chest* 1997. Modifications from Naruke/American Thoracic Society/Lung Cancer Study Group maps.)

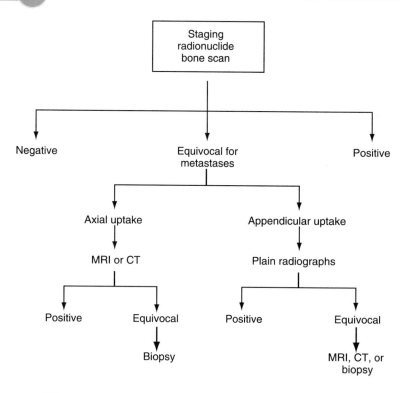

Figure 8–28. An algorithm for the evaluation of bone scan results. Magnetic resonance imaging (MRI) is preferred over computed tomography (CT) unless contraindicated. (From Pearson FG, Cooper JD, Deslauriers J, *et al. Thoracic surgery*, 2nd ed. New York: Churchill Livingstone, 2002:831.)

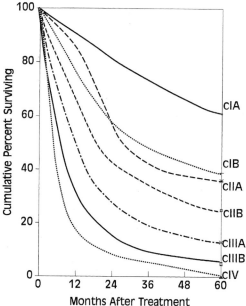

Figure 8–29. Cumulative proportion of patients with non-small-cell lung carcinoma expected to survive 5 years, according to clinical stage. Number of patients: cIA, $n = 675$; cIB, $n = 1130$; cIIA, $n = 26$; cIIB, $n = 329$; cIIIA, $n = 445$; cIIIB, $n = 836$; cIV, $n = 1166$. Overall comparison: $p < 0.05$. Pairwise comparison: cIA versus cIB, $p < 0.05$; cIB versus cIIA, $p < 0.05$; cIIA versus cIIB, $p < 0.05$; cIIB versus cIIIA, $p < 0.05$; cIIIA versus cIIIB, $p < 0.05$; cIIIB versus cIV, $p < 0.05$. (From Mountain CF, Libshitz HI, Hermes KE. *Lung cancer. a handbook for staging, imaging and lymph node classification.* Houston: Mountain & Libshitz, 1999:65.)

'extensive'. This definition of tumor stage relates to whether tumor is confined within a tolerable radiation port. Therefore, limited disease may include supraclavicular node involvement, malignant pleural effusion, recurrent

TABLE 8–11 • TNM (Tumor, Regional Lymph Nodes, Metastasis) by Stage

Stage	TNM Subset
0	Carcinoma *in situ*
IA	T1N0M0
IB	T2N0M0
IIA	T1N1M0
IIB	T2N1M0
	T3N0M0
IIIA	T3N1M0
	T1N2M0
	T2N2M0
	T3N2M0
IIIB	T4N0M0 T4N1M0
	T4N2M0
	T1N3M0 T2N3M0
	T3N3M0 T4N3M0
IV	Any T Any N M1

Staging is not relevant for occult carcinoma, designated TX N0 M0.
From Mountain CF. Revisions in the International Staging System for Lung Cancer. *Chest* 1997;3:1712.

BOX 8–1 TNM (TUMOR, REGIONAL LYMPH NODES, METASTASIS) DESCRIPTORS

Primary Tumor (T)

TX Primary tumor cannot be assessed or tumor proved by the presence of malignant cells in sputum or bronchial washings but not visualized by imaging or bronchoscopy

T0 No evidence of primary tumor

Tis Carcinoma *in situ*

T1 Tumor 3 cm or less in greatest dimension, surrounded by lung or visceral pleura, without bronchoscopic evidence of invasion more proximal than the lobar bronchus* (i.e. not in the main bronchus)

T2 Tumor with any of the following features of size or extent:
    More than 3 cm in greatest dimension involves main bronchus, 2 cm or more distal to the carina
    Invades the visceral pleura
    Associated with atelectasis or obstructive pneumonitis that extends to the hilar region but does not involve the entire lung

T3 Tumor of any size that directly invades any of the following: chest wall (including superior sulcus tumors), diaphragm, mediastinal pleura, or parietal pericardium; or tumor in the main bronchus less than 2 cm distal to the carina but without involvement of the carina; or associated atelectasis or obstructive pneumonitis of the entire lung

T4 Tumor of any size that invades any of the following: mediastinum, heart, great vessels, trachea, esophagus, vertebral body, or carina; or tumor with a malignant pleural or pericardial effusion†; or with satellite tumor nodule(s) within the ipsilateral primary tumor lobe of the lung

Regional Lymph Nodes (N)

NX Regional lymph nodes cannot be assessed

N0 No regional lymph node metastasis

N1 Metastasis to ipsilateral peribronchial and/or ipsilateral hilar lymph nodes and intrapulmonary nodes involved by direct extension of the primary tumor

N2 Metastasis to ipsilateral mediastinal and/or subcarinal lymph node(s)

N3 Metastasis to contralateral mediastinal, contralateral hilar, ipsilateral or contralateral scalene, or supraclavicular lymph node(s)

Distant Metastasis (M)

MX Presence of distant metastasis cannot be assessed

M0 No distant metastasis

M1 Distant metastasis present‡. Specify sites

---

* The uncommon superficial tumor of any size with its invasive component limited to the main bronchus is classified as Ti.

† Most pleural effusions associated with lung cancer are caused by tumor. There are, however, a few patients in whom cytopathologic examination of pleural fluid (on more than one specimen) is negative for tumor, the fluid is nonbloody, and is not an exudate. In such cases in which these elements and clinical judgment dictate that the effusion is not related to the tumor, the patients should be staged T1, T2, or T3, excluding effusion as a staging element.

‡ Separate metastatic tumor nodule(s) in the ipsilateral nonprimary tumor lobe(s) of the lung also are classified M1.
From Mountain CF. Revisions in the International System for Staging Lung Cancer. *Chest* 1997;111:1711.

laryngeal nerve involvement, and superior vena cava obstruction.

Management

Treatment options include surgery for localized disease, chemotherapy for metastatic disease, and radiation therapy for local control in patients whose condition is not amenable to surgery. Radiation therapy and chemotherapy together are better than chemotherapy or radiation therapy alone for primary treatment of advanced-stage lung cancer. Trials evaluating chemotherapy, radiation, and surgery for locally advanced-stage lung cancer are ongoing. In the future, knowledge of molecular changes that predispose to the development of lung cancer may provide strategies for chemoprevention or other treatments directed at genetic alterations in the cancer itself. Many prospective protocols have been initiated through the efforts of oncologists throughout the world, in an attempt to better understand and evaluate various combinations of multidisciplinary treatments.

The most important prognostic factors identified to date are disease stage, performance status, and extent of weight loss. Patients who have lost 5% or more of body weight in the preceding 2–6 months have a poor prognosis, as do nonambulatory patients. Biochemical and hematologic abnormalities are also important prognostic factors and reflect the extent and distribution of systemic disease.

Treatment Options for Non-Small-Cell Carcinoma

Although local and systemic interventions may improve survival rates in these patients, outcome depends on accurate staging before treatment. Anatomic resection of the involved lobe of the lung and mediastinal lymph node dissection provide optimal material for pathologic staging and optimal treatment (local control) for patients with stage I and II lung cancer. In advanced-stage (IIIA) patients, a multidisciplinary approach

(with evaluation and recommendations by the surgeon, the medical oncologist, and radiation oncologist before treatment) provides optimal treatment in a planned and structured manner.

Stage I and II Disease

The different pathologic subtypes of NSCLC respond to treatment in a similar way – that is, treatment does not vary according to the histologic type. Surgical resection is the treatment of choice in early-stage lung cancer. The surgical mortality is 3–4%, generally greater for pneumonectomy and less for lobectomy. Limited resections such as segmentectomies or wedge resections are safer but lead to a higher incidence of local recurrence. The 5-year survival rates for stage I and stage II disease are 60–70% and 40–55% respectively (Table 8–12). Numerous studies have not conclusively shown a survival benefit for postoperative adjuvant treatment with either radiation therapy or systemic chemotherapy or combinations of the two. These approaches continue to be studied in large randomized trials. At present, postoperative chemotherapy or radiation therapy cannot be recommended as stan-

TABLE 8–12 • Selected Series Reporting Postresection 5-Year Survival for Pathologic Stage IA (T1 N0) and Stage IB (T2 N0) Non-Small-Cell Lung Cancer

Report	Dates	T1N0 IA		T2N0 IB	
		n	5-yr	n	5-yr
Williams et al. (1981)	1972–1978	225	80	236	62
Little et al. (1986)*	1974–1984	44	72	47	68
Martini et al. (1986)	1973–1976	50	83	78	65
Roeslin et al. (1987)	1977–1982	108	71	121	43
Naruke et al. (1988)	1962–1986	245	76	327	57
Read et al. (1990)	1966–1988	214	73	158	49
Shimizu et al. (1993)	1973–1989	288 total	75		54
Ichinose et al. (1995)	1981–1988	71	85	80	67
Padilla et al. (1997)†	1969–1993	109	76	45	78
Mountain (1997)	1975–1988	511	67	549	57
Inoue et al. (1998)	1980–1993	480	80	271	65
Tanaka et al. (2000)	1980–1994	208	79	179	66
Van Rens et al. (2000)	1970–1992	404	63	797	46
Jassem et al. (2000)	1991–1995	51	66	220	53

* Limited to complete resection. † Limited to complete resection and small tumors.
  n, number of cases; 5-yr, % actuarial survival at 5 years.
Modified from Locicero J, Ponn R, Daly B. Surgical treatment of nonsmall cell lung cancer. In: Shields T, Locicero J, Ponn R, eds. *General thoracic surgery*. Philadelphia: Lippincott Williams & Wilkins, 200:1323.

dard treatment following complete resection for stage I and II disease. Nevertheless, post-operative radiotherapy may reduce local or regional recurrence and should be considered for patients with macroscopic or microscopic residual disease. In patients with stage I tumors who are physiologically unable to undergo surgery, full-dose irradiation (5900 cGy) may provide an alternative to surgery.

Stage III Disease

Stage III disease is divided into stage IIIA, which is potentially resectable, and stage IIIB, which is considered unresectable. Meta-analyses of randomized clinical trials in inoperable stage III patients have demonstrated that combined modality approaches integrating platinum-based chemotherapy with radiotherapy are superior to radiotherapy alone (Table 8–13). Recent evidence suggests that concurrent administration of chemotherapy and radiation therapy may be superior to sequential administration. Other studies are under way to confirm this finding. Concurrent therapy is more toxic, however, and at present should be reserved for healthy patients with minimal comorbidities. Either neoadjuvant radiation therapy, chemotherapy, or chemotherapy in combination with radiation therapy has been used prior to resection in stage IIIA disease (Table 8–14). Early results from several studies are encouraging. Surgical complications do not appear to be increased by preoperative therapy.

Stage IIIA disease is a heterogeneous group that includes patients with chest wall invasion, mediastinal nodal disease, and direct invasion of mediastinal structures, and certain patients with endobronchial disease. T3N0M0 disease may have a 5-year survival rate of up to 40% with surgery, although the surgical procedure may include chest wall, diaphragm, or pericardial resection (Table 8–15).

Selected patients with mediastinal lymph node involvement (N2M0 disease) may benefit from surgery. Favorable factors include localized, ipsilateral mediastinal adenopathy, and nodes with only microscopic tumor. With complete resection, survival in this group approaches 25–30%. Unfavorable prognostic factors include gross extranodal disease and multiple nodal level involvement. Often it is difficult to judge the extent and character of tumor spread until the time of operation. In this group of patients, strategies to reduce tumor burden preoperatively with chemotherapy and radiation therapy are being investi-

gated. Recent studies indicate increased survival with either chemotherapy or a combination of chemotherapy and radiation therapy before surgery. Following complete resection many patients with N2 disease receive postoperative radiation therapy, although survival benefit has yet to be demonstrated.

Patients with stage IIIB disease generally are considered unresectable, although this is a diverse group and includes those with N3 as well as T4 disease. Treatment with radiation therapy and/or chemotherapy without surgery may improve survival and this approach may also reduce tumor burden so that complete surgical resection is feasible. In some patients with tracheal or carinal involvement, tumor may be resected with tracheobronchial reconstruction techniques. Whether survival is improved needs to be studied further. Some studies have demonstrated equivalent survival between IIIA and IIIB disease because of the diversity of presentations in these two groups.

Stage IV Disease

Disseminated disease occurs in the majority of patients with lung cancer. At the time of presentation, two thirds of patients already have disseminated disease. Each year, approximately 135 000 deaths occur from NSCLC in the USA. The outcome for untreated NSCLC patients with widespread disease is disappointingly predictable, with a median survival time of 4 months and a 1-year survival rate of approximately 10–15%. Palliative treatment (supportive care only or palliative radiation or chemotherapy) is the main option for most patients with advanced unresectable NSCLC. Combination chemotherapy yields superior responses and survival compared with single-agent therapy. Currently, most commonly used regimens are cisplatin-based. In the USA, carboplatin has been substituted for cisplatin in some regimens. Currently, there is no standard chemotherapy regimen for NSCLC. Ongoing trials will help to identify the optimal regimen or regimens.

Treatment Options for Small-Cell Carcinoma

Small-cell lung cancer is assumed to be a systemic disease at the time of presentation. Thus systemic chemotherapy is the treatment modality most commonly employed in these patients. At staging, about one third of

Text continued on page 200

TABLE 8-13 • Phase III Trials of Chemoradiotherapy Versus Radiation Alone

First Author	Year	Type of Patient	n	C vs S*	Regimen†	RR (%)	MS (Months)	Survival 2-Year (%)	3-Year (%)	5-Year (%)	p
Soresi	1988	Inoperable IIIA/IIIB	50		XRT 50.4 Gy	50	11				0.18
			45	C	P per weekly + XRT	64	16				
Mattson	1988	Inoperable, confined to one hemithorax and mediastinal nodes	128	S	Split course XRT 55 Gy	44	10.4	17			NS
			124		CAP×2 → XRT → CAP×1 → XRT → CAP×6	49	11	19			
Dillman	1990	IIIA/IIIB	77	S	XRT 60 Gy	35	9.6	13	10	6	0.012
			78		PVb×2 → XRT 60 Gy	46	13.7	26	24	17	
LeChavalier	1991	Inoperable, no distant metastases, adenocarcinoma excluded	177	S	XRT 65 Gy	35	10	14	4		<0.02
			176		VdLPC×3 → XRT 65 Gy → VdLPC×3	31	12	21	12		
Morton	1991	Inoperable, no distant metastases	58	S	XRT 60 Gy	64	10.4	16		7	NS
			56		MxACL 2 → XRT 60 Gy → MxACL 2	55	10.6	21		5	
Schaake-Koning	1992	Inoperable, no distant metastases	108	C	Split-course XRT 55 Gy	70		13	2		
			98	C	Split-course XRT 55 Gy, P weekly	75		19	13		0.36
			102		Split-course XRT 55 Gy, P daily	85		26	16		0.009
Trovo	1992	IIIA/IIIB	88	C	XRT 45 Gy	59	10.3				NS
			85		XRT 45 Gy, P daily	51	9.97				
Gregor	1993	Inoperable, no distant metastases	39	S	XRT 50 Gy	41	12.3	20			NS
			39		PVd×2 → XRT 50 Gy	36	12.1	20			
			39		Palliative XRT (≤30 Gy)	5	7.9	15			

TABLE 8-13 • Phase III Trials of Chemoradiotherapy Versus Radiation Alone (Continued)

First Author	Year	Type of Patient	n	C vs S*	Regimen†	RR (%)	MS (Months)	Survival 2-Year (%)	3-Year (%)	5-Year (%)	p
Sause	1995	Inoperable II, IIIA/IIIB	152		XRT 60 Gy		11.4	21	11	5	0.04
			152	S	PVb×2 → XRT 60 Gy		13.2	47	25	10	NS
			154		XRT 1.2 Gy twice daily to 69.6 Gy		12	36	21	7	
Jeremic	1995	IIIA/IIIB	61		XRT 1.2 Gy twice daily to 64.8 Gy	63	8	25	6.6	4.9	0.003
			52	C	XRT 1.2 Gy twice daily to 64.8 Gy with CbE weekly	74	18	35	23	21	
			56	C	XRT 1.2 Gy twice daily to 64.8 Gy with CbE weeks 1, 3, 5	62	13	27	16	16	NS
Blanke	1995	Inoperable, no distant metastases	123		XRT to 60–65 Gy	38	11.5	13	3	2	NS
			117	C	XRT to 60–65 Gy with P×3	50	10.8	18	9	5	
Jeremic	1996	IIIA/IIIB	66		XRT 1.2 Gy twice daily to 69.6 Gy	84	14	26	11	9 (4 years)	0.021
			65	C	XRT 1.2 Gy twice daily to 69.6 Gy with CbE daily	92	22	43	23	23 (4 years)	

*Concurrent (C) versus Sequential (S). †A, Adriamycin; C, cyclophosphamide; Cb, carboplatin; E = etoposide; L, lomustine; Mx, methotrexate; P, cisplatin; Vb, vinblastine; Vd, vindesine.
MS, median survival; RR, response rate.

TABLE 8-14 • Phase II Trials of Neoadjuvant Trimodality Therapy

First Author	Year	Type of Patient	n	Regimen*	Complete Resection (%)	Major Pathologic Response (%)	Treatment-Related Mortality Rate (%)	Survival MS (Months)	2-Year (%)	3-Year (%)	5-Year (%)
Faber	1989	Clinical III	85	PF, XRT every other week×4 total; XRT 40 Gy, E added last 29 patients	68	33	7	22.1		40	
Weiden LCSC	1990	Clinical III	85	PF×2 with XRT to 30 Gy	34	9†	8	13	23		
Strauss	1992	IIIA, all but 3 patients had mediastinoscopy; 12% T3N0	41	PFVb×2 + XRT 30 Gy → surgery → PFVb×1 + XRT 30 Gy	59	17	15	15.5	47	22	
Albain SWOG 8805	1995	IIIA(N2), all surgically staged IIIB, all non-T4 tumors surgically staged	75	EP×2 + XRT 45 Gy → surgery → EP×2 + XRT if incomplete resection P×2 + XRT 45 EGy → surgery → EP×2 + XRT if incomplete resection	75	39‡		13	37	27	20 (6 years)
			51		61	19§	12	17	39	24	22 (6 years)
Choi	1997	IIIA(N2) all surgically staged	42	PFVb×2 + XRT (bd) 42 Gy → surgery → PFVb + XRT 12–18 Gy	81	21.5	6.5	25	66	37	37
Eberhardt	1998	IIIA, all surgically staged	52	EP×3 → EP + XRT (bd) 45 Gy → surgery	60			20		36	31 (4 years)
		IIIB, all surgically staged	42	EP×3 → EP + XRT (bd) 45 Gy → surgery	45	26‖	8.5	18		26	26 (4 years)
Rice	1998	IIIA(N2)/ IIIB, all surgically staged	45	PT + XRT (bd) 30 Gy → surgery → PT + XRT (bd) 30–33 Gy	71	31‖	6.6	22	49 (61% IIIA, 17% IIIB)		
Friedel	2000	IIIA(bulky N2)/ IIIB, all surgically staged	93	(84% IIIB) PVd×2 + XRT 36 Gy	53	30 IIIA,64 IIIB‖	6	15			24 (22% IIIA, 24% IIIB)

*P, cisplatin; F, 5-fluorouracil; E, etoposide; C, cyclophosphamide; Vb, vinblastine; T, paclitaxel. ‖ No viable tumor in primary tumor site. Downstaging rate. MS, mean survival.

From Evans TL, Donahue DM, Mathisen DJ, Lynch TJ. Building a better therapy for stage IIIA non-small-cell lung cancer. *Clin Chest Med* 2002;23:202.

TABLE 8-15 • Selected Series Reporting Postresection 5-Year Survival for Tumors Classified as T3 Because of Invasion of the Parietal Pleura or Chest Wall

Report	Dates	Chest Wall Overall		Chest Wall T3N0 IIB		Chest Wall T3N1–N2 IIIA		Chest Wall CR/IR	
		n	5-yr	n	5-yr	n	5-yr	n	5-yr
Piehler et al. (1982)	1960–1980	56	33	26	54	19	7		
Allen et al (1991)	1973–1988	52	26	43	29	N1 9	11		
Casillas et al (1989)	1969–1986	97	23	58	34	N1 16 N2 23	8 6		
Mountain (1990)	1965–1982	31	39						
Watanabe et al. (1991)*	1973–1989	24	43						
Ratto et al. (1991)	1983–1988			14	47	N1 19 N2 22	22 0	CR 45 IR 10	16 0
Albertucci et al. (1992)*	1976–1988	37	30	21	41	N1 9 N2 7	29 0		
McCaughan (1994)	1974–1983	125	NS	45	56	N1 17 N2 42	35 16	CR 77 IR 48	40 0
Downey et al. (1999)	1974–1993	334	NS	100	49*	N1 24 N2 51	27 15	CR 175 IR 94	32 4
Chapelier et al. (2000)*	1981–1998	100	18	All 65 PP, DI – better survival for PP	22	N1 28 N2 7	9 0		
Facciolo et al. (2001)	1990–1999	104	61	All 77 PP 22 DI 70	63 90 54	N2 14	18		
Magdeleinat et al. (2001)	1984–1998	201	21	All 116 PP	25	NI 42 N2 21	21 20	CR 167 PP 66 DI 101 IR 34	24 37 15 13

The negative influence of lymph node metastasis or incomplete resection is apparent.
*Limited to complete resection.

n, number of cases; 5-yr, % survival at 5 years; CR, complete resection; IR, incomplete resection; PP, limited to parietal pleura; DI, deeper invasion; NS, not stated.

Modified from Locicero J, Ponn R, Daly B. Surgical treatment of nonsmall cell lung cancer. In: Shields T, Locicero J, Ponn R, eds. General thoracic surgery. Philadelphia: Lippincott Williams & Wilkins, 2000:1326.

patients will have 'limited' disease and two thirds will have 'extensive' disease.

In most cases, SCLC is sensitive to both chemotherapy and radiation therapy, and a majority of patients with limited disease achieve a complete response to chemotherapy. However, only 15–20% of limited-stage patients and few extensive-stage patients survive 3 years. Even fewer achieve a long-term cure. A number of chemotherapeutic agents are effective in this disease; those that are used most often in varying combinations include cyclophosphamide and doxorubicin and other agents such as vincristine, etoposide, carboplatin or cisplatin, and methotrexate (Table 8–16). Thus far, there has been no significant advantage shown with the use of alternating non-cross-resistant regimens or maintenance therapy after six cycles of initial therapy. Newer approaches include dose escalation of chemotherapy, possibly with autologous hematopoietic stem cell support.

Thoracic radiation therapy used in combination with chemotherapy to control local chest recurrence has been reported to offer a small, but significant disease-free survival benefit (5–15%) in patients with limited disease. However, it may increase the toxicity of chemotherapy and does not have a major benefit in patients with extensive disease.

Combined modality therapy with chemotherapy and concurrent radiotherapy is the accepted standard treatment for limited-stage SCLC. Surgery should be considered only for resection of a solitary pulmonary nodule and must be followed by adjuvant chemotherapy (Table 8–17). In addition, the resection of an unresponsive chest tumor is reasonable, because such lesions may harbor an NSCLC component or may prove to be carcinoid tumor. Addition of radiation to chemotherapy results in a modest but significant improvement in survival compared with chemotherapy alone.

Novel Therapies

Local treatments for airway disease involvement include laser therapy, brachytherapy, and photodynamic therapy. Laser therapy and brachytherapy are useful for the palliation of patients with obstructing airway lesions (Figure 8–30). Photodynamic therapy may be useful in early-stage endobronchial lesions where cure is attempted.

The Nd-YAG laser is used most commonly and the laser fiber is delivered through a rigid or flexible bronchoscope (Table 8–18). Control of endobronchial disease may be accomplished in over 50% of patients. Complications include hemoptysis, perforation, and hypoxemia.

Endobronchial brachytherapy involves the placement of an ionizing radioactive source into the airway through catheters placed adjacent to endobronchial tumors. Placement of the radioactive element is achieved through a high-dose-rate loading system in which a non-radioactive applicator (afterloading catheter) is first placed into the airway and the active source is then later inserted after proper placement of the catheter is verified. This technique eliminates exposure of medical personnel to radiation and allows treatment as an outpatient. Because of the rapid fall-off in radiation dose over a short distance, intense amounts of radiation may be delivered to the primary tumor site with relatively little radiation effect on normal tissues. The majority of patients treated with this technique will have symptomatic improvement in hemoptysis, cough, and dyspnea. Brachytherapy may also be curative in patients with localized endobronchial lesions.

TABLE 8–16 • *Chemotherapy for Small-Cell Lung Cancer*	
Drug	**Dosage and Schedule**
EP	
Etoposide	80–120 mg/m^2 days 1, 2, and 3
Cisplatin	60–90 mg/m^2 over 1–3 d
CAV	
Cyclophosphamide	1000 mg/m^2
Doxorubicin (Adriamycin)	50 mg/m^2
Vincristine	2 mg/m^2

TABLE 8–17 ● Trials of Adjuvant Systemic Chemotherapy in Resected Non-Small-Cell Lung Cancer

Series	n	Stage	Histology	Regimen	Median Survival Time (Months)	Significance	5-Year Survival (%)	Significance
LCSG 772	—	II–III	A, L	CAP				
				i.p. BCG				
LCSC 791	—	Incompletely resected	A, L, S	RT/CAP				
				RT				
LCSG 801	—	T1N1, T2N0	A, L, S	CAP	≈72	NS	≈55	NS
				None	≈72		≈58	
Niiranen	—	I–III	A, L, S	CAP	NA		67	p = 0.05
				None	NA		56	
Teramatsu	—		A, L, S	None			62.6 (3 years)	
				DDP/VDS then UFT			72.5 (3 years)	p = 0.082
				UFT			75.1 (3 years)	p = 0.038
Kimura	11	Curative	NSC	None	—		34.1 (4 years)	
	13			DDP/VDS	—		34.2 (4 years)	
	12			DDP/VDS/LAK/IL2	—		70.9 (4 years)	
	35	Noncurative	NSC	DDP/VDS	—		29.3 (4 years)	
	33			DDP/VDS/LAK/1L2	—		43.1 (4 years)	
Tsuchiya	91	III	NSC	None	No benefit		No benefit	
	90			DDP/VDS				

A, adenocarcinoma; CAP, cyclophosphamide doxorubicin, and cisplatin; DDP, cisplatin; IL2, interleukin-2; L, large-cell carcinoma; LAK, lymphokine-activated killer cells; NSC, non-small-cell carcinoma; RT, radiotherapy; S, squamous-cell carcinoma; UFT, tegafur plus uracil; V, vindesine.
From Roth JA, Ruckdeschel JC, Weisenburger TH. Thoracic oncology, 2nd ed. Philadelphia: WB Saunders, 1995:151.

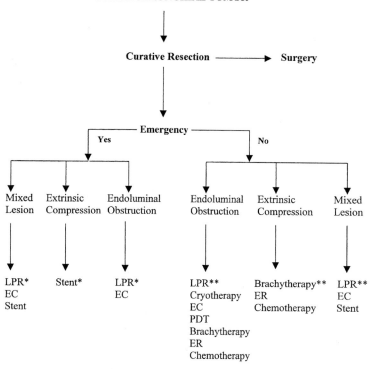

TRACHEOBRONCHIAL TUMOR

Figure 8–30. Algorithm for the management of tracheobronchial obstruction owing to a malignant tumor. Central airway obstruction by primary or metastatic lung cancer is often a medical emergency that requires immediate intervention. Often, curative resection by surgery is impossible owing to the advanced stage of the tumor and associated comorbidities. Therefore, interventional procedures are necessary to re-establish patency of the airway and to avoid the institution of mechanical ventilation as a result of respiratory failure. EC, electrocautery; ER, external beam irradiation; LPR, laser photoresection; PDT, photodynamic therapy. (From Lee P, Kupeli E, Mehta AC. Therapeutic bronchoscopy in lung cancer: laser therapy, electrocautery, brachytherapy, stents, and photodynamic therapy. *Clin Chest Med* 2002;23:242.)

*To be followed by Chemotherapy and/or ER

** Can be used singly or in combination

Photodynamic therapy involves the injection and subsequent uptake and selective retention of a hematoporphyrin derivative into tumor cells (Figure 8–31). This compound is then photoactivated by light at 630 nm to cause cell death. Patients with localized, stage I endobronchial lesions will do very well, with the majority having a complete response of the tumor to phototherapy. Further studies, however, are necessary to determine the long-term efficacy of this approach. Complications of this procedure include light sensitivity up to 2 months following treatment, hemoptysis, and endobronchial obstruction.

Surgical Management

Before considering a patient for surgical resection of a bronchogenic carcinoma, it must be determined that adequate pulmonary reserve exists. Simple spirometry and an arterial blood

TABLE 8-18 • *A Comparison of Laser Types Used in the Tracheobronchial Tree*					
	Carbon Dioxide	**Nd-YAG**	**Argon**	**KTP**	**Diode**
Wavelength (nm)	10 600	1060	488–514	532	805
Bronchoscope system	RB	RB/FB	RB/FB	RB/FB	FB
Tissue absorption	High	Low	Selective High in blood	Selective High in blood	Low
Tissue penetration (mm)	0.1	4	1	1	1–2
Coagulation	Low	High	Medium	Medium	Medium
Cutting effect	High	Low	Low	Low	Low

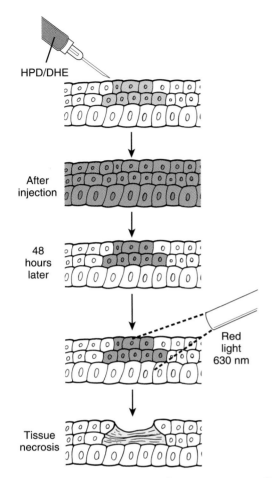

HPD/DHE

After
injection

48
hours
later

Red
light
630 nm

Tissue
necrosis

Figure 8–31. Photodynamic therapy. Tumor cells retain the photosensitizer 48–72 hours after its administration and undergo selective destruction by photoactivation upon exposure to 630 nm wavelength laser light. (Redrawn from Lee P, Kupeli E, Mehta AC. Therapeutic bronchoscopy in lung cancer: laser therapy, electrocautery, brachytherapy, stents, and photodynamic therapy. *Clin Chest Med* 2002; 23:252.)

gas measurement are the only tests routinely required. Patients with a forced expiratory volume in 1 second (FEV_1) of more than 60% predicted or more than 2.0 liters will probably tolerate a pneumonectomy. When pulmonary function does not appear to be evenly distributed between the right and left lungs, quantitative perfusion scanning, which correlates well with regional pulmonary function, may help estimate postoperative pulmonary function. Hypercarbia, unless solely on the basis of a low respiratory drive, is a predictor of poor postoperative outcome, but hypoxemia is not a strong indicator of poor outcome. The roles of exercise testing and pulmonary artery pressure measurement are unclear.

Surgery offers the best chance for curing appropriately staged patients with NSCLC. Patients with stages I–IIIA NSCLC are routinely considered for surgery, with 5-year survival rates ranging from 60–80% for patients with stage I disease to 15–25% for selected patients with stage IIIA disease. Since the late 1960s, operative mortality has dropped from 10–20% to approximately 3%. The incidence of needless thoracotomy, in which a lesion is discovered to be unresectable or inoperable at the time of operation, has decreased from 25% to approximately 5%. The increased use of lung-sparing resections, including sleeve lobectomy, segmentectomy, wedge resection, and thoracoscopic wedge resection, has allowed surgical therapy to be offered to a group of patients with less pulmonary reserve than in the past. Although a prospective trial comparing conventional lobectomy with wedge resection has demonstrated that local recurrence rates are higher with the latter procedure, wedge resection is still an acceptable compromise in patients with diminished pulmonary reserve.

Before a decision for surgical therapy is made in a given patient, three questions must be addressed.

- *Is the cell type NSCLC?* With the exception of peripheral solitary pulmonary nodules without hilar or mediastinal lymphadenopathy, a firm tissue diagnosis should almost always be obtained prior to surgical therapy. Owing to the rarity with which SCLC presents with stage I disease and the likelihood that surgical therapy benefits stage I patients, it may not be necessary to obtain tissue diagnosis for all patients in this group prior to surgical therapy.
- *Is the patient physiologically capable of tolerating resectional surgery?* General medical criteria, such as absence of a recent myocardial infarction, should be applied. In addition, physiologic assessment should determine whether the planned resection will leave the patient with adequate pulmonary reserve.
- *Can the lesion be completely resected?* This answer requires adequate staging with detection of both distant metastases and local lymph node involvement. As surgical therapy provides the best hope for long-term survival in NSCLC, physiologic assessment and staging should be accurate and objective.

Surgical procedures used include pneumonectomy, lobectomy, segmentectomy, wedge resection, and sleeve bronchoplasty. The last three procedures are considered to be parenchyma-sparing techniques helpful in patients with limited lung reserve. Local invasion of chest wall is not a contraindication to resection.

Prevention

Curative therapy in lung cancer is more likely in tumors diagnosed at an early, asymptomatic stage. Given that individuals at high risk for lung cancer can be identified (e.g. heavy smokers), it had been hoped that mass screening of this population through serial chest radiographs and sputum cytology would enable early diagnosis of tumors and allow for curative therapy. This idea led to three large trials at the Mayo Clinic, the Memorial Sloan–Kettering Cancer Center, and Johns Hopkins University in which male smokers over the age of 45 were screened with serial chest radiographs and sputum cytology. Although the trial showed a favorable impact on survival in patients with localized tumors and improved overall survival in both screened and control groups, there was no improvement in survival for the screened group as a whole. Thus currently there is no evidence that mass screening will have a beneficial effect on lung cancer. The use of spiral CT as a screening tool currently is being evaluated.

The most important preventive measure is deterring young individuals from starting to smoke. This public health issue is mainly a social, economic, and political problem. Increasing the cost of tobacco products, through increased taxes, is an effective strategy for keeping people from starting this habit. Negative advertising and measures that make it less socially acceptable and glamorous to smoke are also effective.

Smoking cessation is also an important strategy and results in a gradual decrease in risk for lung cancer over 10–15 years (see Figure 8–6). Approximately 5–20% of patients who enter a smoking cessation program are successful in the long term. Physician input is crucial in this process. Large trials in the 1970s that examined the value of early detection efforts using sputum cytology and chest radiographs as screening tools failed to show a benefit in terms of long-term survival. A shortcoming of these trials is that women and high-risk smokers were not studied. It is possible that early detection may become a viable strategy, espe-

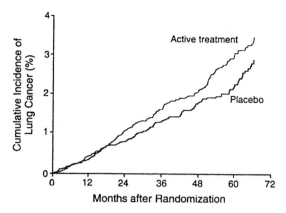

Figure 8–32. Cumulative incidence of lung cancer among participants receiving active treatment (beta-carotene and vitamin A) and those receiving placebo. (From Omenn GS, Goodman GE, Thornquist MD, *et al.* Effects of a combination of beta carotene and vitamin A on lung cancer and cardiovascular disease. *N Engl J Med* 1996;334:1150–1155.)

cially if improved screening tests are developed and high-risk groups are targeted.

Chemoprevention of lung cancer may be possible. The use of 13-*cis*-retinoic acid in patients with laryngeal cancer has been shown to decrease the incidence of second primary lesions in the aerodigestive system. However, the toxicity associated with high doses of this compound is significant. Vitamin A and its derivatives have potent effects on the differentiation of the respiratory epithelium and are logical agents for chemoprevention studies but several trials have demonstrated that dietary supplementation with beta-carotene alone or in combination with vitamin A or vitamin E actually increased rates of lung cancer in a susceptible population (Figure 8–32). These unexpected results emphasize the need for further controlled trials. Additional micronutrients, including selenium, vitamins C and E, and low-dose 13-*cis*-retinoic acid, may have protective effects. Because of the large reservoir of smokers and ex-smokers at risk, chemoprevention has considerable potential.

Key Readings

Curran WJ Jr. Therapy of limited stage small cell lung cancer. *Cancer Treat Res* 2001;105:229–252. *Readable summary of current management of small cell lung cancer.*

Hyer JD, Silvestri G. Diagnosis and staging of lung cancer. *Clin Chest Med* 2000;21:95–106, viii–ix. *Excellent review of the studies that go into staging lung cancer.*

Roth JA, Ruckdeschel JC, Weisenburger TH. *Thoracic oncology*, 2nd ed. Philadelphia: WB Saunders, 1995. *Excellent textbook that has information including everything you would want to know about lung cancer.*

Selected Readings

Arcasoy SM, Jett JR. Superior pulmonary sulcus tumors and Pancoast's syndrome. *N Engl J Med* 1997;337:1370–1376.

Edell ES. Diagnostic tests for lung cancer. *Curr Opin Pulm Med* 1997;3:247–251.

Siefkin AD. Treatment of bronchogenic carcinoma. *Curr Opin Pulm Med* 1995;1:253–264.

Spiliopoulos A, de Perrot M. Four decades of surgery for bronchogenic carcinoma in one centre. *Eur Respir J* 2000;15:543–546.

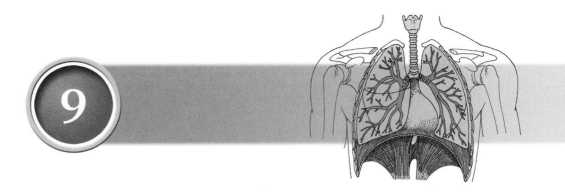

9

Non-Bronchogenic Pulmonary Neoplasms

CARCINOID

SARCOMA

BENIGN LUNG TUMORS

Non-Bronchogenic Pulmonary Neoplasms: Key Points

- Describe the presentation, evaluation, and management of pulmonary carcinoids
- Be familiar with the spectrum of benign lung tumors

Two other malignant tumors of the pulmonary system should be discussed: carcinoid and sarcoma. Carcinoids are a unique category of tumors of neuroendocrine differentiation that are capable on occasion of producing neuropeptides. Pulmonary sarcomas are comparatively rare.

Most benign tumors of the lung are also rare neoplasms. Although many of these lesions present as solitary pulmonary nodules, and occasionally as multiple nodules, slightly fewer than 15% of such nodules are benign neoplasms. The classification of benign tumors remains controversial because of the disagreement regarding the origin and prognosis of some of the most common lesions. A modification of the classification proposed originally by Liebow (1952) seems to be the simplest and most elegant scheme and serves our purposes

well (Box 9–1). The Liebow classification organizes lesions according to their presumed origin, whether epithelial or mesodermal. A number of benign lesions must be classified as unknown in origin and some as inflammatory.

Carcinoid

Lung tumors with neuroendocrine differentiation comprise a diverse group of clinical entities that are linked by their cellular origin. Together they share the capacity to produce a range of neuropeptides (neuron-specific enolase, chromogranin, synaptophysin, serotonin [5-hydroxytryptophan, 5-HT], and bombesin) that are stored within and released from cytoplasmic neuroendocrine granules. Additionally, the cells of these tumors tend to be arranged in orderly

BOX 9–1 LIEBOW CLASSIFICATION OF BENIGN LUNG TUMORS

Epithelial Tumor
- Papilloma
- Polyps

Mesodermal Tumor
- Fibroma
- Lipoma
- Leiomyoma
- Chondroma
- Granular cell tumor
- Sclerosing hemangioma

Origin Unknown
- Hamartoma
- Clear-cell tumor
- Teratoma

Other
- Inflammatory myofibroblastic tumor (i.e. inflammatory pseudotumor)
- Xanthoma
- Amyloid
- Mucosa-associated lymphoid tumor

arrangements such as nests, cords, or rosettes (Figure 9–1).

Typical Bronchial Carcinoid

'Typical' bronchial carcinoid is a well differentiated low-grade malignant neuroendocrine tumor responsible for up to 2% of all lung cancers. There is a slight female predominance and, while peak incidence is in the fifth decade, carcinoids have been described in the first through the ninth decade of life. There are no known predisposing risk factors. Most bronchial carcinoids are found in the central airways, with approximately 75% in lobar bronchi, 10% in main-stem bronchi, and rare tracheal tumors. The remaining tumors, up to 20% in some series, are peripheral lung lesions probably originating in distal airways.

An unusually wide spectrum of clinical presentations has been described in patients with bronchial carcinoid tumors. Carcinoids most often give rise to obstructive or postobstructive symptoms, as would be expected given their endobronchial location. Specifically, patients often complain of wheezing, cough, and dyspnea or recurrent episodes of 'bronchitis' or pneumonia. Hemoptysis is also common, because of the vascular nature of the lesion, and may be the presenting symptom. In addition, a variety of paraneoplastic syndromes have been reported but are rare with this tumor.

The most frequently observed syndromes include the carcinoid syndrome from serotonin secretion, Cushing's syndrome from adrenocorticotropic hormone (ACTH) secretion, and acromegaly from growth-hormone-releasing hormone (GHRH) secretion. The carcinoid syndrome consists of episodic flushing, wheezing, and diarrhea, sometimes accompanied by fibrous thickening of the right-side heart valves. The resulting stenotic and regurgitant valvular lesions can produce significant right-sided heart failure and are believed to result from chemical trauma to the endocardium from circulating serotonin and other biogenic amines normally detoxified by

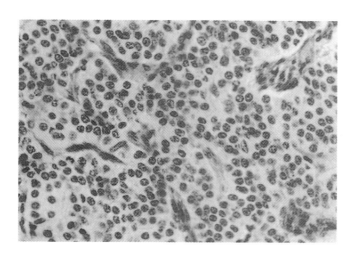

Figure 9–1. Carcinoid. Note the solid organoid architecture, relative cellular uniformity, and delicate fibrovascular stroma. Hematoxylin and eosin, ×1050. (From Roth JA, Ruckdeschel JC, Weisenburger TH. *Thoracic oncology*, 2nd ed. Philadelphia: WB Saunders, 1995:55.)

the liver. The carcinoid syndrome seldom occurs (< 5%) with bronchial tumors and is exceedingly rare in the absence of hepatic metastases. Finally, many patients with carcinoid tumors are completely asymptomatic.

The chest radiograph findings, while nonspecific, may be suggestive of carcinoid. Up to 90% of patients will have abnormal findings on plain chest x-ray. Most often there is evidence of volume loss or complete segmental or lobar atelectasis due to endobronchial obstruction. When the carcinoid tumor is located in the lung periphery, it presents as a solitary pulmonary nodule. While the computed tomography (CT) appearance of carcinoid is also nonspecific, several findings when present should enhance clinical suspicion. Both central and peripheral lesions often have diffuse or punctate calcifications and typically enhance uniformly following administration of intravenous contrast, because of their vascularity. The CT is also occasionally useful for identifying a small peripheral carcinoid in a perplexing patient with ectopic Cushing's syndrome and a normal chest x-ray, or when carcinoid-induced Cushing's syndrome must be distinguished from pituitary-dependent Cushing's syndrome, which can be very difficult on an endocrine basis alone.

Several diagnostic approaches can be considered but flexible fiberoptic bronchoscopy is the most frequently successful. Bronchoscopic examination often reveals a cherry red, fleshy, and smooth endobronchial lesion. Endobronchial biopsy is both safe and effective, with a diagnostic yield of approximately 85%. Concerns regarding hemorrhage following biopsy, due to the vascular nature of these tumors, have probably been overstated, and endobronchial biopsy can be performed safely in most patients if proper technique and precautions are employed. Sputum cytology is rarely diagnostic, since few cells are shed into the tracheobronchial tree owing to the intact mucosal surface overlying most carcinoids. Fine-needle aspiration of either central or peripheral lesions can occasionally provide diagnostic cytologic samples. If the carcinoid syndrome is suspected, elevation of a urinary serotonin metabolite, 5-hydroxyindoleacetic acid, can confirm the presence of a carcinoid tumor.

Histologically, carcinoids appear to arise in the bronchial submucosa from Kulchitsky cells. In general, the tumor cells are small and polygonal, with eosinophilic cytoplasm, finely stippled chromatin and round nuclei.

They are classically grouped into orderly nests. Characteristically, carcinoids will have positive immunohistochemical stains for neuron-specific enolase, chromogranin, synaptophysin, and serotonin. Typical carcinoids, which comprise approximately 90% of all carcinoids, are well differentiated tumors with few mitotic figures and minimal or no necrosis.

The treatment of choice is complete resection, consisting of segmental resection or lobectomy with lymph node removal. A resection margin of 0.5 cm is sufficient, as these tumors invade adjacent tissue less than most other lung cancers. Such procedures have resulted in low recurrence rates and excellent long-term survival. In general, endobronchial resection is not curative because of the submucosal invasion of the tumor; however, there may be a small subset of patients with typical intraluminal carcinoid who can be treated using endobronchial techniques. At present most authorities recommend that endobronchial resection be reserved for palliation in patients not suitable for surgery. Somatostatin receptors are found in up to 80% of carcinoid tumors. Octreotide has recently proven useful in imaging and controlling metastatic carcinoid and the carcinoid syndrome, seen mainly in abdominal carcinoid tumors.

Atypical Bronchial Carcinoids

Atypical carcinoids are much less common, higher-grade tumors that are less well differentiated, with increased mitotic activity, nuclear atypia, and evidence of necrosis. These tumors appear to represent an intermediate group between typical carcinoid tumors and small-cell lung cancers. Clinically, atypical carcinoids occur in an older age group, demonstrate a higher rate of metastasis at presentation, and result in a much lower 5-year survival rate compared to typical carcinoids. This tumor often exhibits immense size and invasion of lung parenchyma, nerves, and pericardium (Figure 9–2). Surgical resection with formal pulmonary resection and mediastinal nodal staging should be performed. There does appear to be a strong correlation with smoking. Whether surgical resection alone is sufficient treatment for the more aggressive atypical carcinoids is a matter of debate. Some authors advocate adjuvant chemotherapy in addition to lobectomy for these tumors but there are no good data supporting this contention. Unfortunately,

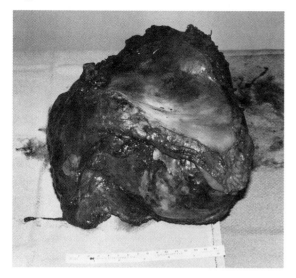

Figure 9–2. Resected atypical carcinoid from a 33-year-old who presented with pleuritic chest pain and shortness of breath. (From Sheppard BB, Follette DM, Meyers FJ. Giant carcinoid tumor of the lung. *Ann Thorac Surg* 1997;63:851–852.)

standard chemotherapy and radiation therapy have generally yielded poor results and resection remains the gold standard. These lesions are clinically identical to 'typical' carcinoids and the diagnosis is made based on histological criteria. The World Health Organization has recently endorsed a new classification of the neuroendocrine lung lesions that includes the entire spectrum of these lesions .

Sarcoma

Pulmonary sarcomas may originate within a main stem or lobar bronchus, peripherally within the pulmonary parenchyma, or from major vessels. By far the most common sarcoma seen within the lung is metastatic from another source; primary sarcomas of the lung comprise a mix of extraordinarily rare lesions. The most prominent of these is AIDS-related Kaposi's sarcoma. Other prominent primary pulmonary sarcomas include malignant fibrous histiocytoma, fibrosarcoma, and leiomyosarcoma. These tumors are usually large, solitary, and may or may not be symptomatic. Chondrosarcoma, liposarcoma, myxosarcoma, rhabdomyosarcoma, synovial sarcoma, neurogenic sarcoma, Ewing's sarcoma, and osteogenic sarcoma also may occur as primary lung neoplasms.

Pulmonary vascular sarcomas are of special interest because of their tendency to mimic chronic thromboembolic disease, sometimes with additional features of weight loss, anemia, and fever. Diagnosis may be facilitated by CT and magnetic resonance imaging (MRI) scans, allowing for occasional surgical cure (Figure 9–3).

Malignant fibrous histiocytoma of the lung is an aggressive sarcoma, usually presenting as a solitary mass. The tumor is characterized by a mixture of fibroblasts and histiocytes in a storiform pattern. Surgery is the treatment of choice, and the role of adjuvant therapy remains undefined. A primary site elsewhere should be ruled out.

Benign Lung Tumors

Benign lung tumors are uncommon, accounting for only 2% of pulmonary neoplasms. Benign lung tumors are classified according to their cell line of origin. Benign pulmonary tumors are symptomatic if they cause bronchial obstruction. Hemoptysis occurs rarely. Most benign lung lesions are detected on routine chest films and require resection to rule out malignancy. A brief overview of the most common neoplasms will be discussed.

Hamartoma

Hamartoma is the most frequent benign neoplasm of the lung. The pathogenesis is currently believed to entail clonal proliferations of mesenchymal elements. Tumors are typically composed of cartilage, fibromyxoid stroma, and adipose tissue, along with incorporated bronchiolar epithelium and less common diverse elements such as bone or hair. Hamartomas occur more frequently in men and the mean age at presentation is in the sixth decade, with only rare detection before the third decade of life. Overall, the prevalence of hamartomas is 0.25% in the general population; however, many cases go unrecognized and are found only at autopsy.

Hamartomas typically present as a solitary pulmonary nodule, usually discovered incidentally on chest films or during the course of a surgical procedure for another indication. Most patients are completely asymptomatic. An exception is the endobronchial hamartoma, which represents less than 20% of cases. Patients with endobronchial hamartomas often complain of cough, dyspnea, wheezing, and

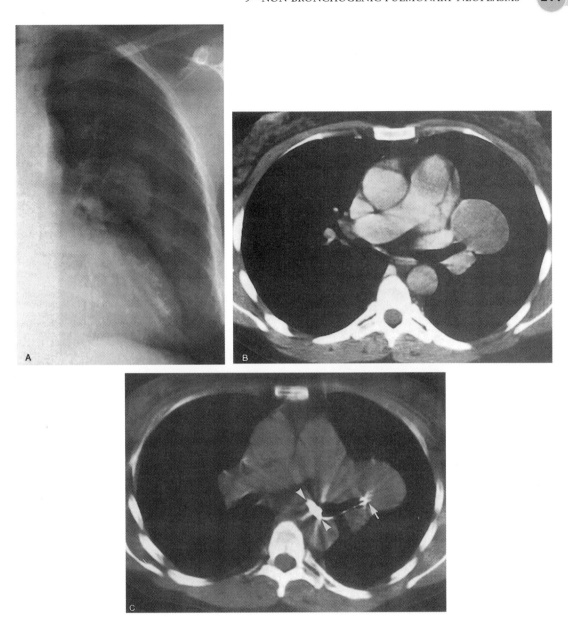

Figure 9–3. Pulmonary sarcoma simulating a bronchogenic cyst in a 26-year-old female 6 years after renal transplantation. **A**, Chest radiograph demonstrates a well-defined, round, 5 cm mass in the left hilum. **B**, Computed tomography (CT) scan shows that the mass is homogeneous and contacts the left upper lobe bronchus. **C**, CT-guided transbronchial biopsy. The end of the bronchoscope (arrowheads) is visible. The tip of the Wang transbronchial biopsy needle (arrow) is shown entering the mass. Cytologic examination demonstrated malignant cells. The diagnosis of pulmonary sarcoma was made from the pneumonectomy specimen. (From Moss AA, Gamsu G, Genant HK. Computed tomography of the body: with magnetic resonance imaging, 2nd ed. Philadelphia: WB Saunders, 1992:198.)

occasionally hemoptysis. The rare mesenchymal cystic variant is also typically symptomatic.

Radiographically, hamartomas are usually solitary, but multiple nodules have been reported in up to 3% of cases. The nodules are typically smooth, lobulated peripheral lesions, approximately 0.5–3 cm in diameter. These tumors grow very slowly, with a mean increase in diameter of 3–5 mm per year, occasionally enlarging to 10 cm in diameter. Classically, hamartomas have an eccentric 'popcorn' calcification pattern. Unfortunately, this is seen by plain chest radiograph in only 10% of cases (Figure 9–4). Calcification can been seen more frequently and to better advantage with CT of the chest (Figure 9–5). These scans may also

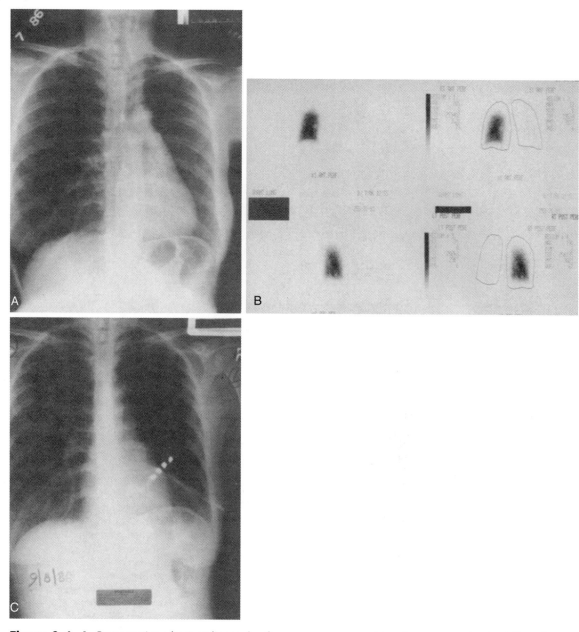

Figure 9–4. A, Preoperative chest radiograph of a young woman with a hamartoma in the left mainstem bronchus. Note the loss of volume evident on the left as manifested by the mediastinal shift and the hyperinflation of the right lung. **B**, Perfusion lung scan of the same patient demonstrating significantly diminished blood flow to the left lung. **C**, Following bronchoscopic removal of the hamartoma, the chest radiograph returns to a completely normal appearance. (From Pearson FG, Cooper JD, Deslauriers J, *et al. Thoracic surgery*, 2nd ed. New York: Churchill Livingstone, 2002:755.)

reveal central fat within the lesion, a distinctive and characteristic finding in hamartoma.

Definitive diagnosis is important to exclude malignancy. However, an argument for close observation can be made in nonsmokers with the classical radiographic features of hamartoma. If a diagnostic workup is pursued, then transthoracic needle aspiration should be con-

sidered, as it has a proven diagnostic yield of greater than 85%.

Biopsy-proven hamartomas can be safely observed without specific therapy. Excision is warranted in symptomatic patients or when lesions demonstrate significant growth. Lung-sparing surgical resection is the treatment of choice, since hamartomas rarely recur. Usually

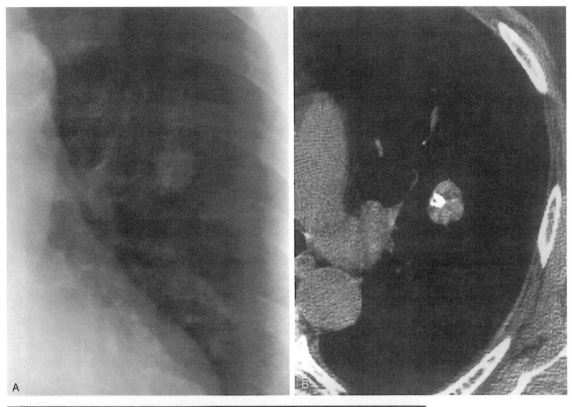

Y\X	358	359	360	361	362	363	364	365	366
297	71	252	183	10	-90	45	63	-4	-34
298	-26	113	82	-24	-86	13	35	30	40
299	80	114	210	89	-63	4	0	28	4
300	267	225	353	162	12	45	60	61	66
301	849	799	548	140	6	10	47	11	7
302	1117	1166	440	-55	-40	-43	-15	14	60
303	367	266	149	-31	-58	-46	-16	22	75
304	24	-40	-50	-50	-7	24	40	20	36
305	-3	-67	-64	-31	23	30	-7	23	31

Figure 9–5. Pulmonary hamartoma. **A,** Chest radiograph shows a 2.5 cm left lung nodule. **B,** High-resolution computed tomography (CT) scan shows the nodule containing dense calcification and adjacent low-density fat. **C,** A region-of-interest chart from within the nodule demonstrates CT numbers up to 1166 H, indicating calcification, and negative numbers as low as −58 H, indicating fat within the nodule. (From Moss AA, Gamsu G, Genant HK. *Computed tomography of the body: with magnetic resonance imaging*, 2nd ed. Philadelphia: WB Saunders, 1992:182.)

these lesions can be enucleated without sacrificing lung parenchyma. No additional adjuvant therapy is required for the typical case.

Clear-Cell Tumor of the Lung

Clear-cell tumors of the lung are rare neoplasms in which patients present with a peripheral solitary pulmonary nodules usually noted incidentally on a plain chest radiograph. Most patients are in their 40s or 50s. Until recently these tumors were universally considered benign, although there is an isolated case report of a patient who died from metastatic clear-cell tumor of the lung.

These tumors bear a resemblance to metastatic renal cell carcinoma. Clear-cell tumors are characterized by sheets and cords of polygonal cells separated by a prominent fibrovascular stroma. The 'clear cells' may indeed have a clear cytoplasm but they often have a granular eosinophilic cytoplasm. Based on their intense periodic-acid–Schiff positivity, the granules are most likely glycogen, and the eosinophilic appearance of the cytoplasm is imparted when granules are present in large numbers. The nuclei are characteristically bland and vary in size; mitoses are usually absent. Although not distinctly encapsulated, the lesions easily 'shell out' of the surrounding lung tissue, are usually peripherally located, and generally are 2 cm or less in size. Immunohistochemical analysis allows for the definitive diagnosis of clear-cell tumors of the lung and their distinction from renal cell carcinomas.

Inflammatory Pseudotumor

Inflammatory pseudotumor (IPT, myofibro-blastic tumor) of the lung is an uncommon lesion of unknown cause. Considerable controversy attends even the most basic questions regarding this entity, such as whether it is a localized inflammatory response or a low-grade primary lung neoplasm. As a result of such uncertainty, various names have been applied to this lesion, including plasma cell granuloma, histiocytoma, xanthoma, and fibroxanthoma; most recently, the term myofibroblastic tumor has been used, emphasizing the low-grade neoplastic behavior of these tumors.

From a clinical standpoint, IPT is remarkably diverse. There is no predisposition of sex or race but most patients are less than 40 years of age. Symptoms have been reported in 20–75% patients with IPT but are truly difficult to estimate given that many asymptomatic patients may never come to medical attention. When present, symptoms may include cough, fever, dyspnea, wheezing, chest pain, or hemoptysis. Radiographically, IPT is an important mimic of bronchogenic carcinoma: it can have mass lesions 1–10 cm in diameter accompanied by hilar and mediastinal adenopathy, pleural effusion, and/or airway involvement with distal atelectasis. The diagnosis is often made via surgical biopsy for suspected lung cancer. Several series have described invasion of other adjacent structures such as pulmonary vessels, diaphragm, pericardium, esophagus, and thoracic vertebrae; a paraneoplastic dermatomyositis-like presentation has also been recognized on occasion.

The etiology of IPT remains controversial. The finding of an antecedent upper respiratory infection in up to one half of all patients has led some to believe that IPT represents an aberrant response to tissue injury. However, the presence of local invasion in up to 50% of cases and evidence of clonal chromosomal abnormalities has led many to support a neoplastic origin.

Treatment is primarily surgical, although some lesions have been known to regress spontaneously. Local recurrence, while uncommon, has been attributed to incomplete excision of the primary lesion. The overall prognosis is excellent; in those few cases where the lesion is not amenable to excision, there may be a role for medical therapy including radiation, chemotherapy, or steroids.

Papilloma

Papillomas are the most common juvenile laryngeal tumor but are rare in adults. Lesions may be single, multiple, or present as diffuse papillomatosis that extends down the tracheobronchial tree into the lungs to obstruct the airway. More proximal lesions consist of squamous cell epithelium on a tissue stalk while more distal papillomas may have lining cells resembling clear cells. Recent data suggest some relationship to human papillomavirus, especially for the squamous-cell type.

In adults, a solitary lesion is typical, presenting as an endobronchial tumor less than 1.5 cm in diameter in a segmental or lobar bronchus. Bronchial papillomas very rarely precede laryngeal or tracheal lesions or develop in their absence. Alternatively, a polypoid inflammatory mass may be seen, related to exuberant granulation tissue secondary to chronic irritation, as from an embedded foreign body. Cellular atypia and the uncertain risk of carcinomatous degeneration have been cited to justify the usual advice for surgical extirpation. Clinically, patients present with chronic cough, hemoptysis, wheeze, and recurrent pneumonia. Although chest radiographs are usually nondiagnostic, the diagnosis is easily made by fiberoptic bronchoscopy and biopsy. Treatment consists of bronchoscopic resection, although the recurrence rate is high. Parenchymal lesions require a sleeve resection to preserve normal lung parenchyma.

Hemangioma

Hemangiomas are benign mesodermal tumors, usually solitary lesions although they present as multiple lesions in one third of cases. The diagnoses of hereditary hemorrhagic telangiectasia and Rendu–Osler–Weber syndrome should be entertained in these patients. Histologically, hemangiomas appear as thin-walled vessels (Figure 9–6). These occur frequently in the trachea or bronchi; however, they do appear in the peripheral lung parenchyma. Individual hemangiomas tend to be sharply circumscribed with a round margin averaging 3 cm in diameter. The interventional radiologist can usually obliterate these lesions with metal coils but occasionally excision is required, depending on the size and location. Endobronchial lesions are best managed by YAG laser therapy followed by radiation therapy on occasion for any residual disease. Endoscopic resection is risky because of the chance of severe bleeding.

Fibroma

Extremely rare, benign fibromas arise from the peripheral lung parenchyma or from the tracheal and bronchial walls. Peripheral fibromas are generally asymptomatic but endobronchial lesions produce symptoms due to obstruction. Endobronchial lesions should be removed bronchoscopically or by YAG laser, if possible. Surgical excision rarely is required.

Chondroma

Chondromas are benign tumors of cartilage chiefly notable for their association with extraadrenal paraganglioma and gastric stromal sarcoma in Carney syndrome. They are slow growing tumors seen mainly in young women. Histologically, the lesion consists of cartilage covered with epithelium without glands. The majority of endobronchial lesions are in the middle third of the tracheobronchial tree adjacent to a large bronchus. Symptoms develop from mass effect on the bronchus. The treatment of choice is endobronchial resection of

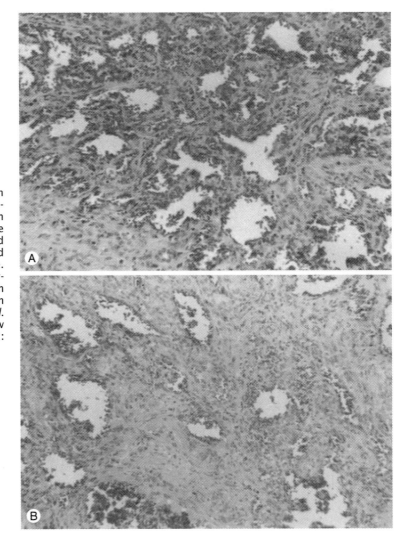

Figure 9–6. A, Histologic section of sclerosing hemangioma demonstrating the vascular pattern marked by the finding of multiple dilated vascular spaces often filled with blood cells and surrounded by tumor cells of fibrous tissue. **B,** Sclerosing hemangioma showing a pattern more consistent with the fibrous type. (From Pearson FG, Cooper JD, Deslauriers J, *et al. Thoracic surgery*, 2nd ed. New York: Churchill Livingstone, 2002: 756.)

those lesions occurring endobronchially and conservative wedge resection of peripheral chondromas.

Lipoma

Benign lipomas occur endobronchially 80% of the time with the remainder in the pulmonary parenchyma. These lesions are slow-growing and histologically benign. Endobronchial lesions are often dumbbell-shaped with a narrow neck lying between the submucosa and lumen position. The majority of intrapleural lipomas lie in the right cardiophrenic angle. Some 90% of these lesions occur in middle-aged men, although they have been noted in females. Therapy consists of tumor removal. Prognosis is excellent.

Leiomyoma

Lung leiomyomas are rare benign tumors. Less than 100 cases have been reported in the literature to date. These tumors are known to occur in the proximal bronchi and parenchyma. Patients typically present in their fourth decade. Surgical resection is the treatment of choice, although laser ablation of endobronchial tumors can be attempted.

Granular Cell Tumor

Granular cell tumors, formerly called myoblastomas and now perhaps more appropriately called schwannomas, may occur as solitary pulmonary nodules or in the trachea or main stem bronchi, occasionally as multiple lesions. Despite the name, skeletal muscle cells are not identified in most myoblastomas. The cells potentially represent granular degeneration of perineural fibroblasts. They occur with equal frequency in both sexes, and the median age of patients with these tumors is 38 years, younger than the typical age of patients with endobronchial malignancies. Patients typically present with cough or other symptoms suggestive of bronchial obstruction; hemoptysis occurs occasionally. Treatment ranges from bronchoscopic removal to open, anatomic resection.

Key Readings

Brambilla E, Lantuejoul S, Sturm N. Divergent differentiation in neuroendocrine lung tumors. *Semin Diagn Pathol* 2000;17:138–148. *Most recent update of the WHO classification.*

Oldham HN Jr. Benign tumors of the lung and bronchus. *Surg Clin North Am* 1980;60:825–834. *Attempt to provide a complete overview of the diverse tumor of the lung.*

Selected Readings

Hansen CP, Holtveg H, Francis D, *et al.* Pulmonary hamartoma. *J Thorac Cardiovasc Surg* 1992;104:674–678.

Gould VE, Warren WH. Epithelial tumors of the lung. *Chest Surg Clin North Am* 2000;10:709–728.

Liebow AA, Castleman B. Benign clear cell tumors of the lung. *Am J Pathol* 1963;43:13a.

Porte HL, Metois DG, Leroy X, *et al.* Surgical treatment of primary sarcoma of the lung. *Eur J Cardio-Thorac Surg* 2000;18:136–142.

Sheppard BB, Follette DM, Meyers FJ. Giant carcinoid tumor of the lung. *Ann Thorac Surg* 1997;63:851–852.

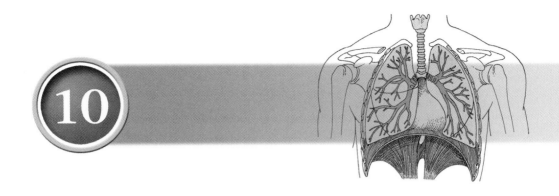

10

Surgery for Emphysema

Sunil Singhal, Joseph Shrager* and Larry R. Kaiser

PATHOPHYSIOLOGY

MEDICAL THERAPY

LUNG VOLUME REDUCTION
SURGERY

TRANSPLANTATION

CONCLUSION

Surgery for Emphysema: Key Points

- Review the pathophysiology of developing emphysema
- Know therapeutic options for patients with emphysema
- Understand the selection criteria requisite to lung volume reduction surgery
- Outline two surgical techniques for lung volume reduction surgery
- List the controversial issues surrounding lung volume reduction surgery

Lung volume reduction surgery (LVRS) is an operation that was initially proposed and abandoned in the late 1950s but was revived as a surgical treatment for patients with severe emphysema – a disease for which there are few other viable therapeutic options. By surgically excising a portion of the diseased lung tissue, the elastic recoil of the remaining lung is improved, resulting in increased expiratory airflow. Respiratory muscles are allowed to

operate at less of a mechanical disadvantage, resulting in increased inspiratory force and decreased dyspnea.

Otto Brantigan was the first to attempt therapeutic resection of pulmonary parenchyma in patients with diffuse, nonbullous emphysema. He noted that all areas of the lungs were not involved equally by the pathologic process and that those areas with the greatest amount of destruction were essentially functionless in terms of gas exchange. Furthermore, he noted that the circumferential pull holding the bronchioles open is significantly impaired in the markedly hyperinflated, emphysematous lung, which is essentially 'stuffed' into an undersized thoracic cavity. Brantigan designed his operation

*The authors thank Joseph B. Shrager, M.D., Chief, Section of General Thoracic Surgery, Hospital of the University of Pennsylvania, Philadelphia, Pennsylvania, for his contribution to this chapter.

of lung reduction to remove functionless lung tissue that was only contributing to volume. To the volume reduction he added a denervation procedure by lysing vagal nerve branches and branches from the sympathetic system. Reduction in lung volume was accomplished by resecting or plicating areas of the lung that were 'most useless as respiratory tissue.' His goal was to reduce the lung volume such that it would match the size of the pleural cavity on full expiration.

Brantigan postulated that, by reducing the lung volume, one could:

- Restore the radial traction on the terminal bronchioles and thereby reduce expiratory airflow obstruction
- Elevate the diaphragm to a more normal anatomic position and contour and thereby improve its function
- Ameliorate hyperexpansion of the rib cage and thus improve intercostal muscle function.

Pathophysiology

Emphysema is best defined in anatomic terms and is recognized pathologically as enlargement of alveoli and destruction of their walls, causing them to become confluent and forming grossly oversized air spaces (Figure 10–1). Emphysema is further characterized as having

an absence of obvious fibrosis, thus differentiating it from primary fibrotic processes that can enlarge airspaces. Centriacinar emphysema, the pattern usually associated with smoking, most commonly involves the upper lobes and the superior segments of the lower lobes and may be quite focal (Figure 10–2). Panacinar emphysema more often affects the basilar segments and is usually seen in patients with alpha-1-antitrypsin deficiency.

Although the distinction can be murky, emphysema is usually distinguished from chronic bronchitis (the other form of chronic obstructive pulmonary disease or COPD; Table 10–1). In so-called 'pure' emphysema the airflow obstruction results from disease of the lung parenchyma and produces the classic 'pink puffer.' In predominant chronic bronchitis, obstruction results from intrinsic disease of the airways and presents clinically as the 'blue bloater.' Certainly, most patients present a combination of these two forms of COPD, demonstrating variable degrees of both airway and alveolar disease. Airway narrowing resulting from the structural abnormalities of

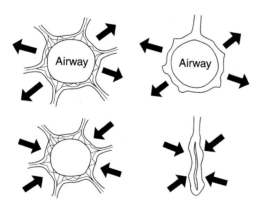

Figure 10–1. Airway collapse leading to flow limitation in emphysematous lungs (right). Normal airway (left) remains patent during expiration (below) because of the tethering forces of intact alveolar walls. Emphysematous airways (right) collapse during expiration (below) because the normal alveolar structures have collapsed. Arrows represent forces on airway during inspiration (above) and expiration (below). (From Hill NS. Current concepts in mechanical ventilation for chronic obstructive pulmonary disease. *Semin Respir Crit Care Med* 1999;20:375–393.)

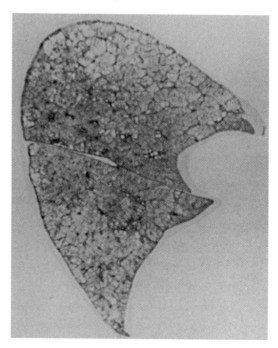

Figure 10–2. Mounted section of inflation-fixed left lung showing centrilobular emphysema. The disruption of respiratory air spaces is present in the basilar segments of the left lower lobe and lingula but is locally most severe in the apical-posterior segment of the upper lobe and superior segment of lower lobe. (From Snider GL. *Clinical pulmonary medicine.* Boston: Little, Brown & Co., 1981.)

TABLE 10-1 • *Diffuse Obstructive Emphysema*

Characteristics (Parameter)	Type A	Type B
Synonyms	Dry emphysema; 'pink puffer'	Wet emphysema; 'blue bloater'
Subjective		
Dyspnea	Severe	Usually severe
Cough	Occasional	Severe
Wheeze	Absent usually	Severe
Sputum	Scant, mucoid	Copious, often purulent
Physical		
Breath sounds	Distant	Rales and wheezes
Cyanosis	None	Frequent
Radiographic findings	Diffuse hyperinflation Bullae	Pulmonary fibrosis
Airway resistance and work of breathing	Severely increased	Severely increased
Maximal breathing capacity and FEV_1	Severely reduced	Severely reduced
Pulmonary volumes		
Vital capacity	Slightly reduced	Severely reduced
Residual volume	Severely increased	Moderately increased
Total lung capacity	Increased	Normal
Blood gases		
Po_2	Slightly reduced	Severely reduced
Pco_2	Slightly reduced	Elevated
Diffusion capacity	Severely reduced	Slightly reduced
Polycythemia	Rare	Frequent
Cor pulmonale	Rare	Frequent
Prognosis for longevity	Fairly good	Quite poor
Pathologic appearance	Usually panacinar	Usually centriacinar

Adapted from Knudson RJ, Gaensler EA. Surgery for emphysema – collective review. *Ann Thorac Surg* 1965;1:332.

emphysema fits nicely into the conceptual framework of how volume reduction surgery might be effective. However, it is difficult to conceptualize how airflow obstruction resulting from intrinsic narrowing of the airways such as that seen in chronic bronchitis might benefit from LVRS. Therefore, there has been rekindled interest recently in distinguishing the respective roles of emphysema and chronic bronchitis in the clinical syndrome of COPD.

Most groups have sought to apply LVRS to patients whose COPD is predominantly of the emphysema type. Both centriacinar and panacinar emphysema are associated with lost of elastin, and possibly collagen, in the lung tissue. Elastin is a rubber-like polymer that is the principal component of the elastic fibers that make up a large part of the extracellular matrix of the lung. From elastin the lung derives the important elastic properties that help determine static lung volumes, are responsible for passive exhalation, and are critical to maintaining patent airways.

According to the most widely held theory of the pathogenesis of emphysema – the proteinase–antiproteinase hypothesis – patients with emphysema have an imbalance between proteinases and antiproteinases in favor of the former. The proteinases are derived from inflammatory cells, which are particularly abundant in smokers. The antiproteinases, particularly alpha-1-antitrypsin, are normally abundant in the lung but may be reduced in emphysema patients. With an imbalance of elastases over anti-elastases and collagenases over anticollagenases, the lung elastin and/or collagen are thought to be reduced, resulting in emphysema (Figure 10–3).

Expiratory airflow obstruction occurs late in the course of the disease and is reflected most accurately in decrements of the forced expiratory volume in 1 second (FEV_1). With loss of elastin, a number of elastic properties that are important to normal airflow are compromised. First, the elastic recoil of the lung, which in normal patients renders quiet exhalation a

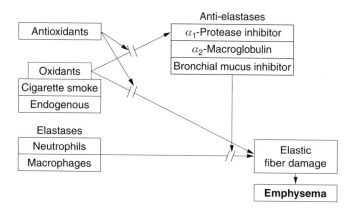

Figure 10–3. Schematic drawing of the elastase–anti-elastase hypothesis of emphysema. The lung is protected from elastolytic damage by alpha-1-protease inhibitor and alpha-2-macroglobulin. Bronchial mucous inhibitor protects the airways. Elastase is derived primarily from neutrophils but macrophages secrete an elastase-like metalloprotease and may ingest and later release neutrophil elastase. Oxidants derived from neutrophils and macrophages or from cigarette smoke may inactivate alpha-1-protease inhibitor and may interfere with lung matrix repair. Endogenous antioxidants such as superoxide dismutase, glutathione, and catalase protect the lung against oxidant injury. (From Snider, GL. Experimental studies on emphysema and chronic bronchial injury. *Eur J Respir Dis* 1986;69(Suppl. 146):17–35.)

passive process, is greatly diminished in severe emphysema. In addition to reducing the driving pressure favoring exhalation, this loss of elastic recoil allows progressive overexpansion of the lung, with increasing residual volume and total lung capacity.

Further, the loss of elastin results in a dramatic loss of mechanical support of the small airways. In normal patients, these airways, 2 mm or less in diameter, are held open by intact surrounding lung parenchyma, which provides radial traction at points where alveolar septae attach to bronchioles. In patients with emphysema, loss of these attachments resulting from the destruction of the extracellular matrix of elastin and collagen is thought

to cause airway narrowing. In addition to having quantitatively less alveolar wall attachments, emphysematous lungs are also thought to exert less radial force on the few remaining attachments, since the hyperexpanded lung is crowded into a relatively undersized thorax and thus is less able to create outwardly directed forces.

In addition to changes in the airways themselves, airflow limitation in emphysema is thought to result also from compromise of the respiratory muscles in these patients. Hyperexpansion of the lung pushes the diaphragm in a caudad direction (Figure 10–4). The curvature of the diaphragm is thereby reduced, forcing its muscle fibers to operate at

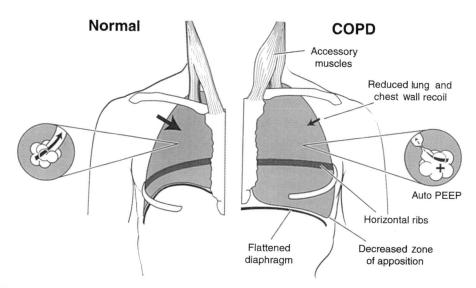

Figure 10–4. Ventilatory dysfunction in chronic obstructive pulmonary disease (COPD). PEEP, positive end-expiratory pressure. (From Hill NS. Current concepts in mechanical ventilation for chronic obstructive pulmonary disease. *Semin Respir Crit Care Med* 1999;20:375:393.)

shorter than normal lengths. Although the hypothesis is controversial, many feel that this causes a decrement in the diaphragm's ability to generate negative intrathoracic pressure. The accessory muscles of respiration and intercostal muscles are similarly, but probably less markedly, forced to operate at an unfavorable position on their length–tension curves. The diaphragm's zone of apposition to the lower ribs decreases in size, reversing the effect of diaphragmatic contraction on the lower rib cage from causing expansion aiding inspiration to create an expiratory force. The overall elastic recoil of the thoracic cage, which is normally directed outward, becomes directed inward because of its overdistention, creating an 'inspiratory elastic load' and further decreasing the efficiency of breathing. Finally, these disadvantaged muscles must work constantly against an increased load created by the increased airflow resistance such that the overall work of breathing is increased.

Emphysema also has deleterious effects on cardiac function. Limitation of cardiac filling by the hyperinflated lung has been demonstrated, such that during exercise the left and/or right ventricles may be compressed, with an elevation of the pulmonary capillary wedge pressure.

The essential concept of LVRS is that, by resecting some amount of emphysematous lung, these pathophysiologic changes demonstrated by emphysematous patients could be positively impacted. Removing the most diseased lung tissue should allow expansion of the remaining tissue to fill the thoracic cavity, thus increasing the elastic recoil of that remaining tissue. This would theoretically increase the radially directed forces on the small airways, improving their pathological narrowing, and increase the driving force for exhalation. The combination of these effects should be to decrease airway resistance and increase airflow.

Reducing the overall lung volume should also improve the performance of the diaphragm and perhaps the other respiratory muscles of emphysema patients. The diaphragm would be allowed to return towards its normal curvature and thus theoretically move more air with each inspiratory sweep. The resting length of the diaphragm and the other respiratory muscles would be returned towards the normal, optimal length and their mechanical disadvantage would be reduced. The abnormal load imposed on the inspiratory muscles by the reversal of chest wall recoil that occurs because of hyperexpan-

sion would also be expected to improve. Since dyspnea in COPD is closely related to respiratory muscle function, these alterations in respiratory muscle physiology might be anticipated to improve dyspnea.

Additional anticipated therapeutic affects of the procedure might include decreased ventilation–perfusion mismatch and improved cardiovascular hemodynamics. If resection is targeted to the most severely affected areas – those with retention of inspired gas and the least perfusion – hypercarbia may be improved. At the same time, shunting in adjacent, atelectatic regions may be reduced, thus improving hypoxia. With regard to the heart, it is possible that right and/or left heart function might be improved following LVRS as a result of recruitment of hypoperfused pulmonary capillaries and reduction of pulmonary artery pressures or by virtue of increased systemic venous return resulting from a reduction in intrathoracic pressures.

Medical Therapy

Smoking cessation and treatment of hypoxia are the only two medical interventions associated with improved disease course and survival. The severity of airflow obstruction as assessed by the postbronchodilator FEV_1 is an important predictor of prognosis. When this value falls below 30% of the predicted normal value, survival is approximately 87% at 1 year, 72% at 2 years, and 59% at 3 years. Smoking cessation reduces the rate of decline in FEV_1. Continuous supplemental oxygen is indicated for all patients with resting P_aO_2 <55 mm Hg or oxygen saturation less than 88%. For patients with secondary polycythemia, cor pulmonale, or pulmonary hypertension, continuous oxygen is indicated when the P_aO_2 is <59 mm Hg or oxygen saturation is <89%. The need for supplemental oxygen must also be addressed during sleep and exertion.

Additional therapeutic goals include relief of airflow obstruction, improvement in exercise tolerance, reduction of symptoms, and improved quality of life. Bronchodilating agents (inhaled beta-agonists and/or ipratropium bromide) represent first line pharmacologic therapy. Administration via metered dose inhaler using a spacer leads to adequate drug delivery while minimizing systemic side effects. If significant symptoms persist, longer-acting agents such as inhaled salmeterol or extended release theophylline may be added to this regimen. Although systemic cortico-steroids are indicated for treatment of acute exacerbations, chronic therapy plays a limited role in the management of emphysema. Approximately 10% of patients may exhibit improvement and it is therefore important to document a response. Systemic corticosteroids are associated with significant side effects and patients who fail to respond should not receive chronic therapy, while dosage in responders should be tapered to the lowest possible level. The role of inhaled cortico-steroids in the treatment of emphysema is a subject of ongoing investigation.

Pulmonary rehabilitation consists of: aerobic and resistive exercise training, education, breathing retraining, energy conservation tech-niques, nutrition, and psychosocial support. Although effects upon survival and pulmonary function have not been demonstrated, pul-monary rehabilitation results in improved exercise performance and reduced symptoms (Figure 10–5). The role of pulmonary rehabili-tation in preparing patients for LVRS or lung transplantation has not been studied, although significantly reduced exercise tolerance has been associated with greater risk of postopera-tive complications in patients undergoing LVRS or lung resection for cancer.

Assessment, treatment, and prevention of comorbid conditions associated with advanced emphysema is also essential. Weight loss is common in advanced emphysema and poor nutritional status is associated with decreased physical performance, respiratory muscle function and overall survival. Nutritional supplementation to achieve weight gain can lead to improvement in these parameters (Figure 10–6). Cachexia or signifi-cant unplanned weight loss should only be attributed to advanced emphysema after other causes have been ruled out. Patients who are postmenopausal or nutritionally comprom-ised or have a history of chronic steroid use should also be evaluated for osteoporosis. All patients should receive vaccination against influenza and pneumococcus.

It should be emphasized that none of the above-described medical therapies for emphy-sema can halt the progressive loss of pulmonary function characteristic of the disease, and patients tend to progress despite these medical interventions. When the disease has progressed to a degree that the patient's quality of life has become unbearable for him/her, the surgical options of LVRS or lung transplantation may be considered in appropriate candidates.

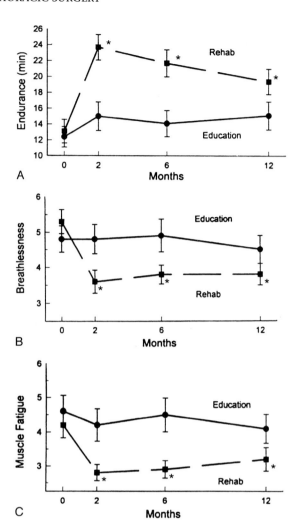

Figure 10–5. Results of treadmill endurance exer-cise tests for patients in the rehabilitation (Rehab) and Education groups at baseline and for 12 months of follow-up. **A**, Exercise endurance time. **B**, Perceived breathlessness rating at the end of exer-cise. **C**, Perceived muscle fatigue rating at the end of exercise. Asterisks indicate $p < 0.05$ for within-group change from baseline; values and error bars repre-sent the mean ± SE. (From Ries AL, Kaplan RM, Limberg TM, *et al*. Effects of pulmonary rehabili-tation of physiologic and psychologic outcomes in patients with chronic obstructive pulmonary dis-ease. *Ann Intern Med* 1995;122:823–832.)

Lung Volume Reduction Surgery

Many groups have expressed opinions about indications and contraindications for LVRS and about which patients are most likely to benefit from the procedure, without providing any objective data to support these opinions. Criteria that have been suggested range from

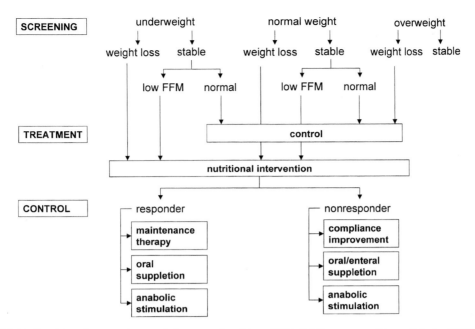

Figure 10–6. Nutritional screening and therapy algorithm. FFM, fat-free mass. (From Schols AMWJ, Wouters EFM. Nutritional abnormalities and supplementation in chronic obstructive pulmonary disease. *Clin Chest Med* 21:759, 2000.)

specific numerical recommendations (e.g. FEV_1 above and pulmonary artery pressures below a certain level) to more subjective evaluations of, for example, a patients' anxiety level (which many groups have suggested predicts a difficult postoperative course) (Table 10–2). Several considerations are reviewed below.

- *P_{CO_2}*. A few studies have specifically addressed the question of patient selection. It is generally agreed that P_aCO_2 of more than 50 mm Hg is predictive of mortality.
- *Inspiratory resistance*. It seems that patients with a greater loss of elastic recoil and greater preservation of airway integrity, as manifest by a lower inspiratory resistance, respond best to lung volume reduction. This would seem to confirm the clinical impression that this is an operation for emphysematous 'pink puffers' rather than for 'blue bloaters' with predominant chronic bronchitis.
- *Heterogeneous disease*. Upper lobe heterogeneous pattern of emphysema on computed tomography (CT) and/or nuclear scan is the best predictor of good outcome, while preoperative FEV_1, residual volume (RV), total lung capacity (TLC), and lung diffusing capacity for carbon monoxide (D_LCO) have no association with outcome.

- *Nutritional status* also has a significant impact on patient outcome, especially in the early postoperative period. Patients who have lost a significant amount of weight, especially women, are not good candidates for operation and, unless they can demonstrate weight gain during the period of pulmonary rehabilitation, they should probably not be offered operation. Body mass index is an accurate determinant of nutritional status in this patient population and preoperative repletion of nutritional deficiencies, if possible, is likely to be beneficial in reducing postoperative morbidity.
- *Six-minute walk distance*. Patients who are so compromised that they cannot cover 500 feet (183 m) in the 6-minute walk test are likely poor candidates for surgery. These patients need to be carefully assessed following pulmonary rehabilitation. If they are able to significantly increase their 6-minute walk distance, they may be candidates for operation. Some of these patients, however, have such significant muscle wasting that they are unable to improve the distance walked, and these patients appear to have a high perioperative mortality.

Careful planning is necessary in preparing for LVRS. Pain management and the ability to cough effectively are particularly important in these patients. Preoperatively, a thoracic

TABLE 10–2 • *Summary of Published Indications and Contraindications for Lung Volume Reduction Surgery*

Features	Indications	Contraindications

Clinical	Age <75 years
	Disability despite maximal medical treatment, including pulmonary rehabilitation
	Ex-smoker (>3–6 months)
		Age >75–80 years
		Comorbid illness with 5-year mortality >50%
		Severe coronary artery disease
		Pulmonary hypertension (PA systolic >45, PA mean >35 mm Hg)
		Severe obesity or cachexia
		Surgical constraints:
		    Previous thoracic procedure
		    Pleurodesis
		    Chest wall deformity

Physiologic	FEV_1 after bronchodilator <35–40% predicted
	Hyperinflation:
	    Increased RV/TLC
	    RV >200%–250%
	    TLC >120% predicted
	    D_LCO <50% predicted
		FEV_1 >50% predicted
		RV <150% predicted
		TLC <100% predicted
		D_LCO <10% predicted
		P_aCO_2 >50–60 mm Hg
		6-minute walk <400 ft after rehabilitation
		Elevated inspiratory resistance

Imaging	Chest x-ray: Hyperinflation CT: Marked emphysema with heterogeneity (upper lobe predominance is ideal) Isotope scan: Target areas for resection	Chest x-ray: No hyperinflation CT: Minimal emphysema; homogeneous, severe emphysema Isotope scan: Absence of target zones

D_LCO, lung diffusing capacity for carbon monoxide; FEV_1, forced expiratory volume in 1 second; PA, pulmonary artery; P_aCO_2, arterial partial pressure of carbon dioxide; RV, residual volume; TLC, total lung capacity.
From Flaherty KR, Martinez FJ. Lung volume reduction surgery for emphysema. *Clin Chest Med* 2000;21:835.

epidural catheter is placed for postoperative analgesia. Induction of anesthesia is a crucial and often dangerous time for patients with severe emphysema. The occasional patient will rapidly deteriorate with the onset of positive pressure ventilation and one needs to rapidly ascertain whether this is from an auto-PEEP phenomenon or a tension pneumothorax. Because of the tenuous nature of the pulmonary parenchyma in these patients, rupture from positive pressure ventilation with an ongoing air leak rapidly results in tension physiology and hemodynamic collapse if not promptly recognized. Any increase in peak airway pressures noted by the anesthesiologist at the time of induction and institution of positive pressure ventilation calls for immediate assessment. The surgeon should always be present at the time of induction when a patient with severe emphysema is anesthetized. The inspiratory:expiratory ratio often needs to be decreased in these patients as a longer expiratory phase usually is necessary to prevent the auto-PEEP phenomenon.

A median sternotomy is performed with complete division of the bone from the sternal notch to the xiphoid process. The skin incision is kept somewhat shorter, from approximately the angle of Louis to 3 cm above the xiphisternal junction, with elevation of flaps to expose the full extent of the bone incision. Care is taken throughout the procedure to handle the sternum gently. Emphysema is a recognized risk factor for sternal infection following heart surgery.

Unilateral ventilation to the side opposite that to be operated upon first – generally the side with the most severe disease as demonstrated on preoperative studies – is begun as the skin incision is made. This provides more time for the lung to deflate, keeping in mind that the most severely diseased areas with the least perfusion remain inflated longer because of the lack of reabsorption atelectasis. Usually, by the time the chest is entered, the areas with the most perfusion are well deflated and the most severely diseased area, usually the apex, remains inflated.

Many of the patients have scattered areas of filmy adhesions, presumably resulting from past inflammatory processes. Attempting to lyse dense adhesions may lead to prolonged air leaks and additional resulting postoperative complications, so prudent judgment must be exercised in these situations. The concept is to reshape the lung with a single large strip and to avoid multiple wedge excisions from various locations. It is possible to take more parenchyma with this single large, linear, oblique strip than with multiple wedge excisions.

In patients who have disease that, by ventilation–perfusion scan, is not localized primarily in the apices, resection of portions of the middle or lower lobes is often required (Figure 10–7). In patients who have minimal function in the right upper lobe, a formal right upper lobectomy may be performed.

How much parenchyma to remove cannot be easily quantified, but an average of 20–30% of the volume on each side is targeted. More is removed, certainly, in hemithoraces containing more diseased lung; less is removed in hemithoraces that contain less severely diseased lung. If too much is resected, postoperative oxygenation may be affected, causing significant difficulties; too little and one fails to accomplish the intent of the operative procedure. These patients are too high-risk not to accomplish what one sets out to do, and that is to reduce the lung volume by resecting nonfunctional lung parenchyma. The 'correct' amount of tissue to be resected is better ascertained after significant experience with the operation.

Control of pain is particularly important in the early postoperative period so that the patient may cough effectively to clear secretions. Mucous plugging can have disastrous consequences in these borderline patients. Secretions may be thick and tenuous and if the patient has any difficulty in clearing secre-

tions a tracheostomy should be placed to facilitate suctioning. Therapeutic bronchoscopy should be performed whenever there is any question that a mucous plug may be present in the proximal airways. Patients should be instructed in use of the incentive spirometer, and postural drainage and chest physiotherapy should be employed when indicated. Bronchospasm must also be managed aggressively usually with inhaled bronchodilators but parenteral steroids may be required to break an acute exacerbation. A rapid tapering schedule should be employed.

Following the initial report of LVRS via median sternotomy, a number of surgeons reasoned that perhaps the procedure could be performed with less morbidity with a video-assisted thoracic surgery (VATS) approach. This would involve a bilateral VATS procedure, and there were those who supported doing both sides under the same anesthetic and others who favored doing one side and bringing the patient back for the other side in 2–3 months. The goal of the operation remains the same whether the procedure is performed via median sternotomy or VATS – to reduce the volume of pulmonary parenchyma by excising nonfunctioning areas that are not contributing significantly to gas exchange. VATS patients are managed postoperatively exactly as if they had undergone LVRS via median sternotomy.

Most thoracic surgeons and pulmonologists would agree that that there is a role for LVRS in the management of selected patients with emphysema, although perhaps more questions have been raised than have been answered. Remaining areas of controversy, aside from the critical issue of patient selection, include issues

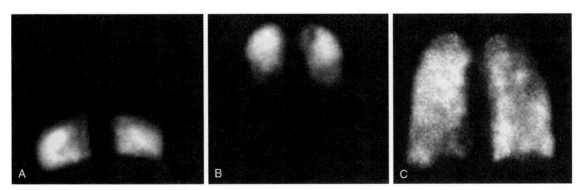

Figure 10–7. Perfusion lung scans, posterior view, of three patients evaluated for lung volume reduction surgery. **A**, Virtually absent perfusion of both upper lung zones, providing 'target areas' for surgical resection. **B**, Virtually absent perfusion of both lower lung zones providing 'target areas' for surgical resection. **C**, Patchy perfusion throughout both lungs: no 'target area' accessible. (From Pearson FG, Cooper JD, Deslauriers J, *et al. Thoracic surgery*, 2nd ed. New York: Churchill Livingstone, 2002:689.)

of surgical technique and approach, the duration of benefit, the question of a survival benefit, and the mechanism of the benefit.

Currently, a controlled clinical trial of the procedure known as the National Emphysema Treatment Trial (NETT) is accruing patients. The NETT will likely serve to confirm the finding of a benefit following LVRS in a more scientifically rigorous fashion while addressing the multitude of completely unanswered questions surrounding the procedure, which we have highlighted.

Patients are being randomized to medical therapy alone versus medical therapy plus LVRS. Both VATS LVRS and LVRS by median sternotomy will be included in the trial. All patients will undergo at least 5 weeks of preoperative and 8 weeks of postoperative pulmonary rehabilitation. While the amount of tissue to be removed is left to the discretion of the surgeon, only stapled excision of tissue is permitted and tissue buttressing of the staple lines is optional.

The two primary objectives of the trial are to determine if LVRS, added to maximal medical therapy, improves survival and if it increases exercise capacity as measured by maximum exercise capacity on a stationary bicycle. Secondary outcome measures have been chosen to learn more about the potential benefits of LVRS, explore proposed mechanisms of improvement, and refine selection criteria. These include measurements of quality of life and utility by questionnaire; and of pulmonary function, pulmonary mechanics, and gas exchange. Additional secondary outcome measures include oxygen requirement, 6-minute walk distance, and right ventricular function. Additional listed objectives include determining those patients who benefit most and those at highest risk, determining the durability of the benefits, and evaluating cost-effectiveness.

In order to be considered for the trial, the patients must have the clinical diagnosis of emphysema and have quit smoking at least 4 months prior to initial assessment. Pulmonary function values post-bronchodilator must be: TLC >110% predicted, RV >220%, FEV_1 <45% (>15% if over age 69), $D_{L}CO$ <70%, and postbronchodilator increase in FEV_1 cannot exceed 30%. P_aO_2 must be greater than 45 mm Hg on room air and P_aCO_2 must be less than 60 mm Hg. Oxygen saturation must be 90% on no more than 6 L/min of supplemental oxygen. Mean pulmonary artery pressure must be below 35 mm Hg and peak below 45 mm Hg.

After pulmonary rehabilitation, patients must be able to achieve a 140 m (460 feet) 6-minute walk distance.

Chest CT must demonstrate, by application of a complex radiologic grading schema, bilateral emphysema of at least moderate severity. Patients with both heterogeneous and homogeneous emphysema will be enrolled but the additional criteria that must be met for a patient with homogeneous emphysema to gain entry into the study are rather stringent.

Essentially, any cardiac abnormality discovered by history or routine electrocardiogram, echocardiogram, stress thallium imaging, or right heart catheterization must be evaluated by a cardiologist. Specific cardiac exclusion criteria include prior coronary artery bypass graft, recent myocardial infarction or congestive heart failure with ejection fraction less than 45%, and a variety of dysrhythmias.

Patients are excluded from consideration for entry into the trial if they do not meet certain body mass criteria or have lost weight immediately prior to their evaluation. Further, patients with giant bullae, bronchiectasis, or a pulmonary nodule, or who have undergone prior volume reduction, are excluded.

The results of the NETT are eagerly anticipated.

Transplantation

Transplantation may be offered when further medical or other surgical therapy is unavailable or inadvisable, expected survival is limited, and significant comorbid medical conditions are absent. Typical age limits are 65 and under for single lung transplantation and 60 and under for bilateral lung transplantation. Patients must be ambulatory, abstinent from smoking, and able to participate in a pulmonary rehabilitation program. Transplantation for emphysema may be considered when the postbronchodilator FEV_1 is below 25% of predicted or significant hypercapnia (P_aCO_2 >55), hypoxemia, or secondary pulmonary hypertension are present. Rapid decline may prompt listing at an earlier time.

Comorbid conditions likely to increase risk or limit survival may preclude transplantation. Absolute contraindications include: significant renal, hepatic, or cardiac dysfunction; severe coronary artery disease; progressive neuromuscular disease; recent active malignancy (excluding basal or squamous cell skin carcinoma); and human immunodeficiency virus or active hepatitis infection (Hepatitis B with positive antigen or Hepatitis C with histologic evidence of liver disease). Additional relative contraindications are: symptomatic osteoporosis; severe musculoskeletal disease; high-dose corticosteroid use (above 20 mg); ventilator dependence; very severe deconditioning; poor nutritional status (<70% of ideal body weight); morbid obesity (>130% ideal body weight); significant psychiatric illness or psychosocial problems; active substance abuse within 6 months; active mycobacterial or fungal infection; or other poorly controlled chronic medical condition.

Pulmonary function testing, chest radiography, quantitative ventilation perfusion, and/or CT scanning are used to assess disease severity and distribution. Assessment of distribution is useful in determining which lung should be replaced in the setting of single lung transplantation and when simultaneously evaluating for LVRS. Exercise testing or 6-minute walk testing determines overall conditioning and oxygen requirements. Echocardiography, radionuclide scanning, and right and left heart catheterization may be performed to assess for pulmonary hypertension, cardiac dysfunction, and coronary artery disease. Additional testing includes: assessment of hepatic and renal function;

lipid profile; viral serologies; blood and tissue typing; measurement of preformed anti-human-leukocyte antibodies; bone densitometry; purified protein derivative of tuberculin (PPD) and anergy testing; and age appropriate screening for malignancy.

Single-lung transplantation is the procedure most commonly performed for emphysema, and it is done via posterolateral thoracotomy or anterolateral muscle-sparing thoracotomy. Ventilation and perfusion of the native lung during implantation usually permits adequate gas exchange and blood flow. After explantation of the native lung, the allograft is implanted by establishing three anastomotic connections. Single-lung transplantation for emphysema creates unique physiologic constraints. Perfusion is preferentially distributed to the allograft because of its lower pulmonary vascular resistance in comparison to the native lung. The combination of increased expiratory airflow resistance and elevated static compliance in the native lung predisposes to hyperinflation of the native lung, particularly in the setting of mechanical ventilation (Figure 10–8). In most cases these relationships do not significantly compromise allograft function or gas exchange. However, when allograft dysfunction necessitates prolonged mechanical ventilation, the compliance differential between native and transplanted lungs is magnified and marked hyperinflation of the native lung may compromise ventilation

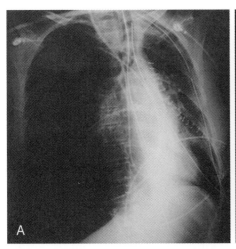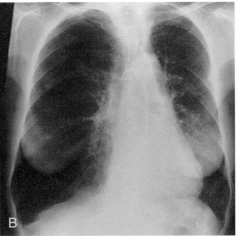

Figure 10–8. A, Postoperative mediastinal shift in a 50-year-old woman after left single-lung transplantation for severe pulmonary emphysema. The native right lung has massively overinflated across the midline, displacing the heart and the transplanted left lung to the left. **B**, Chest radiograph 6 months after left single-lung transplantation. The native right lung remains hyperinflated compared with the transplanted left lung, but there is no mediastinal shift. (From Smiley RM. Postoperative independent lung ventilation in a single-lung transplant recipient. *Anesthesiology* 1991;74:1144–1148.)

of the allograft, leading to hypoxemia, hypercapnia, and hemodynamic compromise. This complication may be managed using independent lung ventilation.

Bilateral lung transplantation is performed via transverse thoracosternotomy, bilateral anterior thoracotomy, or anterolateral muscle sparing thoracotomy incisions. Transplantation is accomplished by a bilateral sequential technique with ventilation and perfusion of one native lung during implantation of the first allograft followed by ventilation and perfusion of the first allograft to permit implantation of the second.

Both single and bilateral lung transplantation produce significant improvement in FEV_1, gas exchange, and exercise tolerance. FEV_1 is usually slightly greater than 50% of predicted after single-lung transplantation and normal or nearly normal after bilateral lung transplantation. Despite this difference in lung function, 6-minute walk distances are only slightly greater after bilateral procedures. Maximum oxygen uptake ($\dot{V}O_{2\ max}$) measured by cardiopulmonary exercise testing ranges from 40% to 60% of predicted with no significant difference between single-lung and bilateral transplant recipients. Reduction in exercise tolerance is not related to ventilatory or gas-exchange factors but more probably to cardiovascular limitations, deconditioning, and skeletal muscle dysfunction due to steroids, cyclosporine, and chronic illness.

Despite careful recipient selection and donor management, complications after lung transplantation are common. Within the perioperative period, infection, primary allograft dysfunction, and surgical complications contribute significantly to mortality. Infection resulting from the requisite immunosuppression is the most common cause of death during the first year and remains a significant cause of mortality in subsequent years. Chronic rejection, however, is the major limitation to long-term survival. Chronic rejection manifests as bronchiolitis obliterans, a fibroproliferative process affecting the small airways and leading to progressive decline in airflow. In contrast to acute rejection, chronic rejection frequently fails to respond to manipulation of immunosuppressive therapy.

Lung transplantation mandates lifelong immunosuppressive therapy. In addition to increasing the risk for infection, this regimen is associated with the development or potentiation of hyperglycemia, hypertension, hyperlipidemia, coronary artery disease, osteoporosis, chronic renal insufficiency, and increased risk of malignancy.

Conclusion

The severity of emphysema may determine the choice of procedure. While LVRS may be offered to patients with FEV_1 less than 45% predicted, lung transplantation is generally not considered until the FEV_1 falls below 25% predicted. More advanced disease with FEV_1 less than 20% predicted or severe homogeneous distribution may warrant transplantation rather than LVRS. The presence of significant pulmonary hypertension or severe chronic bronchitis precludes LVRS but not transplantation. Some patients may be considered simultaneously for both LVRS and transplantation. In this setting, LVRS may improve function sufficiently to permit patients to tolerate the prolonged waiting period until donor organs become available or to actually defer transplantation altogether. Patients who experience ongoing deterioration after LVRS may then undergo transplantation. If lung function deteriorates after transplantation, options are much more limited. The 1-year survival after retransplantation is less than 50% and because of this high risk, retransplantation is rarely considered. Occasionally, progressive hyperinflation of the native lung may compromise allograft function. After exclusion of other causes of late graft dysfunction (e.g. bronchiolitis obliterans, anastomotic stenosis, infection), volume reduction of the native lung has been reported to be of benefit.

To summarize, then, smoking cessation and oxygen therapy for hypoxic patients may improve survival in emphysema, but other medical therapies are palliative and do not dramatically impact the downward course of the disease. When selected patients reach a point of severely limited lifestyle due to their dyspnea, they may consider LVRS or lung transplantation. Transplantation, because of the apparently higher perioperative and long-term morbidity, is generally considered only in patients who are felt to be poor candidates for LVRS or in those whose pulmonary dysfunction is so severe that only transplantation is likely to sufficiently improve them to make an impact on their quality of life. LVRS in well-selected cases, on the other hand, may serve as a 'bridge to transplantation' or obviate the need for transplant entirely.

Key Readings

Brantigan OC, Mueller E. Surgical treatment of pulmonary emphysema. *Am Surgeon* 1957;23:789–804. *Classic paper that started the road to lung volume reduction surgery.*

Cooper JD, Patterson GA, Sundaresan RS, *et al.* Results of 150 consecutive bilateral lung volume reduction procedures in patients with severe emphysema. *J Thorac Cardiovasc Surg* 1996;112:1319–1330. *Written by the father of lung volume reduction surgery at Washington University in St Louis, MO.*

Kaiser LR, Cooper JD, Trulock EP, *et al.* The evolution of single lung transplantation for emphysema. The Washington University Lung Transplant Group. *J Thorac Cardiovasc Surg* 1991;102:333–339. *Description of lung transplantation as an alternative to lung volume reduction surgery.*

National Emphysema Treatment Trial Research Group. Rationale and design of the national emphysema treatment trial (NETT): a prospective, randomized trial of lung volume reduction surgery. *J Thorac Cardiovasc Surg* 1999;118:518–528. *A review of the controversial study that will change lung volume reduction surgery in the future.*

Selected Readings

Bavaria JE, Lotloff R, Palevsky H, *et al.* Bilateral versus single lung transplantation for chronic obstructive pulmonary disease. *J Thorac Cardiovasc Surg* 1997;113:520–527.

Cooper JD, Trulock EP, Triantafillou AN, *et al.* Bilateral pneumonectomy (volume reduction) for chronic obstructive pulmonary disease. *J Thorac Cardiovasc Surg* 1995;109:106–119.

Date H, Goto K, Souda R, *et al.* Bilateral lung volume reduction surgery via median sternotomy for severe pulmonary emphysema. *Ann Thorac Surg* 1998;65:939–942.

Ingenito EP, Evans RB, Loring SH, *et al.* Relation between preoperative inspiratory lung resistance and the outcome of lung-volume-reduction surgery for emphysema. *N Engl J Med* 1998;338:1181–1185.

Levine S, Kaiser L, Leferovich J, Thunov B. Cellular adaptations in the diaphragm in chronic obstructive pulmonary disease. *N Engl J Med* 1997;337:1799–1806.

McCune RJ, Brenner M, Fischel RJ, Gelb AF. Should lung volume reduction for emphysema be unilateral or bilateral? *J Thorac Cardiovasc Surg* 1996;112:1331–1339.

McKenna RJ, Brenner M, Fischel RJ, *et al.* Patient selection criteria for lung volume reduction surgery. *J Thorac Cardiovasc Surg* 1997;114:957–967.

Patterson GA, Cooper JD, Goldman B, *et al.* Technique of successful clinical double-lung transplantation. *Ann Thorac Surg* 1988;45:626–633.

Shrager, JB, Kaiser, LR. Lung volume reduction surgery. *Current Problems in Surgery* 2000;37:253–320.

Sundaresan RS, Shiraishi Y, Trulock EP, *et al.* Single or bilateral lung transplantation for emphysema? *J Thorac Cardiovasc Surg* 1996;112:1485–1494.

Szekely LA, Oelberg DA, Wright C, *et al.* Preoperative predictors of operative morbidity and mortality in COPD patients undergoing bilateral lung volume reduction surgery. *Chest* 1997;111:550–558.

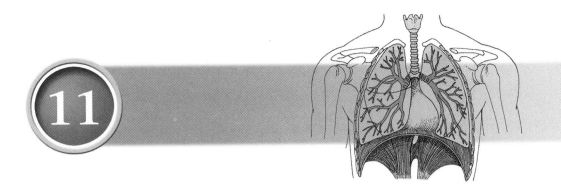

11

Pulmonary Transplantation

SELECTION CRITERIA

DONOR LUNG
CONSIDERATIONS

TRANSPLANTATION

POSTOPERATIVE MANAGEMENT

FUTURE CONSIDERATIONS

Key Points

- Know the indications for lung transplantation
- Know the absolute and relative contraindications for lung transplantation
- Understand optimal conditions to maintain a donor for lung transplantation
- Understand the basic approach in single- and double-lung transplantation
- Name the chief causes of morbidity and mortality after lung transplantation
- Appreciate the current state of lung transplantation and the issues for future success

Transplantation of the lung represents one of the last horizons in solid-organ transplantation. After an initial effort at human pulmonary transplantation in 1963, there was considerable excitement but little activity in this area until 1967, when a flurry of pulmonary transplantations followed the first successful human cardiac transplantation. The longest lung transplantation survivor during this early period lived 10 months, most of that time spent in the hospital. The major problems preventing successful pulmonary trans-

plantation have been failure of the airway anastomosis to heal, infection, and rejection.

Unlike other solid organs, the lung has no systemic arterial supply that can be reconnected. Bronchial arterial anatomy varies greatly, and the size of bronchial arteries, even when they can be identified, precludes direct anastomosis. Therefore, the bronchial anastomosis is ischemic after the operation, and airway dehiscence may occur approximately 3 weeks after transplantation. The combination of anastomotic ischemia and other factors, including the susceptibility of the lung to infection because of its direct contact with the outside environment by the airway, prevented successful transplantation despite the efforts of many investigators.

The first combined heart and lung transplantation was performed successfully in 1981, but the procedure sometimes required removal of an otherwise normal heart from the recipient. Combined cardiac and pulmonary transplantation introduced a series of new problems related to transplanting two organs, including those associated with heart transplantation and especially accelerated coronary artery atherosclerosis. With combined cardiac and pulmonary transplantation, however, healing of the tracheal anastomosis presents less of a problem, probably because the bronchial artery collaterals in the subcarinal space are preserved.

Advances in pharmacology and surgical technique have contributed to success in lung transplantation. Corticosteroids have proved to be detrimental to airway healing, yet cyclosporine does not have this adverse effect. Delaying the administration of maintenance corticosteroids has proved advantageous. Also, wrapping the bronchial anastomosis with a pedicle of gastrocolic omentum results in early capillary ingrowth and revascularization of the airway, promoting healing.

Another significant factor contributing to the improved success of single-lung transplantation was the recognition that careful recipient selection is crucial. Initially, it was felt that the ideal candidate for single-lung transplantation was a patient with end-stage restrictive disease (pulmonary fibrosis), a situation that would lead to preferential ventilation and perfusion of the graft because of the increased compliance and relatively decreased pulmonary vascular resistance of the transplanted lung.

In addition, although almost all previous attempts at pulmonary transplantation involved desperately ill, ventilator-dependent patients, lung replacement in a moribund patient who has already experienced significant nutritional depletion and muscle wasting is likely to fail. It is important to select patients who are ambulatory and to place potential recipients in an intense pretransplantation pulmonary rehabilitation program to increase the likelihood of a successful outcome. Improvement in patient selection may indeed be the single most important factor responsible for the success of pulmonary transplantation, even though indications for pulmonary transplantation have broadened considerably.

Selection Criteria

A patient should be referred for transplantation at a point in the course of the disease at which death is considered likely within several years, so that transplantation would be expected to confer a survival advantage. The patient's perception of an unacceptably poor quality of life is an important additional consideration, but the prognosis must be the overriding impetus for referral. Integrated into the decision must be an anticipated waiting time of up to 2 years, during which the candidate's condition must remain functionally suitable for transplantation. Patients usually have either predominantly obstructive or restrictive disease, although occasionally they may have a mixed defect. Those with end-stage obstructive physiology may demonstrate changes of emphysema, either nonbullous or bullous, or changes secondary to chronic infection (bronchitic). Patients with cystic fibrosis fall into the latter category, their lung disease resulting from the ravages of chronic, persistent infection (bronchiectasis). Patients with cystic fibrosis may also present with a mixed obstructive–restrictive picture. Those with idiopathic pulmonary fibrosis have restrictive physiology. Patients with a congenital deficiency of the alpha-1-antitrypsin protease commonly present with bullous emphysema, most noticeable at the lung bases.

Patients with pulmonary vascular disease are a distinct group. Those with end-stage disease have either primary pulmonary hypertension, a disease of unknown cause, or secondary pulmonary hypertension, resulting from increased pulmonary perfusion caused by a shunt at the cardiac or supracardiac level. When pulmonary vascular resistance increases sufficiently, the resultant increase in pulmonary artery pressure reverses shunt flow from right to left. This condition is known as Eisenmenger syndrome. When shunt reversal occurs, patients are typically considered inoperable because the mortality rate associated with primary cardiac operations is prohibitive. Theoretically, it is feasible to close the cardiac shunt with insertion of a new lung or lungs, thus unloading the right ventricle with a subsequent decrease in pulmonary vascular resistance to normal levels and improvement of right ventricular function.

Because of problems with donor availability, lung transplantation classically has been limited to patients 60–65 years of age or younger who have no other systemic disease and who have no significant coronary artery disease.

BOX 11-1 GENERAL INDICATIONS
FOR LUNG TRANSPLANTATION

- Advanced obstructive, fibrotic, or pulmonary vascular disease with a high risk of death within 2–3 years
- Lack of success or availability of alternative therapies
- Severe functional limitation, but preserved ability to walk
- Less than 60 years old

The criteria used in selecting pulmonary transplant recipients are outlined in Box 11–1.

Candidates for pulmonary transplantation ordinarily have significant functional impairment that interferes with activities of daily living. In patients with restrictive or obstructive disease, abnormal gas exchange is the major problem, and essentially all require supplemental oxygen 24 hours a day. In patients with pulmonary vascular disease, the manifestations of right ventricular failure predominate. These patients may or may not require oxygen.

Disease-specific guidelines for timely referral, which are based on available prognostic indexes, have recently been published (Table 11–1). Of all patients referred for transplanta-

tion evaluation, approximately 30% are ultimately accepted.

Absolute and relative contraindications to lung transplantation are listed in Table 11–2. Relative contraindications include chronic medical conditions such as osteoporosis, hypertension, diabetes mellitus, and coronary artery disease, which may worsen after transplantation and are acceptable in a candidate only if they have not resulted in end-organ damage and are well controlled with standard therapy. Perioperative corticosteroid therapy was once considered an absolute contraindication because it was thought to be associated with impaired bronchial anastomotic healing. Because of improved surgical techniques, transplantation can now be performed safely in patients who receive moderate doses of corticosteroids. Although patients receiving mechanical ventilation have undergone successful transplantation, as a group they have a higher mortality rate.

Donor Lung Considerations

Plain chest radiographs are used to assess potential donor lungs. In addition, bronchoscopy provides a way to examine directly the potential donor organs and to collect material for

TABLE 11-1 • *Disease-Specific Indications for Pulmonary Transplantation*

Chronic obstructive pulmonary disease	FEV_1 <25% of predicted value after bronchodilator therapy Clinically significant hypoxemia, hypercapnia, or pulmonary hypertension; rapid decline in lung function; or frequent severe exacerbations
Idiopathic pulmonary fibrosis therapy	Symptomatic disease unresponsive to medical Vital capacity <60–70% of predicted value Evidence of resting or exercise-induced hypoxemia
Cystic fibrosis	FEV_1 ≤30% of predicted value FEV_1 >30% with rapidly declining lung function, frequent severe exacerbations or progressive weight loss Female sex and age <18 years with FEV_1 <30%*
Primary pulmonary hypertension	NYHA functional class III or IV
Mean pulmonary artery pressure >55 mm Hg	Mean right atrial pressure >15 mm Hg Cardiac index <2 L/min/m²
Failure of medical therapy, especially intravenous epoprostenol, to improve NYHA	functional class or hemodynamic indices
Eisenmenger's syndrome	NYHA functional class III or IV despite optimal medical management

* These factors are associated with a poorer prognosis; therefore, early referral may be indicated.
FEV_1, forced expiratory volume in 1 second; NYHA, New York Heart Association.
Adapted from Arcasoy SM, Kotloff RM. Lung transplantation. N Engl J Med 1999;340;1081–1091.

TABLE 11–2 • *Absolute and Relative Contraindications for Lung Transplantation*

Absolute contraindications	Severe extrapulmonary organ dysfunction including renal insufficiency with a creatinine clearance below 50 mL/min, hepatic dysfunction with coagulopathy or portal hypertension, and left ventricular dysfunction or severe coronary artery disease (consider heart-lung transplantation)
	Acute, critical illness
	Active cancer or recent history of cancer with substantial likelihood of recurrence (except for basal-cell and squamous-cell carcinoma of the skin)
	Active extrapulmonary infection (including infection with HIV, hepatitis B – indicated by the presence of hepatitis B surface antigen – and hepatitis C with evidence of liver disease on biopsy)
	Severe psychiatric illness, noncompliance with therapy, and drug or alcohol dependence
	Active or recent (preceding 3–6 months) cigarette smoking
	Severe malnutrition (<70% of ideal body weight) or marked obesity (>130% of ideal body weight)
	Inability to walk, with poor rehabilitation potential
Relative contraindications	Chronic medical conditions that are poorly controlled or associated with target organ damage
	Daily requirement for more than 20 mg of prednisone (or equivalent)
	Mechanical ventilation (excluding noninvasive ventilation)
	Extensive pleural thickening from prior thoracic surgery or infection

Adapted from Arcasoy SM, Kotioff RM. Lung transplantation. N Engl J Med 1999;340;1081–1091.

culture and Gram stain, the results of which may influence later treatment of the recipient. No other organ has the same risk of infection; a pulmonary infiltrate may preclude the use of a lung. Because all brain-dead patients have endotracheal tubes and are on mechanical ventilation, there is a high likelihood that either the airway is colonized with bacteria or there is ongoing invasive infection. With pulmonary infection, an infiltrate is often present on chest radiography. Even with a clear chest radiograph, purulent secretions preclude using the lungs for transplantation.

Problems with the lungs may begin when the insult that results in brain death occurs, because the patient may aspirate gastric contents. Signs of aspiration may not be evident on the chest radiograph for 24–48 hours, underscoring the importance of bronchoscopy before accepting lungs for transplantation. Characteristic early bronchoscopic evidence of aspiration includes erythematous tracheobronchial mucosa, purulent secretions, and occasionally the presence of food particles.

Major pulmonary contusion resulting from blunt chest trauma also may eliminate lungs from donor consideration, but minor to moderate contusion unilaterally may still allow use of the lungs in a bilateral lung recipient.

Evaluating the full extent of contusion at the time of donor retrieval is often difficult because the interval from injury to determination of brain death and donation may be short. Although the detrimental effect on gas exchange caused by a pulmonary contusion is usually transient, further bleeding into the lung parenchyma could occur if cardiopulmonary bypass is required to perform the transplantation, as would be the case in a recipient with pulmonary hypertension.

Pulmonary edema may occur as a result of massive head injury and may be further complicated by certain donor management protocols (Box 11–2). Traditionally, renal transplantation teams have tried to ensure that adequate urine output is preserved; therefore, they preferentially infuse large volumes of crystalloid solutions. Cardiac transplantation teams prefer to avoid using high doses of inotropic agents to maintain blood pressure and also tend to administer large amounts of crystalloid solutions. The importance of coordinating donor management to prevent 'flooding' of the lungs, which are much more susceptible to the development of edema after significant cerebral insult, cannot be overstated if lungs are to be available for transplantation. Whether such edematous lungs may be 'dried out' when in

BOX 11–2 MANAGEMENT OF DONOR TRANSPLANT PATIENTS THAT MAY HINDER SUCCESSFUL LUNG TRANSPLANTATION

- Maintenance of mean arterial blood pressure above 70 mm Hg
- Preference of inotropic support over massive volumes of crystalloid solution to maintain blood pressure (dopamine 2.5–10 mg/kg/min)
- Replacement of fluid at the rate of the previous hour's urine output plus 100 mL
- Maintenance of normothermia
- Maintenance of positive end-expiratory pressure at 5 cm H_2O
- Frequent endotracheal suctioning
- Gram staining of sputum
- Monitoring of arterial blood gases every 2 hours

place in the recipient remains to be determined. The contribution of pulmonary lymphatics, which of necessity are severed during the donor retrieval at the time of bronchus division, to the clearing of edema in the pulmonary parenchyma is unknown.

Most commonly, lungs are refused after an initial acceptance because the results of bronchoscopy are abnormal or because arterial blood gases deteriorate significantly between the time of acceptance and the time the retrieval team reaches the donor hospital. The size of the donor lungs is less important when the recipient has emphysema, in which each hemithorax is very large, compared with pulmonary fibrosis, in which the hemithorax is contracted. The most important size consideration is a reasonable match between donor and recipient height.

An important area of investigation involves the optimal preservation technique for the ischemic lung. The donor lung must not only remain viable, it must participate actively in gas exchange immediately after implantation. A protocol is employed that uses both a flush technique with cold crystalloid solution and topical cooling to 4 °C by immersion. After removal of the donor heart, leaving a cuff of left atrium around the pulmonary veins, the lungs are removed by dividing the trachea above the carina and the pulmonary artery just proximal to the bifurcation.

The maximal safe interval for the lung to remain ischemic even when cooled has not been defined. Based on empiric observation, 6 hours has been selected as the limit. This time constraint places limits on the distance that may be traveled to procure lungs. The limits of donor lung ischemia have been expanded because of bilateral, sequential

lung replacement. The second lung to be implanted is perforce ischemic for a longer time because the lungs are not implanted simultaneously. Although donor lung dysfunction occasionally occurs (5–10% incidence), it is usually reversible.

It is believed that lung injury results not only from the ischemic insult but from reperfusion of the ischemic organ. Several experimental models of acute lung injury implicate oxygen free radicals as a factor in the genesis of reperfusion injury. A significant early increase in lung permeability is seen after an ischemic period followed by reperfusion. Permeability improves within several hours. Changes in the contralateral, nonischemic lung are presumably due to substances released during reperfusion of the ischemic lung. Efforts are directed at identifying techniques to attenuate the reperfusion injury.

Most experimental studies in lung preservation to date have been empiric, evaluating the effects of various techniques on subsequent lung function. Further progress requires a more detailed understanding of events at the cellular level during ischemia and reperfusion so that a rational approach to reduce or eliminate these changes may evolve. Satisfactory preservation techniques must protect not only cell structure and metabolism but the functional integrity of the lung as a whole to maintain normal gas exchange. Methods of preservation that allow for a prolonged ischemic time must also preserve the viability and microcirculation of the airway to prevent subsequent complications of airway healing. It would serve no useful purpose to extend the ischemic time only to have the airway fail to heal because of thrombosis in small vessels. Given the ability safely to preserve livers and kidneys for 24 hours or longer, it seems likely that donor lung preservation times will be extended in the near future.

Transplantation

Whether one lung or both lungs are replaced depends on recipient factors (Table 11–3), including the cause of the end-stage pulmonary disease, as well as donor lung availability. Patients with chronic infection, such as those with cystic fibrosis, require replacement of both lungs. Patients with restrictive physiology (pulmonary fibrosis) do well with single-lung replacement. The situation in patients with end-stage obstructive disease, specifically emphysema, offers considerably more variability. Early in the pulmonary transplantation experience, it became evident that problems resulted from leaving the native emphysematous lung *in situ*. Air trapping in the remaining native lung, with resultant mediastinal shift, significantly crowded the transplanted lung, resulting in poor expansion and minimal function. Ventilation preferentially went to the overly compliant native lung, whereas most of the perfusion went to the newly transplanted lung, creating a significant ventilation/perfusion mismatch that further worsened an already precarious situation.

Despite these concerns, single-lung transplantation is not only an acceptable operation for patients with emphysema, it may be the operation of choice for patients older than 50 years of age. Data demonstrate improved forced expiratory volume in 1 second (FEV_1) and 6-minute walk results in patients with emphysema undergoing single- versus double-lung transplantation at 1 year, although long-term survival is better following transplantation of two lungs. From a donor standpoint, single-lung transplantation, when acceptable, is a more efficient use of donor organs. The decision to use single-lung transplantation for emphysema evolved mainly from experience with the original *en bloc* double-lung operation, which involved a tracheal anastomosis and routine cardiopulmonary bypass and resulted in significant perioperative cardiac morbidity and mortality.

Replacement of both lungs was greatly simplified by the development and refinement of the bilateral, sequential lung transplantation procedure. A bilateral thoracosternotomy incision ('clamshell' procedure) or bilateral anterior thoracotomies without sternal division permits easier completion of the recipient pneumonectomies than is achieved using median sternotomy, and replacing the lungs sequentially usually avoids the need for cardiopulmonary bypass. Even previous chest operations are not contraindications to this procedure. This operation replaced *en bloc* double-lung procedures and heart-lung transplantation as the operation of choice for patients with end-stage pulmonary disease who need both lungs and for those with pulmonary vascular disease.

In patients with pulmonary hypertension, it has not been determined whether it is preferable to replace one or both lungs. Originally, single-lung transplantation was chosen because replacing one lung allowed adequate unloading of the right ventricle with immediate improvement in right ventricular function and normalization of pulmonary artery pressures (Table 11–4). However, replacing both lungs in this patient population offers a better margin of safety in the perioperative period and results in better hemodynamics in the long term. Whether replacement of both lungs is absolutely required remains to be determined but currently it is the preferred method in most transplantation centers for patients with pulmonary hypertension, despite donor limitations.

TABLE 11–3 • *Indications for Pulmonary Transplantation*		
	Single Lung (%)	**Double Lung (%)**
Emphysema	45.1	19.4
Alpha-1-antitrypsin deficiency	10.7	10.7
Cystis fibrosis	2.1	32.8
Idiopathic pulmonary fibrosis	21.9	7.3
Primary pulmonary hypertension	4.7	9.9
Retransplantation	2.8	2.2

Data from Hosenpud JD, Bennett LE, Keck BM, *et al*. The Registry of the International Society for Heart and Lung Transplantation: fifteenth official report – 1999. *J Heart Lung Transplant* 1999;18:611–626.

TABLE 11–4 • *Hemodynamic Characteristics for Single-Lung Transplantation in Patients with Pulmonary Hypertension*

Measurement	Pretransplantation	Post-transplantation
Pulmonary artery pressure		
Mean	58 mm Hg	16 mm Hg
Systolic	94 mm Hg	28 mm Hg
Right ventricular ejection fraction	25%	52%
Cardiac output	4 L/min	7 L/min
Pulmonary vascular resistance	1302 dyn/cm^5/s	161 dyn/cm^5/s

Single-Lung Transplantation

The performance of the donor operation does not vary because the attempt is always made to use both lungs, either for single-lung replacement on two recipients or for distribution to another transplantation medical center. This practice provides the most efficient use of limited donor organs. In the recipient operation, a standard posterolateral or muscle-sparing axillary thoracotomy is performed, with dissection of the hilar structures as usual for a pneumonectomy (Figure 11–1). The dissection mobilizes the main pulmonary artery, both superior and inferior pulmonary veins, and the main stem bronchus. When the donor lung arrives in the operating room, the recipient pneumonec-

tomy is performed by dividing the hilar vessels as far distally as possible and the bronchus at the level of the upper lobe take-off.

The implantation operation begins with construction of an anastomosis between the donor and recipient bronchus (Figure 11–1). This anastomosis is followed by left atrial cuff anastomosis. The pulmonary artery anastomosis is usually performed last. The bronchial anastomosis, formerly wrapped with a pedicle of gastrocolic omentum, now is either wrapped with a piece of pericardial fat or left unwrapped because the telescoping anastomosis offers an added margin of safety for bronchial healing. Once the vascular anastomoses are constructed, clamps are removed and blood flow is reestablished as the lung is inflated. The chest is closed

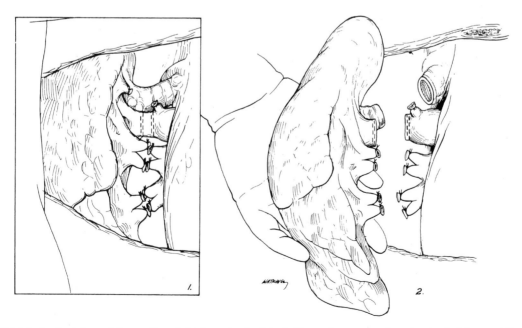

Figure 11–1. Excision of the native right lung is depicted. The pulmonary artery is stapled beyond its first upper lobe branch. Pulmonary veins are divided between ligatures, and the bronchus is transected just proximal to the upper lobe orifice. (From Shields TW. *General thoracic surgery.* Philadelphia: Lea & Febiger, 1994.)

in standard fashion. Either the right or left lung may be transplanted. The decision about which side to transplant is based on both donor lung availability and recipient perfusion lung scan data. If one lung receives most of the perfusion, the opposite lung is transplanted.

Double-Lung Transplantation

The technique of double-lung transplantation has evolved considerably since the late 1980s. The favored approach is essentially bilateral, sequential lung replacement. With the patient in the supine position, this operation is performed through either a bilateral thoracosternotomy incision that includes anterolateral thoracotomies and a transverse sternotomy (Figure 11–2), or bilateral anterior thoracotomies without sternal division. The bilateral thoracosternotomy incision provides excellent access to both hemithoraces, facilitating dissection and mobilization of hilar structures. This exposure is particularly important in recipients with diffuse or dense adhesions between the

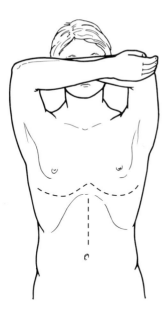

Figure 11–2. The position of the patient on the operating table before the start of the bilateral, sequential pulmonary transplantation operation. The chest incision, a bilateral thoracosternotomy, is seen, as is the separate midline incision used to expose the omentum. The sternum is divided transversely and the fifth intercostal space on each side is entered. (Redrawn from Kaiser LR. Pulmonary transplantation. In: Greenfield LJ, Lillimoe KD, Mulholland MW, *et al. Surgery: scientific principles and practice*, 2nd ed. Philadelphia: Lippincott-Ran, 1996.)

visceral and parietal pleural surfaces, as is often seen in patients with cystic fibrosis.

Although both lungs are replaced, the operation can usually be performed without cardiopulmonary bypass, although some surgeons prefer the routine use of bypass. By first replacing the lung with the least function, oxygenation and ventilation are maintained by the lung that receives the major fraction of perfusion. If the patient is unable to tolerate single-lung ventilation because of inadequate gas exchange or rising pulmonary artery pressures with right ventricular dysfunction, cardiopulmonary bypass is mandatory. The donor lungs are separated as for single-lung transplantation, leaving a cuff of left atrium around the pulmonary veins on each side. The recipient pneumonectomy is carried out with the patient maintained on one-lung ventilation. Each donor lung is implanted using essentially the same technique as described for single-lung transplantation. The bronchial anastomosis is completed first, followed by the left atrial and then the pulmonary arterial anastomoses. Flow and ventilation are restored to the newly implanted lung, and this lung then supports the patient while the opposite lung is removed and the second lung is implanted. Although all cardiac output is going through the newly implanted lung once the opposite pulmonary artery is ligated, clinically significant pulmonary edema has not been a problem. Both thoracotomies are then closed, and the sternum is approximated with wire sutures.

Other than procedures performed in patients with pulmonary hypertension, essentially all of these procedures are done without the need for cardiopulmonary bypass. The operation has afforded the opportunity to compare function between lungs with different ischemic times. Lungs may remain ischemic for 7–9 hours and still actively participate in gas exchange. Immediate postoperative perfusion scans usually show that the lung with the longer ischemic time receives less of the perfusion initially, although perfusion normalizes between the two lungs by 24–48 hours.

Postoperative Management

Immunosuppression is initiated in the immediate perioperative period and continued for the rest of the recipient's life. Standard regimens consist of cyclosporine or tacrolimus, azathioprine or mycophenolate mofetil, and prednisone. Some centers also use antilymphocyte antibody preparations during the induction phase, but there is no convincing evidence that this approach diminishes the incidence of acute or chronic rejection. Two important issues regarding standard immunosuppressive therapy are the myriad side effects associated with these agents and the numerous interactions with other commonly prescribed medications.

Complications resulting from pulmonary transplantation occur frequently, may be severe, and occasionally result in death (Box 11–3). Intraoperative complications include technical problems with the vascular or bronchial anastomoses, injury to the phrenic or recurrent laryngeal nerves, and myocardial infarction. Postoperative complications include primary graft dysfunction, infection, and problems with airway healing, rejection, and bronchiolitis obliterans. Intraabdominal complications are not uncommon. Wound infection is noted rarely, although overriding of the sternal edges after double-lung transplantation is not uncommon.

Causes of recipient death can be categorized according to the time frame in which they occur. Early deaths (<90 days post-transplantation) most commonly result from bacterial infection. Primary donor organ failure accounts for the next largest group of deaths, followed by heart failure. Rejection accounts for only 6% of deaths in the early post-transplantation period. Hemorrhage and airway dehiscence each are responsible for 6% of early postoperative deaths. Infection accounts for approximately one third of late deaths (>90 days) post-transplantation. A similar percentage results from manifestations of chronic rejection and bronchiolitis obliterans. Respiratory failure and malignancy are the next most common causes of late mortality,

each accounting for approximately 6% of deaths. Despite major strides made in operative and early postoperative care, the complications resulting from chronic immunosuppression continue to plague the transplant recipient.

Primary Graft Dysfunction

Mild, transient pulmonary edema is a common feature of the freshly transplanted allograft. In approximately 15% of cases, the injury is sufficiently severe to cause a form of acute respiratory distress syndrome termed primary graft failure. Primary graft failure is presumed to reflect ischemia–reperfusion injury, but surgical trauma and lymphatic disruption may be contributing factors. The diagnosis rests on the presence of widespread infiltrates on chest radiographs and severe hypoxemia within 72 hours after the transplantation and the exclusion of other causes of graft dysfunction, such as volume overload, pneumonia, rejection, occlusion of the venous anastomosis, and aspiration. Treatment is supportive, relying principally on conventional mechanical ventilation. Independent lung ventilation, inhaled nitric oxide, and extracorporeal membrane oxygenation have been used as adjunctive measures. Mortality rates of up to 60% have been reported and, among those who survive, the recovery period is often protracted but achievement of normal allograft function is possible. The results of emergency retransplantation in such cases have been poor.

Rejection

With few exceptions, acute rejection episodes occur soon after transplantation, usually between post-transplantation days 5 and 7. Usually, two or three rejection episodes occur within the first month. Mild temperature elevation, perihilar fluffy infiltrates, or a minimal decrease in blood oxygenation as measured by arterial oxygen tension may herald rejection. Because rejection occurs so frequently during this period, the distinction between infection and rejection may be difficult. Often, the distinguishing factor between these two entities is that rejection responds positively to the administration of corticosteroids. Treatment of early rejection episodes involves the use of bolus corticosteroid administration given on three consecutive days. Within 12–18 hours after the first corticosteroid dose, symptoms relating to

BOX 11–3 POTENTIAL COMPLICATIONS OF LUNG TRANSPLANTATION

- Technical complications
  - Vascular anastomosis
  - Bronchial anastomosis
  - Phrenic nerve injury
- Primary graft dysfunction
- Infection
- Airway healing complications
- Rejection
- Bronchiolitis obliterans
- Wound infection

rejection usually resolve, including clearing of infiltrates on chest radiograph.

The utility of transbronchial biopsy to diagnose and monitor rejection after cardiopulmonary transplantation is substantial, but the number of biopsies required to maximize specificity is large. One group recommends obtaining 18 separate transbronchial biopsy specimens to achieve 95% specificity. The risks and potential complications of transbronchial lung biopsy do not justify their routine performance because suspected rejection episodes respond so well to corticosteroids. Transbronchial lung biopsy can be used when the issue of rejection versus infection is not resolved after steroid administration. Flexible bronchoscopy can be performed at the bedside, and six to 10 separate biopsies can be obtained under fluoroscopic guidance. When symptoms or signs of rejection persist despite adequate treatment, open lung biopsy may be considered.

Infection

Infection in the post-transplantation period continues to be a significant cause of morbidity as well as mortality (Box 11–4). Bacterial pneumonia usually responds to appropriate antibiotic therapy, and patients are maintained on specific antibiotics as dictated by sputum culture and results of bronchial washings obtained at bronchoscopy. Antibiotic administration is particularly important if one predominant organism is grown from the donor lung cultures obtained at organ harvest. If a specific organism is grown from donor bronchial washings, the recipient is maintained on an appropriate antibiotic or combination of antibiotics for at least 1 week. The most common organism recovered from donor bronchial washings is *Staphylococcus*

aureus. In a series of 32 transplantations, this organism was recovered from donors 11 times and subsequently from four transplant recipients. Other commonly recovered pathogens include *Enterobacter* species and *Candida albicans*. The presence of organisms cultured from donor bronchial washings, however, does not absolutely predict the development of invasive infection in recipients. Invasive infection develops in less than half of recipients from whom organisms are recovered.

The second most significant pathogen is cytomegalovirus (CMV). The diagnosis of CMV is usually made from culture of bronchoalveolar lavage fluid or tissue obtained from transbronchial lung biopsy. In the pulmonary transplantation population, CMV pneumonitis is the predominant form of CMV infection, although CMV enteritis and retinitis also occur. Approximately half of lung recipients acquire documented CMV infection. Ganciclovir has proved particularly effective and is the drug of choice for CMV infection in this circumstance. The drug is well tolerated in most patients, with neutropenia accounting for most of the toxicity.

The mortality rate from life-threatening CMV infections treated with ganciclovir has been reported at 10%, far better than the 40% or greater mortality rate reported before this agent was available. Major difficulties with life-threatening CMV infection have occurred in CMV-negative recipients who have received a lung from a CMV-positive donor (primary infection) or in recipients who are already CMV-positive (secondary infection). Current practice is to attempt to place only a CMV-negative donor lung in a CMV-negative recipient, but this often proves to be unrealistic given the shortage of donor organs. Despite initial concerns, data from the St Louis International Lung Transplant Registry fail to demonstrate any survival advantage at 1 or 2 years post-transplantation by avoiding donor-recipient CMV mismatching. Cytolytic therapy, especially with OKT3, is associated with an increased risk and severity of CMV infection. CMV prophylaxis with ganciclovir is used for CMV-positive recipients or for recipients who receive a lung from a CMV-positive donor.

Airway Complications

A major concern after pulmonary transplantation is healing of the airway anastomosis. During the early pulmonary transplantation

BOX 11–4 INFECTIOUS SOURCES IN THE POST-TRANSPLANT PERIOD

- Bacterial pneumonia
  - *Staphylococcus aureus*
  - *Streptococcus pneumoniae*
  - *Enterobacter* species
- Viral infection
  - CMV
  - HSV
- Other
  - *Candida albicans*

experience, problems with airway healing resulted in a significant percentage of deaths. Partial bronchial dehiscences often heal without sequelae. The use of a telescoping bronchial anastomosis and other techniques obviates the need for the omental pedicle wrap, allows for immediate use of corticosteroids, and has essentially eliminated anastomosis healing problems.

Bronchiolitis Obliterans

Approximately 50% or more of pulmonary transplant recipients develop progressive deterioration in pulmonary function because of bronchiolitis obliterans. The lesion is characterized histologically by progressive small airway destruction, filling of these small airways with an inflammatory exudate, and, finally, fibrosis. Bronchiolitis obliterans is first manifest clinically by a subtle decrease in pulmonary function reflected in a decreased FEV_1. This complication is likely a form of chronic rejection, although its exact etiology remains unknown. A good animal model of bronchiolitis obliterans does not exist, making study of this entity difficult. If diagnosed early, enhancing immunosuppression may either halt the process or slow progression. It has been hypothesized that the development of bronchiolitis obliterans in cardiopulmonary transplant recipients is related to an A2 antigen mismatch. Others postulate that CMV infection may be implicated. Once diagnosed, it is imperative to increase immunosuppression to prevent what is usually an insidiously progressive disorder. In patients who have bronchiolitis obliterans and then undergo retransplantation, the lesion redevelops in the newly transplanted lungs. The disorder remains a major problem for patients surviving for more than 2 years post-transplantation and essentially is responsible for 5-year survival rates for lung transplantation being less than 50%.

Future Considerations

Pulmonary transplantation has slowly evolved from an experimental therapy. The number of these operations performed is still small compared with other solid-organ replacements. Donor availability is still a major issue and will probably continue to be an obstacle. Lung volume reduction surgery, as an alternative to transplantation or to delay transplantation in patients with emphysema seems to be a viable option. Definition of a role for lung reduction therapy is an important consideration because emphysema is the most common indication for lung transplantation. Questions about long-term follow-up and preservation of lung function also remain to be answered. Living donor lung transplantation using either one (child) or two lobes, one each from two donors, has become an option for certain patients. Pulmonary transplantation has joined other solid-organ transplantations as a viable alternative in patients with end-stage disease. Cost considerations and managed care are likely to have a significant impact on transplantation at the beginning of the 21st century.

Key Readings

Arcasoy SM, Kotloff RM. Lung transplantation. *N Engl J Med* 1999;340:1081–1091. *An up to date review of where lung transplantation stands at the turn of the century.*

DeMeo DL, Ginns LC. Clinical status of lung transplantation. *Transplantation* 2001;72:1713–1724. *Better review of some of the pharmacology of lung transplantation.*

Selected Readings

Barr ML, Baker CJ, Schenkel FA, *et al*. Living donor lung transplantation: selection, technique, and outcome. *Transplant Proc* 2001;33: 3527–3532.

Kaiser LR. Pulmonary transplantation. In: Greenfield LJ, Lillimoe KD, Mulholland MW, *et al. Surgery: scientific principles and practice*, 2nd ed. Philadelphia: Lippincott-Raven, 1996.

Maurer JR, Frost AE, Estenne M, *et al*. International guidelines for the selection of lung transplant candidates. The International Society for Heart and Lung Transplantation, the American Thoracic Society, the American Society of Transplant Physicians, the European Respiratory Society. *J Heart Lung Transplant* 1998;17:703–709.

Sulica R, Teirstein A, Padilla ML. Lung transplantation in interstitial lung disease. *Curr Opin Pulm Med* 2001;7: 314–322.

Trulock EP. Lung transplantation for primary pulmonary hypertension. *Clin Chest Med* 2001;22:583–593.

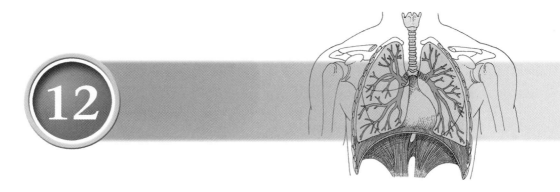

12

Chest Wall Disorders

PECTUS EXCAVATUM   POLAND'S SYNDROME
PECTUS CARINATUM   CHEST WALL TUMORS

Chest Wall Disorders: Key Points

- ○ Describe the etiology and pathophysiology of pectus excavatum
- ○ Understand the issues that are involved in the decision to operate on patients with pectus excavatum
- ○ Name the features of Poland's syndrome
- ○ Understand the classification of chest wall tumors
- ○ Have a plan to diagnose and treat a typical chest wall mass

Pectus Excavatum

Pectus excavatum is the most common congenital deformity of the sternum, occurring in 1:400 children. Symptoms vary from a mild manifestation to significant depression of the sternum.

The etiology is unknown and does not follow any particular family inheritance or neonatal exposure history. There is an increased familial incidence and male bias but the deformity is not inherited in a strictly mendelian fashion. Some 40% of patients have a family history of chest wall deformity. Pectus excavatum is present at birth or within the first year of life in the majority of

children. Marfan's syndrome should be ruled out in all patients with pectus excavatum, particularly if they have accompanying scoliosis.

The defect arises from a deformity in the costal cartilage that causes it to form in a concave fashion, thus depressing the sternum (Figure 12–1). The degree of depression increases from the sternomanubrial joint to the xiphoid process. Often the right side is more depressed than the left, and the sternum may be rotated as well. The heart can be displaced to the left in severe cases (Figure 12–2). Occasionally there is an anterior indentation of the right ventricle. A systolic ejection murmur is sometimes described due to the proximity

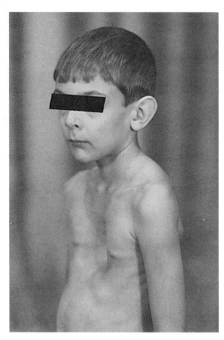

Figure 12–1. A 5-year-old boy with severe pectus excavatum. (From Robicsek F. Surgical treatment of pectus excavatum. *Chest Surg Clin North Am* 2000;10:277–296.)

between the sternum and the pulmonary artery, which produces a flow murmur effect. The defect is usually present at birth and increases with time. Many children have accompanying scoliosis so they should be

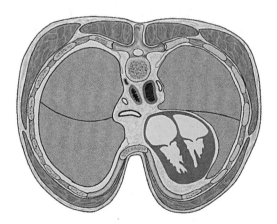

Figure 12–2. Cross-section of the thorax in pectus excavatum deformity. Note the decreased space between the sternum and the vertebra and the shifting of the heart into the left hemithorax. (From Robicsek F. Surgical treatment of pectus excavatum. *Chest Surg Clin North Am* 2000;10:277–296.)

evaluated for both. Pectus excavatum is associated with congenital heart disease in 2% of patients.

In most patients, the primary indication for correction is cosmetic. Children on entering grade school begin to have a negative self-image associated with the chest wall abnormality. Patients rarely have respiratory or cardiovascular compromise. Older patients admit to occasional respiratory difficulty, cardiac-related symptoms and palpitations, which are brought out in those who are involved in highly competitive athletics. Although there is not necessarily any physiological impairment, many patients admit to an increased level of activity after surgical repair. Several studies have attempted to discover if there is a true physiological impairment in pectus excavatum. No report has demonstrated support for this. Often the study size is small or the degree of improvement between preoperative and postoperative is quite variable, dependent on the degree of the patients conditioning.

The main issue to be resolved is the timing of the surgical procedure. Ideally the operation should be done before the age of 5; however, the operation can be done at any age. If the child is symptomatic, an operation before 5 years of age is warranted. Similarly, as a patient moves into late adolescence and young adulthood, surgical intervention is not always necessary. Patients at this end may psychologically attribute chest pain to their pectus anomaly.

The general principle of operative management is an appreciation that the real problem lies with deformed costal cartilages and that the sternal depression is a result of this. Overgrowth of the costal cartilages is responsible for this chest wall distortion. Repair of the pectus excavatum relies on correcting the surgical depression and maintaining the sternum in its corrected position (Figure 12–3). Several techniques exist such as sternal eversion performed with an aggressive resection of abnormal cartilages and the use of Marlex mesh to support the sternum in its corrected position (Figure 12–4). The Ravitch repair uses a transverse incision placed below the nipples and placement of a steel bar to support the sternum in the proper location (Figure 12–5). Alternatively, others have instituted a minimally invasive procedure with placement of a convex steel bar under the sternum through a small lateral thoracic

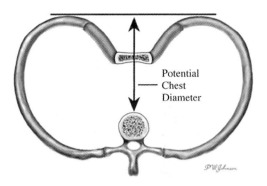

Figure 12–3. The limit of how far anteriorly the sternum can be raised by most conventional surgical techniques designed to correct pectus excavatum. (From Robicsek F. Surgical treatment of pectus excavatum. *Chest Surg Clin North Am* 2000;10: 277–296.)

incision (Nuss procedure). Currently our preferred approach in adolescents uses a modification of the Ravitch technique with modern orthopedic fixation appliances (plates and

screws). Cosmetic results are satisfactory in 80–90% of cases.

Despite the approach taken, the major complication is recurrence. Pneumothorax follows as the second most common concern, with wound infection third. Recurrence can be quite problematic and difficult to predict, although it occurs in approximately 10% of patients. Patients with Marfan's syndrome or poor muscular development are most at risk of recurrence.

Pectus Carinatum

Pectus carinatum, 'pigeon breast', the second most common anomaly of the chest wall, is significantly less common than pectus excavatum but is characterized by protrusion of the sternum caused by an upward curve in the lower costal cartilages, generally the fourth to the eighth cartilage (Figure 12–6). Again, there is an increased family incidence suggesting a genetic bias. Pectus carinatum occurs in excess

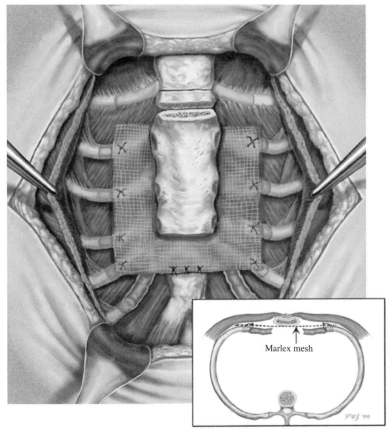

Figure 12–4. Repair of pectus excavatum using a Marlex 'hammock.' After transfer wedge sternotomy and resection of the deformed cartilages and detachment of the xiphoid process the sternum is maintained in its corrected position by suturing a sheath of Marlex mesh taut under it. The insert shows the process in lateral cross-section. (From Robicsek F. Surgical treatment of pectus excavatum. *Chest Surg Clin North Am* 2000;10:277–296.)

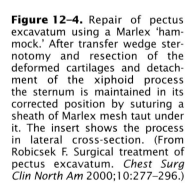

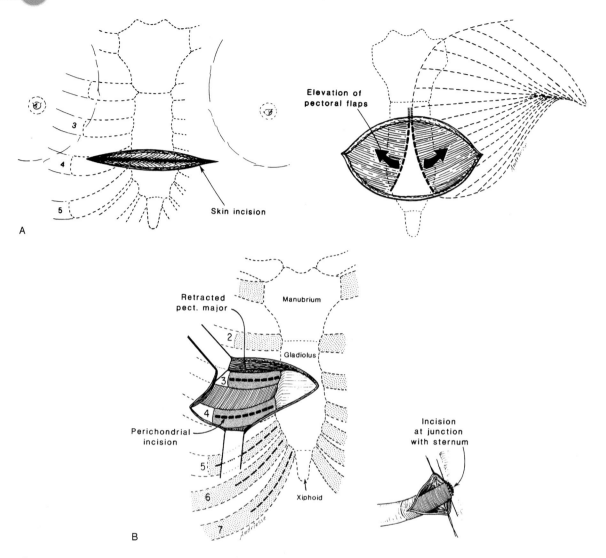

Figure 12–5. A, A transverse incision is placed below and well within the nipples at the site of the future inframammary crease. The pectoralis major muscle is detached from the sternum along with the portions of the pectoralis minor and serratus anterior muscles and retracted forward and laterally to expose the depressed costal cartilages (usually the third to seventh). **B,** Subperichondrial resection of the costal cartilages is achieved by incising the perichondrium anteriorly. It is then dissected from the costal cartilages in the bloodless plane between the perichondrium and the costal cartilage. Cutting the perichondrium 90° in each direction at its junction with the sternum (inset) facilitates visualization of the back wall of the costal cartilage.

of three times more frequently in males than females.

Pectus carinatum typically is present at birth but unlike pectus excavatum does not present until the child approaches puberty (Figure 12–7). This defect is evident through clothing. Symptoms are present, including cardiac arrhythmias and exertional dyspnea. These difficulties arise because the chest has difficulty expanding during inspiration because of reduced flexibility of the chest caused by the anteriorly displaced sternum and defective cartilages. Scoliosis is a common associated abnormality.

The psychological effects of pectus carinatum are quite pronounced. Children and young adults are self conscious, shy, and tend to walk slightly bent to conceal their anomaly. The pathogenesis of pectus carinatum is unknown. Theories suggested include sternal

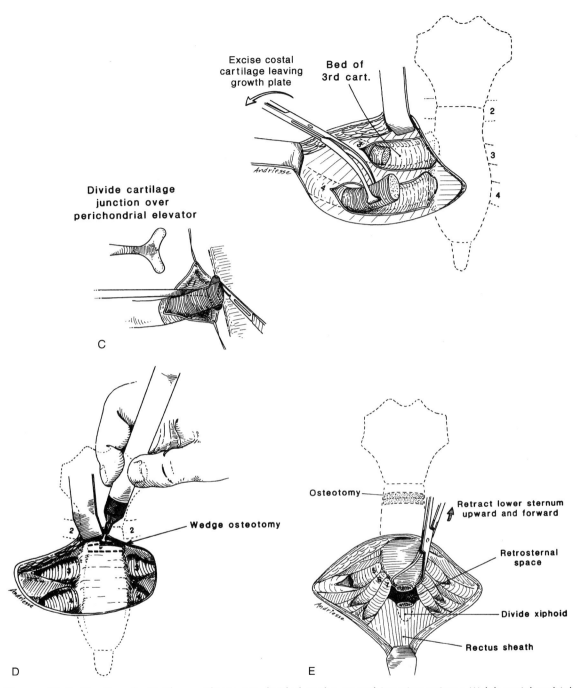

Figure 12–5. Continued. **C**, The cartilages are divided at the sternal junction using a Welch perichondrial elevator held posteriorly to elevate the cartilage and protect the mediastinum (inset). The divided cartilage is then held with an Allis clamp and elevated; the costal cartilage is then excised, preserving a margin on the rib to protect the costochondrial junction and the longitudinal growth plate. **D**, The sternal osteotomy is created above the level of the last deformed cartilage and the posterior angulation of the sternum, generally the third cartilage but occasionally the second. Two transverse sternal osteotomies are created 2–4 mm apart through the anterior cortex using a Hall air drill. **E**, The base of the sternum and the rectus muscle flap are elevated with two towel clips, and the xiphoid can be divided from the sternum with electrocautery, allowing entry into the retrosternal space. This step is not necessary with the use of a retrosternal strut. Preservation of the attachment of the sheaths and xiphoid avoids an unsightly depression, which can occur below the sternum.

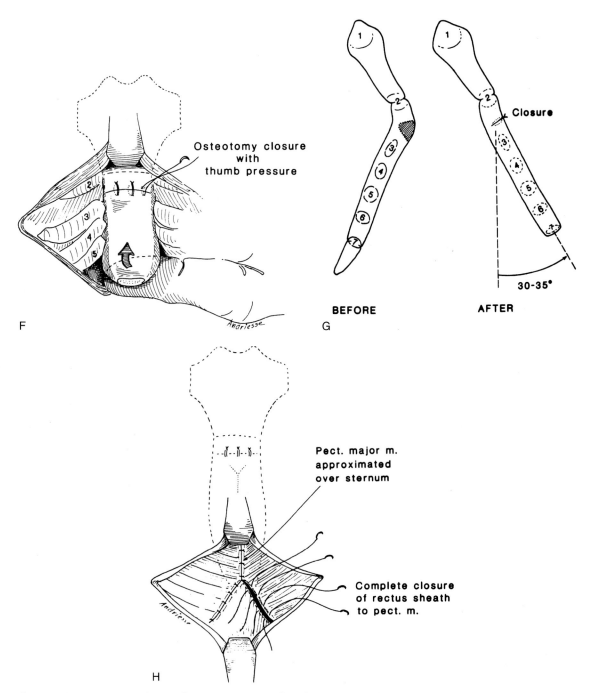

Figure 12–5. Continued. **F,** The osteotomy is closed with several heavy silk sutures as the sternum is being elevated with the assistant's thumb if a strut is not used. **G,** Correction of the abnormal position of the sternum is achieved by creation of a wedge-shaped osteotomy, which is then closed, bringing the sternum anteriorly into an overcorrected position. **H,** The pectoral muscle flaps are secured to the midline of the sternum while being advanced to provide coverage of the entire sternum. The rectus muscle flap is then joined to the pectoral muscle flaps.

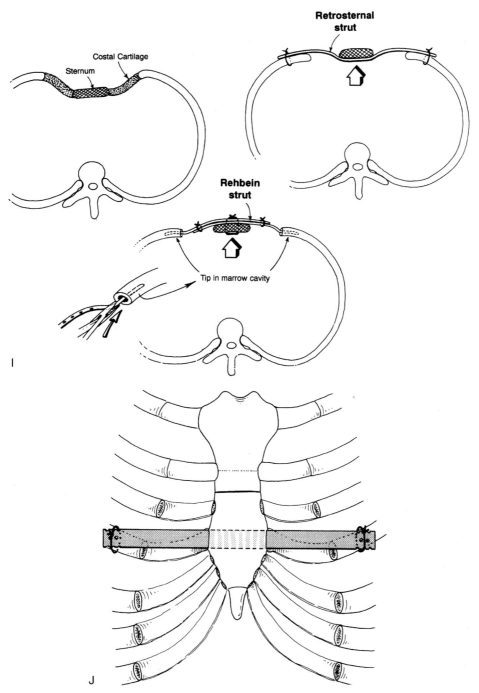

Figure 12–5. Continued. **I,** Demonstration of the use of both retrosternal struts and Rehbein struts. The Rehbein struts are inserted into the marrow cavity (inset) of the third and fourth ribs and are then joined to each other medially to create a metal arch anterior to the sternum. The sternum is sewn to the arch to secure it in its new forward position. The retrosternal strut is placed behind the sternum and is secured to the rib ends laterally to prevent migration. **J,** Anterior depiction of the retrosternal struts (V. Mueller). The perichondrial sheath to either the third or fourth rib is divided from its junction with the sternum, and the retrosternal space is bluntly dissected to allow passage of the strut behind the sternum. It is secured with two pericostal sutures laterally to prevent migration. (**A–H** from Shamberger RC, Welch KJ. Surgical repair of pectus excavatum. *J Pediatr Surg* 1988;23:615; **I–J** from Shamberger RC. Chest wall deformities. In: Shields TW, ed. *General thoracic surgery,* 4th ed. Baltimore: Williams & Wilkins, 1994.)

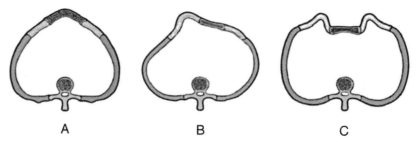

Figure 12–6. Different anatomical types of pectus carinatum. **A**, Keel chest (keel chest either with sternal elongation or sternum elevatum). **B**, Asymmetrical pectus carinatum. **C**, Bilateral protrusion of the costal cartilages. (From Robicsek F. Surgical treatment of pectus excavatum. *Chest Surg Clin North Am* 2000; 10:277–296.)

displacement caused by hypoplasia of its attachment to the center of the diaphragm with compensatory hypertrophy of the lateral muscular compartment. Other theories suggest that the primary problem is not diaphragmatic but due to excessive cartilaginous elongation of the ribs. If the sternum is pushed inward, pectus excavatum develops; if it is pushed outward, pectus carinatum results.

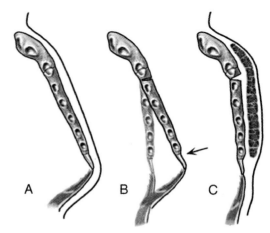

Figure 12–8. Surgical repair of pectus elevatum. **A**, The anatomy of the deformity. **B**, After transverse sternotomy the sternum is pushed down. **C**, The corrected position of the sternum is maintained by uniting the detached pectoralis muscles pre-sternally. (From Robicsek F. Surgical treatment of pectus excavatum. *Chest Surg Clin North Am* 2000;10:277–296.)

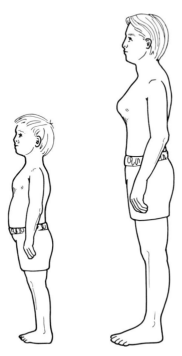

Figure 12–7. The pectus carinatum deformity becomes more visible in larger children because of the disappearance of the natural pot belly of the infant. (Redrawn from Robicsek F. Surgical treatment of pectus excavatum. *Chest Surg Clin North Am* 2000;10:277–296.)

Conservative treatment for pectus carinatum is ineffective. Repair is performed through a submammary incision and the principles of pectus excavatum repair are similar. Sternal portions of all involved costal cartilages need to be subperiosteally resected (Figures 12–8 and 12–9).

Poland's Syndrome

In 1841, Poland described congenital absence of the breast or nipple, hypoplasia of subcutaneous tissue, pectoralis major and minor muscles, and occasionally absence of costal cartilages or ribs 2,3, and 4 or 3,4, and 5. The

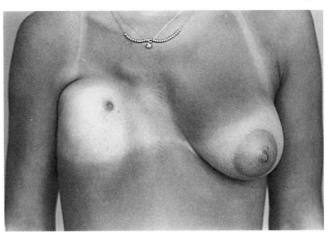

Figure 12–9. A 15-year-old girl with Poland's syndrome, showing absence of the breast with a vestigial nipple, absence of the pectoralis major and minor muscles, and chest wall deformity with absence of costal cartilages and the second, third and fourth anterior ribs. (From Urschel HC Jr. Poland's syndrome. *Chest Surg Clin North Am* 2000;10:393–403.)

disease incidence is 1:30 000, with a slightly higher incidence in females.

This syndrome often involves the chest wall and breasts. The extent of thoracic involvement may range from hypoplasia of the sternal head of the pectoralis major and minor muscles with normal underlying ribs to complete absence of the anterior portions of the second to fifth ribs and cartilages (Figure 12–9). Breast involvement can range from mild hypoplasia to complete absence of the breast (Figure 12–10). Hand deformities and syndactyly are commonly present. The chest wall defect is often associated with a lung hernia.

Symptoms are unilateral, allowing ease of reconstruction. The right side is more commonly affected than the left. The diagnosis is easily established from the lack of breast tissue, axillary fold, and chest wall deformity. Single-stage reconstructions are now performed that aim to stabilize the chest wall and simultaneously perform breast augmentation. Chest wall defects are repaired with Marlex mesh and the breast prosthesis is placed directly on the mesh (Figure 12–11). A myocutaneous flap of latissimus dorsi is transferred to cover the prosthesis (Figures 12–12 and 12–13) Results are excellent.

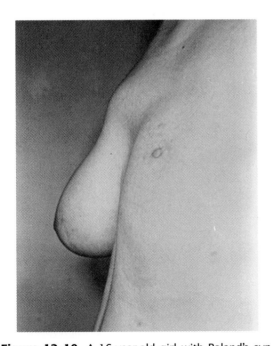

Figure 12–10. A 16-year-old girl with Poland's syndrome, showing absence of the breast with a vestigial nipple, absence of the pectoralis major and minor muscles, normal cartilages and ribs on the left side, and a pectus carinatum defect on the right side. (From Urschel HC Jr. Poland's syndrome. *Chest Surg Clin North Am* 2000;10:393–403.)

Chest Wall Tumors

Primary chest wall tumors account for 5% of all thoracic neoplasms and 1–2% of all primary tumors (Table 12–1). Most chest wall resections are undertaken for metastatic tumors or pulmonary tumors with local chest wall invasion. Most (85%) primary chest wall tumors occur in the ribs. Primary bony chest tumors represent 8% of all bony tumors. Half of all primary chest wall tumors are benign.

The most frequent benign chest wall tumors are osteochondroma, chondroma, and fibrous dysplasia, which together represent 60–70%

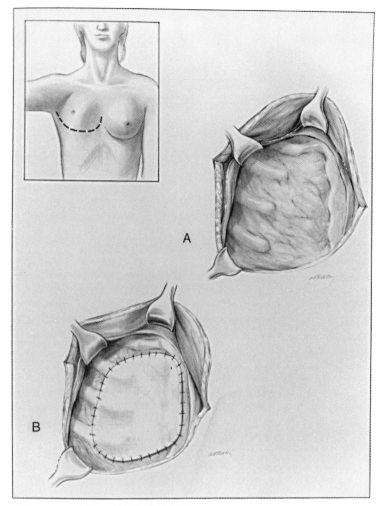

Figure 12–11. A, An incision is made from the axilla underneath the involved breast to the sternum. Flaps are raised similar to those for a pectus excavation repair between the subcutaneous tissue and what would be the pectoralis muscle layer. In most cases, the muscles and costicartilages are absent. The defect may also involve an absence of the second, third, and fourth ribs. **B,** The chest wall is usually reconstructed with either Marlex or Prolene mesh or a methomethacrylate plate. These are sutured to the edge of the chest wall defect with interrupted 0 Prolene sutures to stabilize the chest wall. **C,** Reconstruction of anterior cartilage and rib defect with a double layer of Marlex mesh covered with a thin layer of artificial dura mater. (From Urschel HC Jr. Poland's syndrome. *Chest Surg Clin North Am* 2000;10: 393–403.)

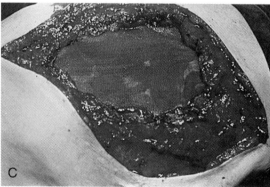

of all benign rib tumors. Osteochondroma accounts for 50% of all nonmalignant rib tumors. They are usually asymptomatic and are found incidentally during radiographic evaluation for another process. Chondromas arise from cartilaginous tissue at the sternocostal junction. Many authorities prefer to consider fibrous dysplasia a developmental disorder or hamartoma. Typically, fibrous dysplasia appears in the lateral or posterior tract of the ribs.

Among soft tissue tumors, the desmoid is considered by some to be benign fibromatosis and by others to be a low-grade fibrosarcoma.

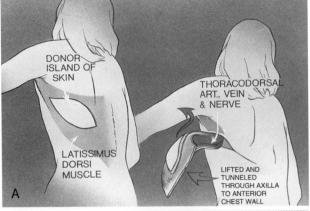

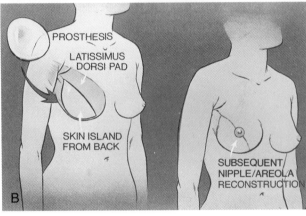

Figure 12–12. **A**, Dorsal view of myocutaneous flap construction with preservation of the thoracodorsal neurovascular pedicle, transfer of the latissimus flap through an axillary tunnel, and suture of the anterior chest wall skin to the island (paddle) of the transplant. **B**, Frontal view of myocutaneous flap construction with preservation of the thoracodorsal neurovascular pedicle, transfer of the latissimus flap through an axillary tunnel, and suture of the anterior chest wall skin to the island (paddle) of the transplant. ART, artery. (From Urschel HC Jr. Poland's syndrome. *Chest Surg Clin North Am* 2000;10:393–403.)

From the surgical point of view, it is treated as a primary malignant chest wall tumor and therefore must be resected with adequate margins to avoid local recurrence.

More than half of malignant tumors of the chest wall are metastatic lesions from distant organs or invasion from contiguous structures such as breast, lung, pleura, or mediastinum. Primary malignant neoplasms include tumors arising from the soft tissues as well as cartilaginous and bony tissue, sarcoma being the most common primary malignant tumor of the chest wall. Multiple myeloma and solitary plasmacytoma are the main pathologic bony malignant tumors of the chest wall (Figure 12–14).

Chondrosarcoma is the most common primary bone chest wall sarcoma, usually arising in the anterior tract of ribs and less frequently from the sternum, scapula, or clavicle (Figure 12–15). The grade is strictly correlated with the prognosis. Clinical and radiologic features of well differentiated chondrosarcoma can be confused with chondroma; therefore, a histologic diagnosis is required to assess for malignancy and avoid local recurrence with a consequently poorer chance of survival.

In general, soft tissue chest wall tumors are initially asymptomatic and present as a mass. When the tumor spreads to involve surrounding tissue, pain appears. Patients with soft tissue tumors frequently present without pain whereas patients with bony tumors frequently have pain. Fever is sometimes found as a systemic symptom. With cartilaginous and bone tumors, by comparison, pain is often the first sign of disease, and the tumor may be discovered on a standard chest radiograph. The advent of computed tomography and magnetic resonance imaging (MRI) has allowed precise localization of the lesion, evaluation of contiguous organ involvement, determination of the spread of breast and lung carcinoma to the thoracic wall, and detection of pulmonary

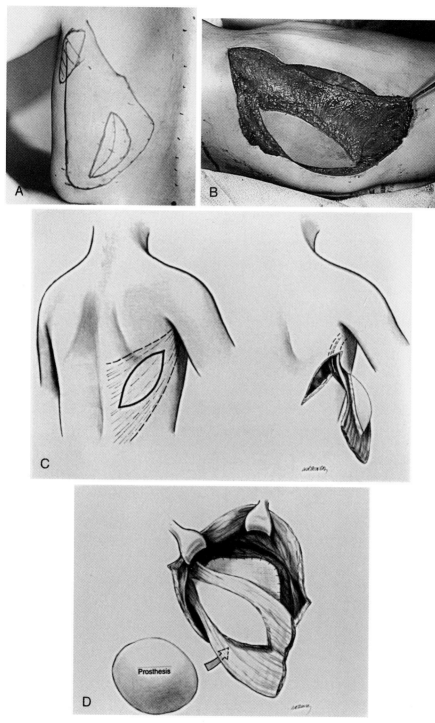

Figure 12–13. A, Preoperative mapping of myocutaneous flap. **B,** Myocutaneous flap construction with division of muscle attachments except for those needed to preserve the neurovascular bundle in the axilla. The flap is ready for transfer through the tunnel. **C,** Following the chest wall reconstruction, the patient is placed in the lateral position for dissection of the latissimus dorsi muscle flap. The skin and subcutaneous tissue with the latissimus dorsi muscle are freed posteriorly. **D,** The neurovascular bundle of the thoracoabdominal vessels is preserved as the blood and nerve supply for the cutaneous muscular flap, which is pulled through the axilla anteriorly. The skin, subcutaneous tissue, and muscle flap are brought through the axilla to cover the reconstructed chest wall. The posterior incision is closed with interrupted #1 Neurlon sutures and 2-0 Vicryl sutures in the subcutaneous tissue and skin clips in the skin. A prosthesis of either silicone or reconstructed muscle is placed under the breast between the reconstructed chest wall and the muscle flap of the latissimus dorsi.

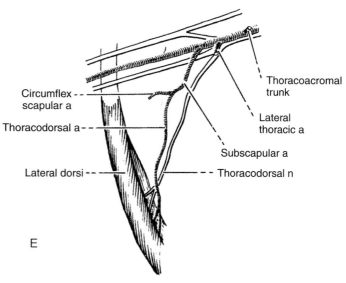

Figure 12–13. Continued. **E**, Vascular pedicle to myocutaneous flap. **F**, The myocutaneous flap, in position anteriorly over the chest wall reconstruction, is sutured to the chest wall in anticipation of insertion of a breast prosthesis beneath the flap. a, artery; n, nerve. (From Urschel HC Jr. Poland's syndrome. *Chest Surg Clin North Am* 2000;10:393–403.)

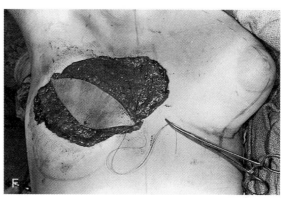

metastases. MRI provides multiplanar imaging and high-contrast resolution, which may make it the modality of choice to evaluate chest wall and spinal involvement. Vertebral body invasion with spinal cord involvement is best demonstrated by MRI. Radionuclide bone scanning should be performed before any major resection is carried out in a patient with a primary malignant chest wall tumor.

The most frequent primary malignant tumors also have characteristic radiographic features. Chondrosarcoma arises from a rib and presents with characteristic calcifications (Figure 12–16). Bone chest wall plasmacytoma is often part of a systemic disease and presents as a well defined lytic lesion with associated extrapleural soft tissue masses.

To determine the best treatment plan it is essential to choose a correct diagnostic procedure for the individual patient: fine-needle aspiration, incisional or excisional biopsy, or immediate chest wall resection. In general, however, excisional biopsy is preferable to needle or incisional biopsy. Excisional biopsy should be utilized for small lesions less than 2 cm or definitive resection of an uncertain radiologic and pathologic entity such as rib neoplasm. Incisional biopsy is indicated if the lesion is greater than 2 cm, needle biopsy is inconclusive, and neoadjuvant treatment is required for a large neoplasm. The biopsy should be made with a transverse incision which can be easily excised when skin flaps are used at a later operation (Figure 12–17). Such an invasive

TABLE 12–1 • *Classification of Chest Wall Tumors*

Benign Tumors of Bone

Bony	Osteoid osteoma
Cartilage	Enchondroma Osteochondroma
Fibrous	Fibrous dysplasia
Vascular	Hemangioma
Marrow	Eosinophilic granuloma
Osteoclast	Giant cell tumor Aneurysmal bone cyst

Benign Tumors of Soft Tissue

Fibrous	Probably do not exist
Adipose	Lipoma and its variations
Neural	Schwann cell (neurinoma, neurilemoma) Neurofibroma
Muscle	Vascular leiomyoma

Malignant Tumors of Bone

Bone	Osteosarcoma
Cartilage	Chondrosarcoma
Fibrous	Malignant fibrous histiocytoma
Vascular	Hemangiosarcoma
Marrow	Plasmacytoma
? cell	Ewing's sarcoma

Malignant Tumors of Soft Tissue

Fibrous	Desmoid Fibrosarcoma
Fibrohistiocytic	Malignant fibrous histiocytoma
Adipose	Liposarcoma
Neural	Neurofibrosarcoma Schwann cell sarcoma Askin's tumor
Muscle	Rhabdomyosarcoma

From Faber LP, Somers J, Templeton AC. Chest wall tumors. *Curr Prob Surg* 1995;32:661–747.

diagnostic procedure may potentially seed malignant cells, so flaps and deep sampling must be avoided.

The treatment of chest wall tumors varies according to the specific tumor. Benign tumors are treated by simple excision and malignant tumors are generally treated with wide excision. The exceptions to the rule are solitary plasmocytomas, which are treated with radiation therapy, and Ewing's sarcoma, which is treated by chemotherapy followed by radiation and surgical resection (Figure 12–18). The ability of thoracic surgeons to perform wide resection of the thoracic wall and to close the defect successfully at the same operating procedure, without significant mortality and limited morbidity, firmly established the role of surgery in the management of primary malignant chest wall tumors.

Data concerning treatments and results of therapy are sparse. Positive margins are the most important risk factor for local recurrence and have a considerable impact on

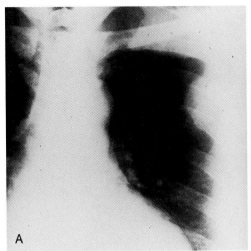

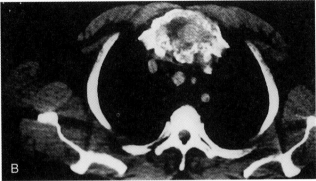

Figure 12–14. A, Posteroanterior chest radiograph showing a mass in the chest wall on the lateral aspect of the left pleura. Note that the mass encroaches on the pleural space. It is contiguous with the chest wall structures. Even though the mass had radiographic characteristics suggestive of a chondrosarcoma, on excision it was found to be a plasmocytoma. **B,** Computed tomography scan showing a large irregular mass that has replaced the entire manubrium of the sternum. Note that it displaces the great vessels posteriorly. This mass, which was a rapidly enlarging neoplasm of the sternum, was thought to be a chondrosarcoma. Pathologic examination confirmed that it was a plasmocytoma. (From Pearson FG, Cooper JD, Deslauriers J, ed. *Thoracic surgery*, 2nd ed. New York: Churchill Livingstone, 2002:1342.)

disease-free and overall survival. It is recommended that a margin of at least 4 cm of normal tissue be obtained when wide resection for malignant tumors of the chest wall is performed (Figure 12–19). The role of adjuvant chemotherapy in the management of thoracic wall primary sarcomas is still unclear. The use of preoperative chemotherapy and radiotherapy should be explored in patients with chest wall tumors that carry a significantly low 5-year survival, such as osteosarcomas. For primary chest wall malignant tumors, radical resection is the treatment of choice, except for solitary plasmacytomas, where biopsy followed by radiation therapy appears to be a valid alternative. For small chest wall tumors, such as Ewing's sarcoma and Askin's tumor, surgery is part of a multimodality

Figure 12–15. A characteristic field from a histologic section of a chondrosarcoma. The histologic characteristics of this tumor include a cartilaginous neoplasm, which has anaplastic cells with one or more bizarre, hyperchromatic nuclei. This malignant neoplasm is also known to have frequent variations in the grade of tumor cells present through the presenting mass (H & E, ×200). (Pearson FG, Cooper JD, Deslauriers J, ed. *Thoracic surgery*, 2nd ed. New York: Churchill Livingstone, 2002:1421.)

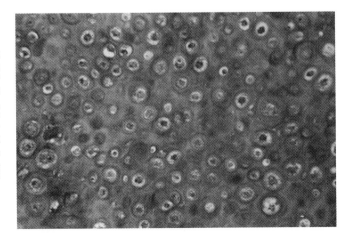

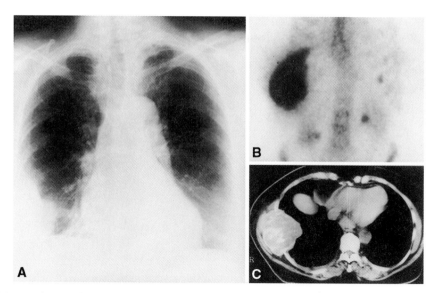

Figure 12–16. A, Chest radiograph, **B,** bone scan and **C,** computed tomography image of right lateral chest wall chondrosarcoma, demonstrating intralesional calcification (**A** and **C**) and extrathoracic involvement (**B**). (From Cameron JL, ed. *Current surgical therapy,* 7th ed. St Louis: Mosby, 2001:752.)

approach that includes chemotherapy and radiotherapy.

Wide surgical resection with adequate margins is no longer limited by the size of the chest wall defect, and surgery may be considered the best option for most primary malignant tumors. Nowadays successful management cannot be precluded by tumor size, site, or contiguous structure involvement; and concurrent reconstruction with prosthetic materials and myocutaneous flaps is a feasible treatment. The strategy of reconstruction must be based on the extent of the soft tissue and skeletal defects (Box 12–1). The potentially available combinations of myocutaneous flaps and prosthetic materials are numerous, and the best option is based on the characteristics of the individual's disease.

Full-thickness resection must include an adequate margin of normal tissue because a radical surgical procedure is the key to successful management. Most authors recommend excision of 2–4 cm from the macroscopic tumor

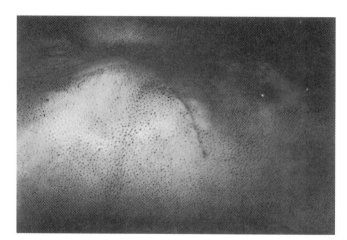

Figure 12–17. Transversely placed previous biopsy of chest wall sarcoma. Transverse orientation lends itself to easier excision in raising the skin flaps at time of definitive resection. (From Roth JA, Ruckdeschel JC, Weisenburger TH, ed. *Thoracic oncology,* 2nd ed. Philadelphia: WB Saunders, 1995:523.)

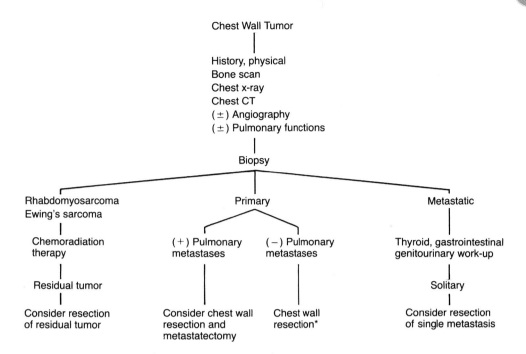

Chest Wall Tumor

History, physical
Bone scan
Chest x-ray
Chest CT
($\pm$) Angiography
($\pm$) Pulmonary functions

Biopsy

Rhabdomyosarcoma
Ewing's sarcoma

Chemoradiation
therapy

Residual tumor

Consider resection
of residual tumor

Primary

(+) Pulmonary
metastases

Consider chest wall
resection and
metastatectomy

(−) Pulmonary
metastases

Chest wall
resection*

Metastatic

Thyroid, gastrointestinal
genitourinary work-up

Solitary

Consider resection
of single metastasis

*If chest wall lesion is too large to ensure negative margins,
consider primary radiation therapy or preoperative best-choice
chemotherapy with tumor resection after objective response.

Figure 12-18. Diagnosis and staging of chest wall neoplasms. (From Roth JA, Ruckdeschel JC, Weisenburger TH, ed. *Thoracic oncology*, 2nd ed. Philadelphia: WB Saunders, 1995:524.)

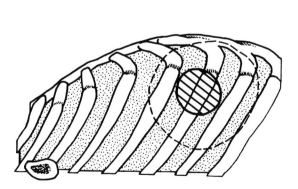

Figure 12-19. Diagrammatic representation of the extent of resection necessary for chest wall tumors. The resection should include one normal rib cephalad and caudad to the tumor and 4–5 cm of grossly normal tissue laterally. (From El-Tamer M, Chaglassian T, Martini N. Resection and debridement of chest-wall tumors and general aspects of reconstruction. *Surg Clin North Am* 1989;69: 947–964.)

BOX 12-1 FACTORS TO CONSIDER
FOR RECONSTRUCTION OF
CHEST WALL DEFECTS

Location
Size
Depth
   • Partial thickness
   • Full thickness
Duration
Condition of local tissue
   • Irradiation
   • Infection
   • Residual tumor
   • Scarring
General condition of patient
Chemotherapy
Corticosteroids
Chronic infection
Life-style and type of work
Prognosis

From Sabiston DC, Spencer FC. *Surgery of the chest*, 6th ed. Philadelphia: WB Saunders, 1995:517.

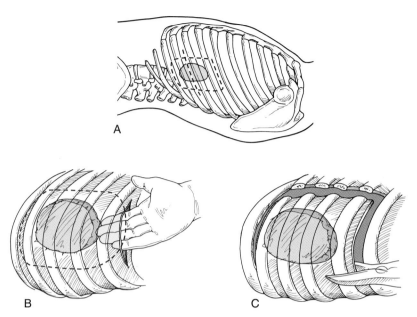

Figure 12–20. A, The chest wall tumor originates from the anterolateral chest wall. The skin incision is made over the lesion and flaps are developed accordingly. The anticipated resection margins are outlined. **B**, The chest cavity is entered at least one interspace above the planned border of resection. The tumor is palpated within the chest to distinguish the extent of gross disease. The line of resection is outlined with the electro-cautery on the skeletal surface. **C**, A 2 cm section of rib is removed with each incised rib to facilitate mobility of the chest wall. This maneuver is particularly helpful for tumors that abut the spine or sternum. (Redrawn from Cameron JL, ed. *Current surgical therapy*, 7th ed. St Louis: Mosby, 2001:755–756.)

TABLE 12–2 • *Choice of Flaps for Reconstruction of Full-Thickness Defects of the Chest Wall*

Muscle	Neurovascular Supply	Origin	Insertion
Latissimus dorsi	Primary: thoracodorsal nerve, artery, and vein Secondary: artery to serratus anterior	T6–S3, posterior crest of ileum	Intratubular groove of the humerus
Pectoralis major	Primary: thoracoabdominal nerve, artery, and vein Secondary: internal mammary and intercostal arteries	Sternum, clavicle, ribs 1–7	Tricipital groove of humerus
Rectus abdominis	Primary: superior and inferior epigastric arteries	Pubic crest	Rib cartilage of ribs 5–7, xiphoid
Serratus anterior	Primary: serratus branch of thoracodorsal artery Secondary: long thoracic artery	Outer surface and superior border of ribs 8–10; intercostal fascia	Scapula tip
External oblique	Primary: lower thoracic intercostal artery, nerve, and vein	External surface and inferior border of ribs 4–12	Iliac crest, lower abdominal process
Trapezius	Primary: transverse cervical artery, nerve, and vein Secondary: occipital branches and intercostal perforators	Occipital bone, C7–T12 spinous processes	Posterior and lateral third of clavicle, acromion, superior lip of scapular spine

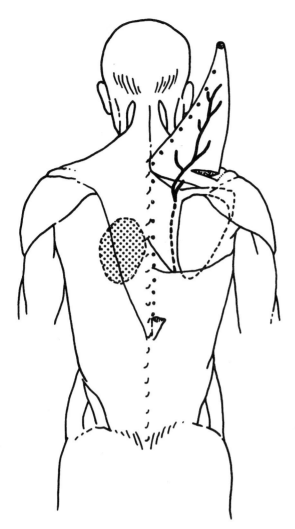

margin, whereas others believe that excision should include all involved bone and a 4 cm margin of normal tissue on all sides (Figure 12–20 and Table 12–2).

The size and site of the neoplasm influence the strategy for skeletal reconstruction, which is a necessary procedure for sternum and anterior and lateral defects. In contrast, posterior defects may not require reconstruction when covered by the scapula without any risk of inward rotation or if stabilized by adjacent muscles (Figure 12–21). Some authors maintain that partial sternal and posterior defects require less stabilization than anterior and lateral ones, which cause paradoxical respiration.

Resections less than 5 cm of diameter usually do not require stabilization, with rigid prosthetic replacement and soft tissue being enough. When the defect is larger, the thoracic wall solidity must be reconstituted. Various synthetic materials are available: Marlex mesh, Vicryl mesh (Ethicon®), polytetrafluoroethylene (PTFE) patch, and Prolene mesh are well tolerated.

Figure 12–21. Trapezius flap: left side demonstrates the design of the cutaneous element; right side shows the flap after elevation. Notice that the muscular branches of the dorsal scapular artery may arise under the rhomboid minor. A back cut over the lateral edge of the flap increases its mobility. (From El-Tamer M, Chaglassian T, Martini N. Resection and debridement of chest-wall tumors and general aspects of reconstruction. *Surg Clin North Am* 1989;69:947–964.)

Selected Readings

El-Tamer M, Chaglassian T, Martini N. Resection and debridement of chest-wall tumors and general aspects of reconstruction. *Surg Clin North Am* 1989;69:947–964.

Faber LP, Somers J, Templeton AC. Chest wall tumors. *Curr Prob Surg* 1995;32:661–747.

Haller JA Jr. Complications of surgery for pectus excavatum. *Chest Surg Clin North Am* 2000;10: 415–426.

Incarbone M, Pastorino U. Surgical treatment of chest wall tumors. *World J Surg* 2001;25:218–230.

Morshuis WJ, Mulder H, Wapperom G, *et al*. Pectus excavatum. A clinical study with long-term postoperative follow-up. *Eur J Cardio-Thorac Surg* 1992;6:318–328.

Robicsek F. Surgical treatment of pectus carinatum. *Chest Surg Clin North Am* 2000;10:357–376.

Robicsek F. Surgical treatment of pectus excavatum. *Chest Surg Clin North Am* 2000;10:277–296.

Urschel HC Jr. Poland's syndrome. *Chest Surg Clin North Am* 2000;10:393–403.

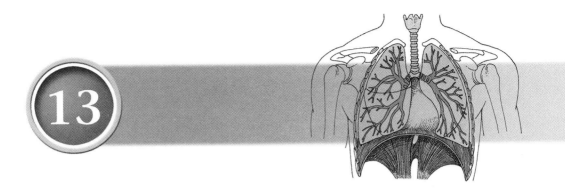

13

Trachea

Trachea: Key Points

- Understand the anatomy of common congenital tracheal lesions
- Describe the development of postintubation injuries and how they should be managed
- Know the management of acquired tracheoesophageal fistulas
- Know the choices in radiographic evaluation of the trachea
- Know the histological types of tracheal neoplasms

Anatomy

The trachea is a cartilaginous and membranous airway extending from the lower part of the larynx, on a level with the C6 vertebra, to the upper border of the T5 vertebra, where it divides into the two bronchi, one for each lung. The trachea is somewhat elliptical but flattened posteriorly (Figure 13–1). It is about 11 cm in length and 2–2.5 cm in diameter (Figure 13–2).

The anterior surface of the trachea is convex and is covered in the neck by the thyroid isthmus, the sternothyroid and sternohyoid muscles, the cervical fascia, and the anastomosing branches between the anterior jugular veins. In the thorax, the trachea is covered by the manubrium, the remains of the thymus, the left innominate vein, the aortic arch, the innominate and left common carotid arteries, and the deep cardiac plexus. The esophagus lies contiguous to the membranous, or posterior, aspect. Laterally, in the neck, it borders the common carotid arteries, the right and left lobes of the thyroid gland, the inferior thyroid

263

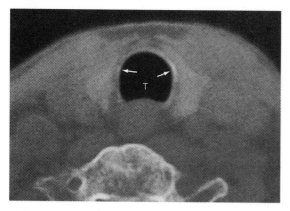

Figure 13–1. Normal extrathoracic trachea. Computed tomography shows a normal horseshoe-shaped trachea (T). The posterior tracheal membrane bulges slightly into the tracheal air column. Anteriorly, a calcified tracheal cartilage is visible *(arrows)*. (From Moss AA, Gamsu G, Genant HK. *Computed tomography of the body*, 2nd ed. Philadelphia: WB Saunders, 1992:3.)

trachea are the left recurrent nerve, the aortic arch, and the left common carotid and subclavian arteries.

The trachea is composed of incomplete rings of hyaline cartilage, fibrous tissue, muscular fibers, mucous membrane, and glands. There are 16–20 tracheal cartilages, which form rings around the anterior two thirds of the circumference of the trachea. The ring does not extend posteriorly. Instead the trachea is supported by fibrous tissue and nonstriated muscular fibers. The cartilages are placed horizontally above each other, separated by narrow intervals. They measure about 4 mm in depth and 1 mm in thickness. Their outer surfaces are flattened in a vertical direction but the internal surfaces are convex. The cartilages are thicker in the middle than at the margins. Two or more of the cartilages often unite and they are sometimes bifurcated at their ends. They are highly elastic but may become calcified in advanced life. In the right main bronchus the cartilages vary in number from six to eight; in the left, from nine to 12. They are shorter and narrower than those of

arteries, and the recurrent nerves. In the thorax, it lies in the superior mediastinum and borders the right pleura, the right vagus, and the innominate artery. On the left side of the

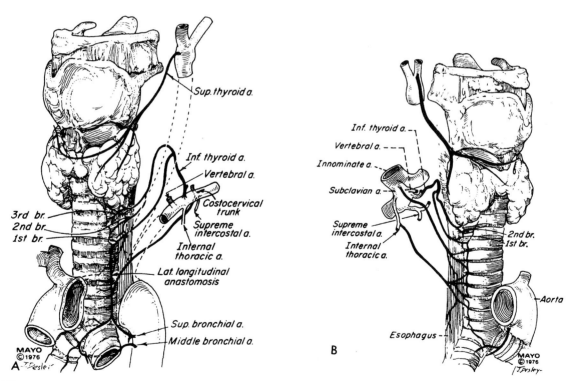

Figure 13–2. A, Left anterior view of arteries supplying the trachea. In this specimen, the lateral longitudinal anastomosis links branches of the inferior thyroid, costocervical trunk, and bronchial arteries. **B,** Right anterior view of vessels supplying the trachea. In this specimen, the lateral longitudinal anastomosis links branches from the inferior thyroid, the subclavian, the internal thoracic, and the superior bronchial arteries. (From Salassa JR, Pearson BW, Payne WS. Gross and microscopic blood supply of the trachea. *Ann Thorac Surg* 1977;24:100. Reprinted with permission from the Society of Thoracic Surgeons.)

the trachea but have the same shape and arrangement.

The first cartilage is broader than the rest and is often divided at one end; it is connected by the cricotracheal ligament to the lower border of the cricoid cartilage. The last cartilage is thick and broad in the middle and curves inferiorly and posteriorly between the two bronchi. It ends on each side in an imperfect ring that encloses the take-off of the bronchus. The cartilage above the last is somewhat broader than the others at its center.

The muscular tissue consists of two layers of nonstriated muscle, longitudinal and transverse. The longitudinal fibers are external and consist of a few scattered bundles. The transverse fibers are internal and form a thin layer that extends transversely between the ends of the cartilages.

The mucous membrane is continuous from the larynx to the bronchi. It consists of areolar and lymphoid tissue and presents a well marked basement membrane, supporting a stratified epithelium. The surface layer is columnar and ciliated, while the deeper layers are composed of oval or rounded cells. Beneath the basement membrane there is a distinct layer of longitudinal elastic fibers with a small amount of intervening areolar tissue. The submucous layer is composed of a loose meshwork of connective tissue, containing large blood vessels, nerves, and mucous glands.

Diagnosis

Obstructing (intraluminal) tracheal lesions often are recognized late despite a prolonged period of symptoms. Most patients are initially given the presumptive diagnosis of adult-onset asthma.

Several methods can be used to study the trachea and evaluate masses, stenosis, and vascular abnormalities. In addition to usual posteroanterior and lateral chest films, oblique views are taken to show the full extent of the trachea with the mediastinal structures rotated to one side. Lateral cervical films, with swallowing to raise the larynx, give excellent information about laryngotracheal relationships, especially at the stomal level (Figures 13–3, 13–4). Radiopaque markers placed on the skin at the level of a tracheostomy can help pinpoint exact surface relationships to tracheal lesions.

Fluoroscopy is also used to determine the function of the larynx, the location of abnormalities, and the presence of cartilage thin-

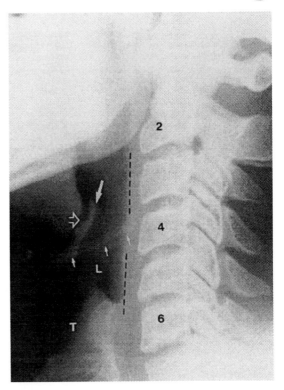

Figure 13–3. Normal anatomy: soft tissue structures of the neck, lateral view. Air outlines the key anatomic structures of the upper airways. The epiglottis is well-defined (large arrow), as are the anterior and posterior margins of the hypopharynx and the larynx (L). The vallecula (open arrow) lies anterior to the epiglottis. The hyoid bone (small arrows) overlies the base of the epiglottis. Note the width of the anterior cervical tissues, normally less than 7 mm at C2 and 21 mm at the C5–C6 level (dotted lines). T, trachea. (From Meholic A, Ketai L, Lofgren R. *Fundamentals of chest radiology.* Philadelphia: WB Saunders, 1996:40.)

ning. Contrast studies are rarely indicated except with tracheoesophageal fistula, and this is better shown by barium esophagogram (Figure 13–5).

Computed tomography (CT) is used to evaluate extramural extension to adjacent structures (Figure 13–6). Most importantly, CT adds information about mediastinal extent of tumor. It is of little use in assessing benign stenosis except in the case of external compression from goiters, vascular rings, or histoplasmosis.

Bronchoscopic examination is a standard part of tracheal evaluation. If possible, endoscopy should be avoided until time of surgery to avoid precipitating an acute event in an uncontrolled setting. The bronchoscopy is done with the patient under general anesthesia,

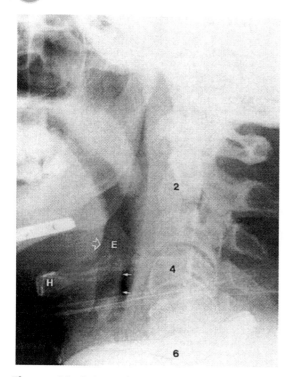

Figure 13–4. Lateral cervical soft tissue: acute epiglottitis. The bulbous epiglottis (thumb shape) is consistent with acute epiglottitis (compare with the normal epiglottis shown in Figure 13–4). **E**, epiglottis; **H**, hyoid bone; small arrows, arytenoepiglottic folds; open arrow, vallecula. (From Meholic A, Ketai L, Lofgren R. *Fundamentals of chest radiology.* Philadelphia: WB Saunders, 1996:42.)

permitting unhurried, atraumatic examination and manipulation. In general, biopsy of lesions should also be avoided until this time because of the unknown vascularity of many airway tumors. Esophagoscopy is also performed when neoplasms are examined. Rigid bronchoscopy under general anesthesia using pediatric bronchoscopes serially can be used to dilate severe stenosis for emergency relief.

Congenital Lesions

The most frequent abnormalities which have been described in the pediatric population are tracheomalacia, congenital stenosis, tracheoesophageal fistulas, and vascular rings.

Tracheomalacia

Tracheomalacia represents the inability of the cartilages to keep the airway open during respiration (Figure 13–7). Primary tracheomalacia is an inherent cartilage abnormality. Secondary tracheomalacia is due to external pressure exerted on the airway from esophageal atresia or vascular abnormalities. Patients present with a full spectrum of symptoms. Some patients have expiratory wheeze whereas others with severe disease can have both inspiratory and expiratory stridor. Bronchoscopy is the most reliable means of diagnosing children with tracheomalacia.

Most children have a spontaneous resolution of symptoms without treatment. Severe tracheomalacia may require a tracheostomy. A long tracheostomy cannula can help stent open the airway lumen. Stents are also available to splay open the trachea; however, they can develop extensive granulation into the tissue, making removal difficult (Figure 13–8).

Congenital Stenosis

Congenital stenosis is a broad category describing a variety of tracheal abnormalities including webs and narrowing of the airway. Congenital stenosis of the trachea is grouped into three categories: generalized hypoplasia (30%), funnel-like stenosis (20%), and segmental stenosis (50%) (Figure 13–9). The bronchi are usually not involved. In progressive narrowing of the trachea, the cartilage rings get progressively smaller in diameter moving down to the carina. In diseases with segmental stenosis of the trachea, the C-shaped cartilage rings are usually completely closed around and not open on the posterior aspect.

Most infants with congenital stenoses are not symptomatic at birth, although the majority do have symptoms within the first month of life. Diagnosis is based on a high degree of suspicion in infants with respiratory distress. Inspiratory and expiratory stridor can often be audible, in addition to wheezing and use of accessory respiratory muscles. Neonates have feeding difficulties and failure of normal development. Air tracheograms and bronchoscopy can be used to obtain detailed information about airway anatomy.

Congenital tracheal stenoses are frequently associated with other anomalies. Lower tracheal stenosis can be seen in association with an aberrant left pulmonary artery (Figure 13–10). In cases with a 'pulmonary artery sling', the left pulmonary artery originates from the proximal portion of the right artery and passes behind the trachea to the left lung. The importance of vascular compression of the tracheal wall is an important

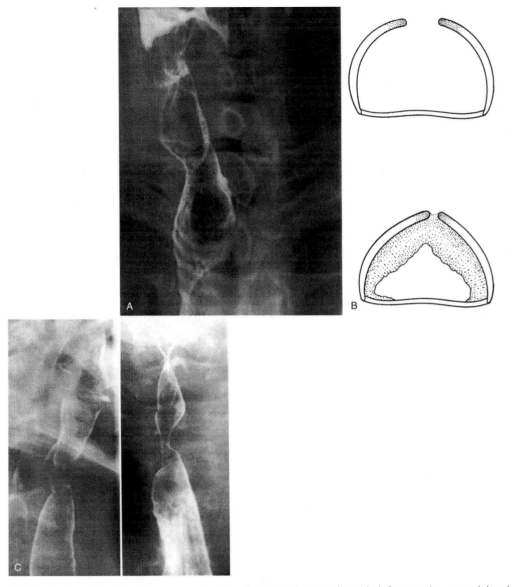

Figure 13–5. A, A contrast tracheogram showing the typical anterolateral defect at the stomal level after tracheostomy. This relatively mild lesion was asymptomatic. **B**, This diagram illustrates the mechanism of stomal stenosis. A variable segment of cartilage is lost anteriorly (top); with healing, the remaining margins fall together and form scar tissue in the anterolateral parts of the trachea. The membranous trachea is relatively preserved, and a triangular stenosis results. **C**, A contrast tracheogram illustrating a severe stomal stenosis. (From Pearson FG, Cooper JD, Deslauriers J. *Thoracic surgery*, 2nd ed. New York: Churchill Livingstone, 2002:304.)

part of tracheal stenosis pathophysiology. Congenital stenosis of the trachea usually manifests in the lower part of the airway. These lesions often require urgent definitive repair and cannot be bypassed. High tracheal or laryngeal lesions often allow delay or staging after tracheostomy.

Surgical repair of congenital tracheal lesions is risky. Postoperative edema can result in total obstructions. Attempts at stenting open the air-

way with an endotracheal tube can damage the anastomoses. Dilatation of the airway is rarely successful and is more likely to crack the trachea, resulting in formation of granulation tissue. Conservative methods are the treatment of choice. Tracheal webs are removed via a bronchoscope by biopsy forceps. Alternatively, an infant can be given a tracheostomy until old enough to undergo definitive repair and re-anastomosis. Sleeve resection and incision

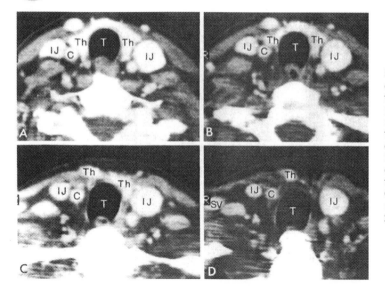

Figure 13–6. Normal extrathoracic trachea. **A–D,** Sequential scans through the lower neck. The middle and lower poles of the thyroid gland (Th) are anterior and lateral to the horseshoe-shaped trachea (T). The right carotid artery (C) courses from anterior to posterior. The internal jugular veins (IJ) and right subclavian vein (SV) are anterolateral to the trachea. (From Moss AA, Gamsu G, Genant HK. *Computed tomography of the body,* 2nd ed. Philadelphia: WB Saunders, 1992:4.)

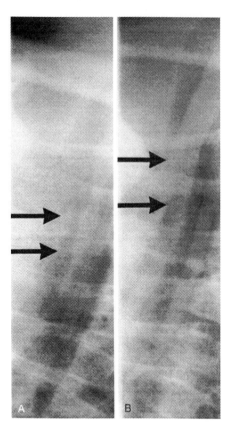

Figure 13–7. Lateral chest films in a 2-month-old child with tracheomalacia. Note the tracheal air shadow. **A,** During inspiration, a slight indentation related to the aorta is seen on the anterior wall of the trachea (between arrows). **B,** During expiration, the tracheal air shadow disappears in this same region (between arrows) as the trachea collapses. (From Pearson FG, Cooper JD, Deslauriers J. *Thoracic surgery,* 2nd ed. New York: Churchill Livingstone, 2002:288.)

with tracheoplasty are also viable options (Figure 13–11).

Congenital Tracheoesophageal Fistula

Tracheoesophageal fistulas (TEF) occur in 1:4000 births, slightly more commonly in males. The embryology of TEF is poorly understood. A global disturbance in embryogenesis causes well-characterized anomalies in vertebral, anal, cardiac, renal, and limb systems (VACTERL) at the same time as esophageal atresias with tracheoesophageal fistulas.

Tracheoesophageal fistulas have been classified into five broad categories:

- *Type A.* Isolated esophageal atresia without TEF (5%) (Figure 13–12). In this scenario, there is complete absence of a portion of the esophagus without any connection between the two lumens.
- *Type B.* Esophageal atresia with proximal fistula: A rare entity that occurs when a short fistula connects the upper esophagus to the trachea with a luminal discontinuity.
- *Type C.* Esophageal atresia with a distal TEF (85%) (Figure 13–13). The proximal esophagus is dilated and thickened and ends at the level of T3. The blood supply to the upper esophagus is from the thyrocervical trunk on both sides. The esophagus often shares a common wall with the posterior aspect of the trachea. The fistula occurs along the lower back wall of the trachea, along the soft, noncartilaginous

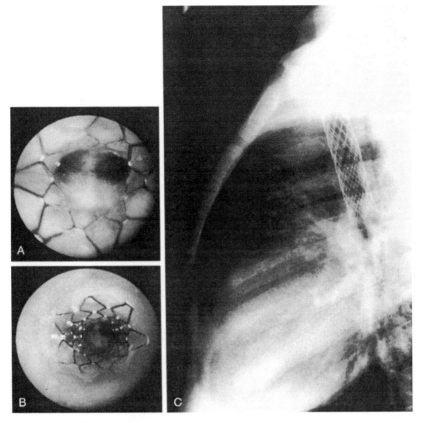

Figure 13–8. A, This 3-month-old was born with esophageal atresia and tracheoesophageal fistula. Because of dying spells and confirmed tracheomalacia, two overlapping Palmaz stents were inserted in the trachea. The illustration shows the expanded stent above the carina. **B**, This illustration was taken at the proximal end of the stent. **C**, Post-stenting lateral chest radiograph. (From Pearson FG, Cooper JD, Deslauriers J. *Thoracic surgery*, 2nd ed. New York: Churchill Livingstone, 2002:290.)

membranous wall. This site is close to the carina. The blood supply to the lower esophagus is segmental.

- *Type D*. Esophageal atresia with a proximal and distal fistula (Figure 13–14). Also rare, these are similar to Type C TEF. There is a fistula from the distal trachea to the esophagus. In addition, there is a proximal fistula adjoining the proximal trachea to the esophagus.
- *Type E*. Isolated TEF without esophageal atresia (5%) (Figure 13–15). The trachea and esophagus are linked by a short fistula, termed the H-type fistula, without loss of either lumen.

Tracheoesophageal fistulas are evident soon after birth and present with excessive secretions, difficulty in swallowing, and inability to eat. If a distal TEF is present, gastric secretions gain access to the respiratory tract, leading to pneumonitis and progressive respiratory failure. Severe hypoxia can require mechanical ventilation.

The diagnosis can be quickly attained by attempting to place an orogastric tube. Chest radiography will demonstrate coiling of the tube in the proximal esophagus. Air in the abdomen confirms the presence of a distal TEF (Figure 13–16). A gasless abdomen, on the other hand, suggests complete atresia. Further studies, although often not necessary, can be performed using dilute barium.

Next, the infant should be evaluated for potential other congenital abnormalities. Radiographs of the chest and abdomen can assess vertebral or rib abnormalities. Echocardiography can evaluate cardiac problems and renal ultrasonography can suggest abdominal pathology.

Management of infants with TEF depends on the status of two things: the severity of associated anomalies and the overall physiological state of the infant. A healthy

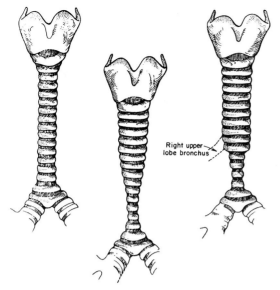

Figure 13–9. Types of congenital tracheal stenosis. Type 1 (left): generalized hypoplasia of the trachea. The larynx is of normal caliber. The bronchi may be stenotic or not. Type 2 (center): funnel-like narrowing. This may occur in the upper or lower trachea. Type 3 (right): segmental stenosis that may be accompanied by bronchial anomalies. This is a type of stenosis that is also seen with 'pulmonary artery sling.' (From Cantrell JR, Guild HR. Congenital stenosis of the trachea. *Am J Surg* 1964; 108:297.)

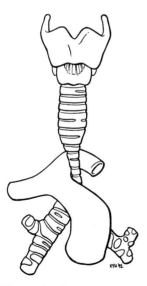

Figure 13–10. Tracheal stenosis is associated with aberrant left pulmonary artery (sling) in 50% of cases. Repair of the sling will not correct the intrinsic tracheal problem. (From Pearson FG, Cooper JD, Deslauriers J. *Thoracic surgery*, 2nd ed. New York: Churchill Livingstone, 2002:293.)

near-term or full-term infant with a stable cardiovascular system and no significant respiratory problems should undergo early repair. Early repair minimizes the time during which the child may aspirate gastric contents. These patients should undergo take-down of the TEF with primary anastomosis with the atretic end of the esophagus.

In the event that the patients have several comorbid events, symptomatic control should be obtained by a decompression gastrostomy tube and placement of a Fogarty balloon catheter into the fistula. The balloon occlusion can be maintained for days or weeks while the patient stabilizes from a cardiopulmonary stand point.

Occasionally patients will have a long esophageal atresia, which will prevent primary anastomosis. A gastrostomy should be placed and repair delayed until a primary repair can be performed.

Vascular Rings

Vascular rings can cause tracheal compromise due to compression of the airway, not to inherent abnormalities in the trachea. Vascular abnormalities that cause problems include double aortic arch, right aortic arch with patent ductus arteriosus or ligamentum arteriosum, aberrant subclavian artery, and abnormal innominate artery.

The double aortic arch is the most common complete vascular ring that causes tracheoesophageal compression. Patients present in the first months of life with symptoms of stridor, respiratory distress, and a cough. The ascending aorta divides into two arches that pass around the trachea and esophagus and join posteriorly to form the descending aorta (Figure 13–17). The carotid and subclavian arteries originate symmetrically and separately from each arch. The tight, constricting ring that forms compresses the trachea and the esophagus. The diagnosis can be suspected on a chest radiograph because the location of the aortic arch in relation to the trachea is indeterminate. A barium esophagogram is the most reliable study for diagnosis of vascular rings. CT scanning is also a reliable method of diagnosing vascular abnormalities. All infants with a double aortic arch should be operated on. A narrowed trachea, when further compromised by mucosal edema from even a mild upper respiratory infection, can cause sudden respiratory arrest. For a double aortic arch, a

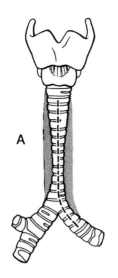
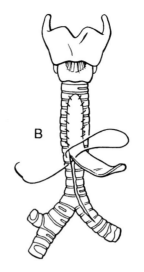
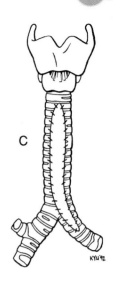

Figure 13–11. General technique of tracheoplasty. **A**, The stenotic segment of trachea is opened longitudinally to an airway of normal diameter superiorly and inferiorly. **B**, Tissue selected for grafting is sutured to the defect with running or interrupted sutures of absorbable material. **C**, Completed tracheoplasty. (From Pearson FG, Cooper JD, Deslauriers J. *Thoracic surgery*, 2nd ed. New York: Churchill Livingstone, 2002:296.)

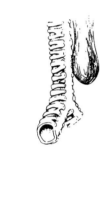
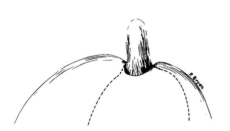

Figure 13–12. Isolated esophageal atresia. (No tracheoesophageal fistula is present.) (From Ashcraft KW. *Pediatric surgery*, 3rd ed. Philadelphia: WB Saunders, 2000:350.)

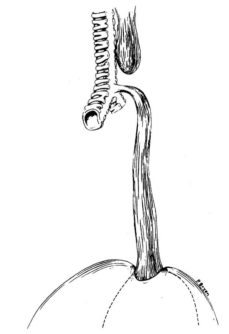

Figure 13–13. Esophageal atresia with distal tracheoesophageal fistula. (From Ashcraft KW. *Pediatric surgery*, 3rd ed. Philadelphia: WB Saunders, 2000:350.)

left thoracotomy approach is recommended. The vascular ring caused by the double aortic arch is released by dividing the lesser of the two arches, usually where it inserts into the descending aorta. The ligamentum arteriosum is also divided. Careful dissection is then per-

formed around the trachea and esophagus to lyse any residual adhesive bands.

The right aortic arch with a ligamentum arteriosum completing the vascular ring is almost as common as a double aortic arch. It is the most common constricting disease of the

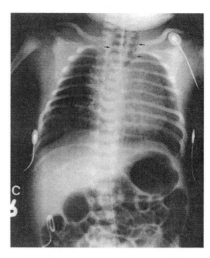

Figure 13–16. Chest radiograph demonstrates a dilated proximal esophageal pouch *(arrows)*. A catheter extends to the lower end of the pouch at the level of the third thoracic vertebra, indicating esophageal atresia. The presence of gas in the stomach indicates a distal TEF. A generous amount of small bowel gas is noted. (From Ashcraft KW, Holder TM. *Pediatric surgery*, 2nd ed. Philadelphia: WB Saunders, 1993:254.)

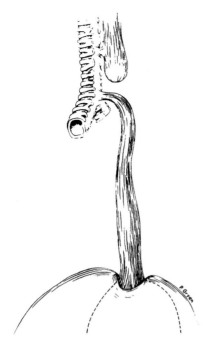

Figure 13–14. Esophageal atresia with proximal and distal tracheoesophageal fistulas. (From Ashcraft KW. *Pediatric surgery*, 3rd ed. Philadelphia: WB Saunders, 2000:352.)

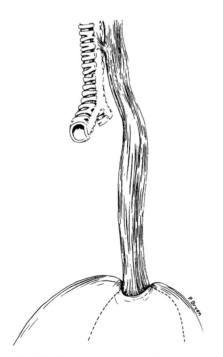

Figure 13–15. H-type tracheoesophageal fistula. No esophageal atresia is present. (From Ashcraft KW. *Pediatric surgery*, 3rd ed. Philadelphia: WB Saunders, 2000:351.)

incomplete rings. The ring is usually not as tight and children do not present until later in life, 6–12 months of age. The right aortic arch with a left descending aorta may cause anterior tracheal compression from the left subclavian and carotid arteries. Infants present similarly with stridor and respiratory distress. In addition, dysphagia may be present. Again, the best radiographic study is the barium esophagogram. A left thoracotomy with muscle-sparing approach is recommended. The ring is released by dividing the ligamentum between vascular clamps and oversewing the stumps. Adhesive bands are lysed.

Innominate artery compression syndrome results from anterior compression of the trachea by the innominate artery. There is usually a normal left aortic arch. The innominate artery appears to originate somewhat more posteriorly and leftward on the aortic arch than usual. Infants present with stridor, respiratory distress, cyanosis, and apnea with feeding. The infant may hold the head hyperextended to splint the trachea and improve breathing. Apnea or cyanosis may be precipitated by swallowing a bolus of food, which presses on the soft posterior trachea with the innominate artery compressing the anterior trachea. Symptoms attributable to innominate artery compression have been identified as late as adolescence. Diagnosis is made with

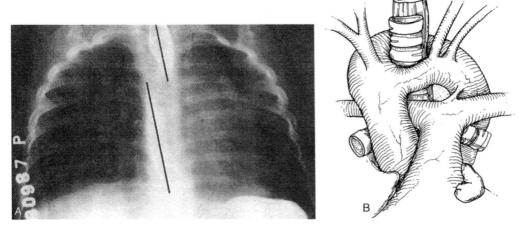

Figure 13–17. A, A double aortic arch demonstrated by barium esophagram. The axes of the proximal and distal portions of the esophagus are offset by the presence of a complete vascular ring. **B,** The double arch as drawn is usually narrowest on the left branch and is best approached for division through a left thoracotomy. (From Ashcraft KW, Holder TM. *Pediatric surgery*, 2nd ed. Philadelphia: WB Saunders, 1993:245.)

rigid bronchoscopy, which demonstrates a pulsatile anterior compression of the trachea extending from left to right, with at least a 70% obstruction of the tracheal lumen. Anterior compression of the tracheal wall by the bronchoscope may compress the innominate artery and temporarily obliterate the right radial pulse. The diagnosis is usually confirmed by CT scan. For an innominate artery suspension a right thoracotomy approach is taken. The innominate artery is secured to the posterior periosteum of the sternum to lift the innominate artery away from the trachea. The symptoms of stridor, dyspnea on exertion, and cyanotic episodes improve by altering the arterial-tracheal anatomy.

A pulmonary artery sling is a rare vascular anomaly in which the left pulmonary artery originates from the right pulmonary artery and encircles the right main stem bronchus and distal trachea before coursing anterior to the esophagus and descending aorta to enter the hilum of the left lung. Infants present within the first months of life with respiratory distress, particularly if there are associated complete tracheal rings. Surgical intervention should be undertaken as soon as the diagnosis is made because of the tenuous respiratory status. Pulmonary artery reimplantation alone is associated with high mortality because the tracheal stenosis is often intrinsic, resulting from complete tracheal rings. For repair of pulmonary artery sling a median sternotomy and extracorporeal circulation is recommended.

Acquired Tracheoesophageal Fistulas

Although rare, when they do occur, acquired tracheoesophageal fistulas can be quite devastating. Their etiology is quite variable – neoplastic, traumatic, infections, and iatrogenic. TEFs due to tumors can result from necrosis of tumor involving both the trachea and the esophagus or from radiation treatments. Advanced lesions can be difficult to cure and often have a poor outcome.

Most iatrogenic TEFs are due to erosion of the tracheal and esophageal walls by tracheostomy or endotracheal tubes. Typically they occur from posterior wall ulceration due to compression and ischemia from an overinflated cuff. TEF formation is usually slow and progressive. Fibrous adhesions produce a well epithelialized tract without mediastinal contamination. TEF can cause significant morbidity, including flow of esophageal contents (saliva, food) into the trachea. Gastroesophageal reflux can cause respiratory distress, congestion, infection, pneumonia, and atelectasis.

Patients typically present with food in the airway and cough on swallowing, especially with liquids. Recurrent pneumonias can be devastating. Gastric distention is one of the worrisome complications of ventilatory support for patients with a TEF. A barium swallow is the study of choice and has 70% sensitivity. All barium swallows should be followed by evaluation to rule out distal stenosis. Bronchoscopy is also effective but is limited to subtle fistulas.

Surgery is the curative treatment of TEF and should not be delayed. There is little room for expectant observation. Severe bronchopulmonary complications can cause severe morbidity. The surgical incision depends on the site of the lesion. High TEF can be performed via a left neck incision. A partial sternotomy can be added for exposure. Only a fistula located below the fourth or fifth intercostal space will require a right thoracotomy.

Closure of the esophagus is performed in two layers – the inner layer approximates the mucosa and submucosa; the outer layer brings together the esophageal muscle. Closure of the trachea can be difficult and should be done in a single layer. Tracheal closures should avoid airway narrowing. Particular care should be taken along the posterior membranous wall near the TEF stoma. Recurrence can be avoided by avoiding contact between the esophageal and tracheal suture lines and complete drainage

of the mediastinal space. Strap muscle interposition is the best available material to separate the two lumens. Large TEFs (>4 cm in length) can often make primary closure impossible, particularly if there is significant local necrosis or infection. In this case, the treatment of choice is total esophageal exclusion with a cervical esophagostomy.

Postintubation Injury

The management of iatrogenic tracheal injuries from intubation has evolved significantly over the past several decades. The endotracheal tube can produce various injuries due to pressure necrosis even after 48 hours (Figure 13–18). Factors such as hypotension and prolonged administration of steroids can contribute. Injury at the laryngeal level can occur as a result of glottic edema, vocal cord granulomas, erosions over the arytenoids, formation of granulation tissue, and polypoid obstructions. Anything from erosion of nasal cartilages to

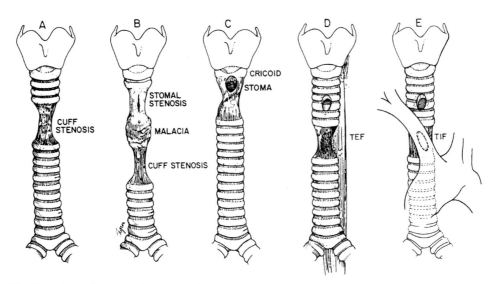

Figure 13–18. Principal postintubation tracheal lesions. **A,** Lesion at the cuff site in a patient who has been treated with an endotracheal tube alone. The lesion is high in the trachea and is circumferential. Sometimes the external tracheal surfaces look almost normal. **B,** Lesions that occur with tracheostomy tubes. At the stomal level, anterolateral stenosis is seen. At the cuff level, which is lower than with an endotracheal tube, circumferential cuff stenosis occurs. The segment between is often inflamed and malacic. Malacia may also occur at cuff level. **C,** Damage to the subglottic larynx. A high tracheostomy or one that erodes back by virtue of the patient's anatomy may damage the inferior cricoid and produce a low subglottic stenosis as well as an upper tracheal injury. **D,** Tracheoesophageal fistula. The level of fistulization is usually where the cuff has eroded posteriorly. There is also usually severe circumferential damage at this level by the cuff. Occasionally, angulation of the tube may produce erosion from the tip. **E,** Tracheo-innominate-artery fistula. A high-pressure cuff frequently rests on the trachea directly behind the innominate artery. Erosion may occur, although rarely. The more common innominate artery injury is from a low tracheostomy in which the inner portion of the curve of the tube rests in proximity to the artery and causes direct erosion. Laryngeal injuries due to endotracheal tubes or cricothyroidostomy are not shown. (From Grillo HC. Surgical treatment of postintubation tracheal injuries. *J Thorac Cardiovasc Surg* 1979;78:860.)

laryngeal edema is possible. Most laryngeal lesions both in children and adults are reversible with time. Vocal cords can become inflamed and irritated. Granulomas can result in the posterior commissure of the larynx. This can cause fusion of opposing sides and voice changes. If irritation of the cricoid cartilage by the endotracheal tube occurs, subglottic stenosis can result. Subglottic stenosis often requires a more complex procedure because of the proximity to the vocal cords and the recurrent laryngeal nerves.

Endotracheal tube and tracheostomy injuries are serious complications of instrumentation of the trachea. There are two potential areas of injury: stomal lesions and cuff lesions. Stomal injuries occur at the site of the stoma: in the trachea with a tracheostomy or in the subglottic larynx with cricothyroidotomy. Endotracheal tubes can produce equally damaging injuries. Proximal injuries from endotracheal tubes include glottic granulomas, anterior and posterior commissural stenosis, and posterior arytenoid erosion. Intraluminal granulomas rarely cause obstruction while the tracheostomy tube is in place; however, severe respiratory compromise can occur on tube removal. The granulomas tend to grow on the cephalad aspect of the tracheostomy tube. Injuries to the subglottic larynx at the level of the cricoid can be particularly difficult to repair.

At the tracheostomy stoma, there is a high incidence of granuloma. A granuloma can be easily removed bronchoscopically. Small deformities are without consequence; however, loss of a significant portion of the tracheal wall can produce significant strictures. Many times the anterior wall of the trachea will be severely damaged with little erosion of the posterior wall. Factors that can play a role in predicting the degree of injury include the size of the initial stoma when created, tissue hygiene and development of infection, and use of a connecting system to the tracheostomy, which can cause pressure erosion along the airway. Special care should be taken to avoid injuring the first cartilaginous ring. Such injury can lead to erosion and inflammatory change in the cricoid cartilage and the subglottic larynx. Severe subglottic stenosis can often not be corrected (Figure 13–19). Alternatively, if placed too low, a tracheostomy can erode into the innominate artery.

Cuff injuries cause pressure necrosis so the mucosa overlying the cartilage is initially destroyed. The bared cartilages become necrotic and ultimately slough. Attempts at

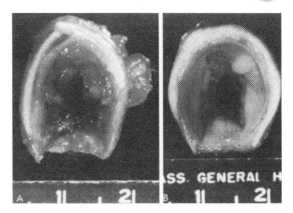

Figure 13–19. Stenosis at the stomal site. Surgical specimens. **A,** The roughly triangular shape of the stenosis is evident with the apex anteriorly. The principal cicatricial and granulomatous changes are anterolateral. In this case of a relatively fresh stricture, there are some granulations posteriorly as well. **B,** A more 'mature' stomal stricture shows the same triangular narrowing with firm cicatricial changes in the anterolateral wall. The membranous wall is relatively intact, although it is squeezed together by the lateral processes. (From Sabiston DC Jr, Spencer FC. *Surgery of the chest*, 6th ed. Philadelphia: WB Saunders, 1996:413.)

repair following full-thickness damage to the tracheal wall lead only to scar formation. Because the erosion is circumferential, the resultant strictures are also (Figure 13–20).

Persistent pressure necrosis from ventilatory tubes can develop into a tracheoesophageal fistula or tracheo-innominate-artery fistula. These lesions have a high mortality risk. Tracheoesophageal fistulas manifest by increasing difficulty in ventilating the patient, gastric dilation, or large quantities of secretions in the tracheobronchial tree. Tracheoesophageal fistulas occur most commonly in patients who have a ventilating cuff in the trachea for a long period of time along with a feeding tube in the esophagus. The two foreign bodies compress the common wall between the trachea and esophagus, leading to inflammation, perforation, and epithelialization. Patients occasionally develop pneumonitis, pneumonia, or abscesses. Tracheo-innominate-artery fistulas present as sudden massive hemorrhage into the tracheobronchial tree. Emergency control can be obtained by inserting an endotracheal tube with inflation of a high-pressure cuff to tamponade the opening. Alternatively, direct digital pressure can be used through the stoma for emergency control.

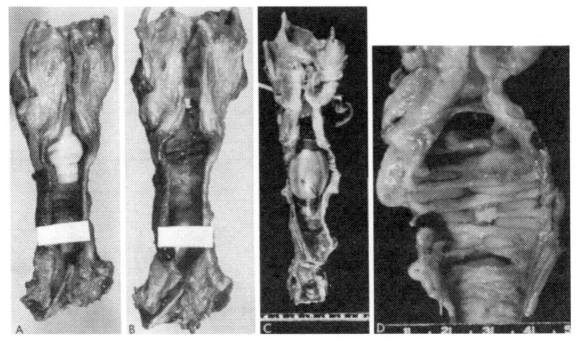

Figure 13–20. Injury due to cuffed tracheostomy tubes of prior design that produced high intracuff pressures. **A**, Autopsy specimen of a patient who had received ventilatory treatment with a Portex tube in place. The wall is thinned at the site of the cuff. There is tracheitis below it. **B**, Beneath the cuff there has been mucosal erosion baring the tracheal cartilages. **C**, Another trachea with an inlying metal tracheostomy tube and standard rubber cuff. **D**, Detail shows not only baring of cartilage but also evidence of missing fragments. (From Cooper JD, Grillo HC. The evolution of tracheal injury due to ventilatory assistance through cuffed tubes: a pathologic study. *Ann Surg* 1969;196:334.)

Tracheomalacia is another consequence of intubation injury. The region between the stoma and the cuff is at highest risk because there is pooling of secretions in this area, which can lead to inflammatory changes. This can translate into cartilage thinning and can form a pseudo-obstruction. The trachea is more prone to collapse in this region, particularly after a maximal respiratory effort.

Most injuries to the trachea become a problem due to airway obstruction. Patients present with dyspnea, wheezing, and stridor. Hemoptysis does not occur. In most instances, the obstruction appears only after extubation, because the tube splints a cuff stenosis or potential stomal stenosis as long as it remains in place. This disease entity is extremely under-diagnosed and is usually mislabeled as asthma. Any time that a patient has a prolonged intubation, or multiple intubations over several years, the diagnosis of tracheal stenosis should be considered. Symptoms appear between 1 week and 2 months after extubation. Often, symptoms are not initially obvious during the patient's recovery time, especially because the patient is not very active. However, there is sig-

nificant disease in peak flow rates in going from an airway diameter of 8 mm to 4 mm.

Evaluating tracheal anatomy can be best performed with single radiographs and fluoroscopy. Bronchoscopy is useful; however, the procedure can precipitate acute decompensation. Therefore, it should be avoided until the patient is in the operating room and sedated under general anesthesia.

Before undertaking repair of a postintubation tracheal lesion, the anatomy and functional status of the larynx should be determined. If a patient is taking high-dose steroids, repair should be delayed until s/he can be weaned off them. All sources of systemic or local inflammation should be allowed to resolve. Direct examination followed by fluoroscopy should be employed. Synchronous lesions are known to develop, especially in the setting of an intensive-care patient who undergoes a long initial endotracheal intubation followed by a prolonged tracheostomy.

Management of these tracheal lesions can be a complex problem. Fully developed stenotic lesions with a high degree of obstruction in patients who have been extubated and who are no longer receiving ventilatory support should be treated surgically whenever possible. Subglottic tracheal lesions require complex repairs and often require staged procedures. An attempt can be made to manage a patient conservatively by dilatation of the stenosis, placement of a new tracheostomy, and the insertion of a splinting tracheostomy tube through the stenosis. Stricture dilation can be the initial therapeutic maneuver; however, the procedure carries a significant degree of risk of airway perforation and respiratory compromise due to temporary balloon occlusion.

If the tracheal lesion is accessible in the neck and there is no existing stoma, a new stoma should be placed at the level of resection to avoid multiple injuries. Intraluminal granulomas can be prolapsed out of the tracheostomy stoma with a bronchoscope for external excision. Endoscopic resection with laser excision has been used for thin, web-like stenoses of the subglottic larynx and trachea.

Most segmental resections can be performed safely in a controlled, well prepared setting (Figure 13–21). A high-frequency jet ventilation device should be available. A low collar incision in the neck offers adequate exposure for most postintubation tracheal strictures and for higher segmental strictures. The tracheal blood supply is located posterolaterally just anterior to the tracheoesophageal groove; therefore, extensive lateral or circumferential dissection should be avoided. Furthermore, the proximity of the recurrent laryngeal nerve necessitates that dissection be carried out close to the tracheal wall. There is significant variability in the amount of tracheal resection that a patient can tolerate. Infants and children tend to tolerate significant mobilization and resection because of the greater mobility and elasticity of the child's tracheobronchial tree.

Neoplasms

Tracheal masses are rare (Table 13–1). Tracheal cancer is rarer. Tracheal tumors are 100 times less common than bronchial tumors and constitute only 2% of all upper respiratory tract tumors. Malignant tumors are more common than benign pathology. Squamous cell carcinoma and adenoid cystic carcinoma have been reported to be the two most common pathologies. Other variants include carcinoid, carcinosarcoma, basal cell adenoma, fibroma, hemangioma, chon-

droma, chondrosarcoma, leiomyoma, neurofibroma, and paraganglioma.

Typically, tracheal cancers present in one of several ways, varying from dyspnea on exertion to respiratory obstruction due to accumulation of secretions. The most characteristic symptom is inspiratory dyspnea, found in 80% of patients. Wheezing becomes apparent as the airway narrows. As a result of obstruction, some patients present with repeat bouts of pneumonitis or pneumonia that responds to antibiotics. A persistent cough could also suggest tracheal masses. Most often, there is history of slowly progressive dyspnea on exertion. Hemoptysis occurs in approximately 25% of patients, more commonly in patients with squamous cell carcinoma. A change in voice or hoarseness can be related to paralysis of the vocal cord resulting from invasion of the recurrent laryngeal nerve or to direct extension of an upper tracheal tumor into the larynx. Dysphagia is an uncommon symptom that indicates esophageal compression by a large bulky tumor.

The most common benign tumors of the trachea are chondroma, papilloma, fibroma, and hemangioma. Benign tumors most often occur in the upper one third of the trachea in children and are more common in the lower one third in adults, frequently arising from the membranous portion of the trachea.

Chondromas histologically duplicate normal cartilage and can exhibit vascular invasion. Endoscopically, a chondroma appears as a firm, white nodule projecting into the tracheal lumen. The tumor occurs 4:1 in men to women and is more common in adults than children. No definite etiology for this lesion has been described. A chondroma occurs more frequently in the larynx than in the trachea. Biopsy of the lesion can be difficult because of the firm consistency. Vascularity is minimal and the lesion can be easily removed via a bronchoscope.

A solitary papilloma of the trachea is rare but has been noted to occur in adults. A solitary benign papilloma is easily removed through the bronchoscope and the base of the tumor can be ablated by laser. Juvenile laryngotracheal papillomatosis is common in children and more common than adult solitary papillomas. These account for 60% of benign tracheal tumors in children. They have been linked with the Human papillomavirus types 6 and 11. Papillomatosis more commonly involves the larynx, but it is found in the tracheobronchial tree in 20% of patients. Although it is benign, the recurrence rate is as high as 90%.

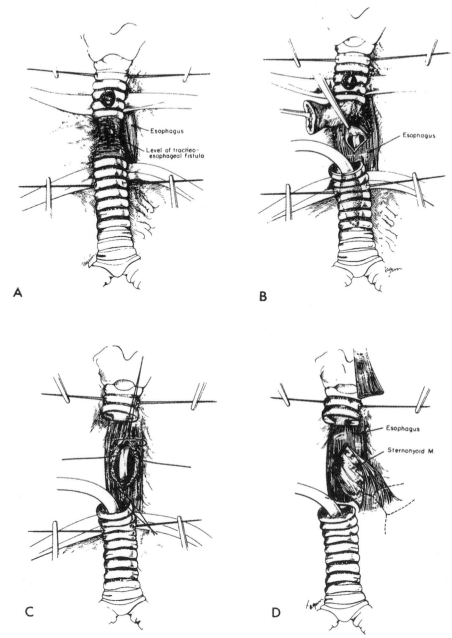

Figure 13–21. Postintubation tracheoesophageal fistula. **A,** Dissection has been extended to expose the trachea in the midline. This dissection remains close to the trachea and esophagus to avoid injury to the recurrent laryngeal nerves; these nerves are not exposed. Stay sutures are placed above and below the lines of planned resection. Although it is not always necessary to resect the segment of trachea that contains the stoma, this is often so close to the area of injury that the trachea below is of too poor quality to be used successfully for anastomosis. Tapes have been passed around the trachea above and below the fistula but care is taken not to dissect excessive lengths of trachea circumferentially. **B,** The trachea is transected and the patient is intubated across the operative field. With the proximal end of the divided trachea elevated, the area of the fistula can be identified. The esophagus is entered at the lowermost border of the fistula. The edges of the fistula are then excised elliptically by continuing upward on both sides (*dotted lines*). **C,** The trachea has been excised above the level of the stoma. The fistula in the esophagus is closed using fine interrupted sutures that invert the mucosa and a second layer is made with Lembert's sutures. **D,** The sternohyoid muscle is detached superiorly, and a pedicle is inserted across the esophageal closure. This is carefully sutured into place with 4-0 silk to cover the closure completely. End-to-end tracheal repair is performed. (From Grillo HC, Moncure AC, McEnany MT. Repair of inflammatory transesophageal fistula. *Ann Thorac Surg* 1976;22:112. Reprinted with permission from the Society of Thoracic Surgeons.)

TABLE 13-1 • *Causes of a Tracheal Mass*

Inflammatory granuloma	Post-traumatic
	Tuberculosis
	Fungus
	Wegener's granulomatosis
	Scleroma
	Laryngeal papillomatosis
Benign neoplasms	Chondroma, hamartoma
	Squamous cell papilloma
	Fibroma
	Hemangioma
	Granular cell myoblastoma
	Leiomyoma
	Others (neurilemoma, lipoma, fibrous histiocytoma, benign mixed tumors)
Malignant neoplasms	Squamous cell carcinoma
	Adenoid cystic carcinoma (cylindroma)
	Adenocarcinoma
	Sarcoma
	Carcinoid
	Other (pseudosarcoma, oat cell carcinoma, lymphoma, plasmacytoma, melanoma, hemangioendothelioma)
Invasion from adjacent neoplasm	Thyroid
	Lung
	Esophagus
Metastasis from distant site	Breast
	Colon
	Genitourinary
	Melanoma
Extrinsic compression	Neoplasm
	Aneurysm
	Vascular ring
Idiopathic	Goiter
	Amyloid
	Tracheopathia osteochondroplastica

Fibromas account for 20% of benign tumors in adults. These can be easily removed by bronchoscopy followed by laser ablation of the base of the tumor. Local recurrence is unusual but, if it does occur, segmental tracheal resection is indicated.

Squamous cell carcinoma of the trachea can present as a well localized lesion of the exophytic type or as an ulcerating lesion. Lesions have been described in multifocal regions as well as superficial infiltrating histology. They most commonly occur in the distal one third of the trachea along the posterior wall (Figure 13–22). It occurs with a male:female ratio of 4:1, typically in men between 50 and 60 years of age, and accounts for 50% of all primary tracheal malignancies. Most patients are heavy smokers. Patients will often have a secondary primary tumor in the larynx or lung. Based on the results from small series, spread is suspected to occur to regional lymph nodes followed by direct mediastinal invasion. Limitations to resectability include an excessive longitudinal extent of the tumor leaving insufficient trachea for reconstruction, invasion of critical mediastinal structures, and distant metastasis.

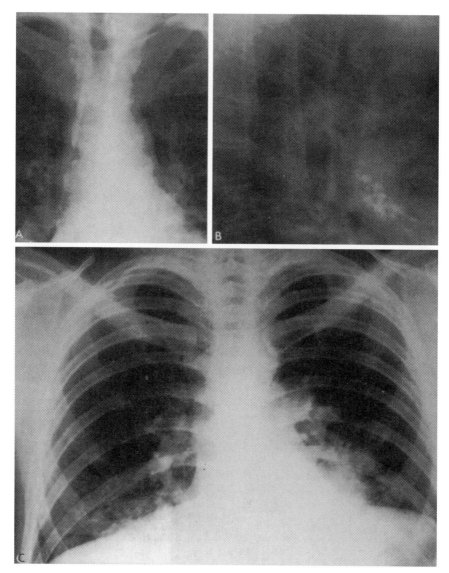

Figure 13–22. Neoplasms in the trachea. **A, B,** Details of posteroanterior and lateral chest films of a patient with a squamous-cell carcinoma of the lower trachea. This lesion, which produced relatively high-grade obstruction, might be overlooked on a cursory examination of the chest film because the lung fields are clear. **C,** Chest film shows bilateral pneumonitis that has recurred several times in a young patient.

Adenoid cystic carcinoma is a slow-growing neoplasm that behaves in an indolent fashion. It is the most common primary tumor of the trachea. Tobacco exposure is not a risk factor. It tends to compress mediastinal structures without invasion but with poorly defined margins. In contrast to squamous cell carcinoma, adenoid cystic carcinomas tend to occur in the upper one third of the trachea. However, they infiltrate the airway submucosally for longer distances than is grossly apparent. Perineural spread is common. The tumor pushes adjacent mediastinal structures aside rather than directly invading them. The initial operation should be aggressive in debulking the tumor. These patients should be followed for the rest of their life. Adenoid cystic carcinomas do spread to regional lymph nodes and occasionally metastasize to the lung or distant organs.

Uncommon malignant tracheal tumors include carcinoid, tracheal adenocarcinoma, and small-cell carcinoma. Secondary tumors also involve the trachea. Direct extension into the trachea occurs from cancers of the thyroid, larynx, lung, and esophagus. Mediastinal

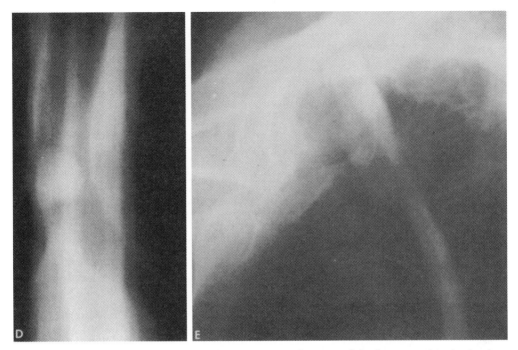

Figure 13–22. Continued. **D**, The lesion is shown. Carcinoid tumor of the lower trachea is clearly revealed in this detail of a laminogram of the lower trachea and carina. **E**, Squamous cell carcinoma of the lower trachea. This detail of a spot film taken during fluoroscopy with a swallow of barium outlines the lesion, which narrows the tracheal lumen and slightly indents the esophagus by extrinsic pressure. (**A, B**, from Grillo HC. Circumferential resection and reconstruction of mediastinal and cervical trachea. *Ann Surg* 1965;162:374. **C–E**, from Sabiston DC Jr, Spencer FC. *Surgery of the chest*, 6th ed. Philadelphia: WB Saunders, 1996: 423, 424.)

tumors may directly invade the trachea; the most common is lymphoma. Metastasis to the trachea is uncommon, but breast cancer, melanoma, and sarcomas have all been found in the trachea.

Several diagnostic tools are available to the thoracic surgeon attempting to define the presence and extent of the tumor. Chest radiographs with varying penetration can expose tracheal masses. CT is less helpful than contrast studies of the trachea in revealing invasion of the lumen. Endoscopy is mandatory, but risky. Instrumentation of tracheal lesions always risks sudden respiratory collapse due to bleeding, inflammation, and bronchospasm. The larynx should be examined carefully. The vocal cord function should be evaluated and fluoroscopic and radiographic examination should be performed. The region that needs to be corrected must be carefully delineated because this will affect the incision of choice. Synchronous lesions, both tumor and stenosis, should be ruled out.

All primary tracheal malignant tumors should be resected whenever feasible. For benign tumors, an endoscopic approach can be performed, however, open operation is warranted for malignant masses. Surgical procedures for malignant tracheal tumors are typically radical operations. Segmental resection and reconstructions performed in a single stage offers the best chance of cure or extended palliation for squamous-cell carcinoma and adenoid cystic cancer. If the tumor is large and requires urgent management secondary to obstruction, an endoscopic procedure to debulk the tumor should be performed prior to elective open surgery. The majority of these patients should have postoperative radiation. Palliation therapy with or without chemotherapy often is the treatment of choice for patients with unresectable tracheal malignant neoplasms.

Surgical approach depends on tumor location. Lesions of the upper half of the trachea are best approached via an anterior collar incision and a vertical partial sternal division if necessary (Figure 13–23). An inflatable bag is placed beneath the shoulders to provide cervical extension (Figure 13–24). Lesions of the lower half of the trachea should be approached through a right posterolateral

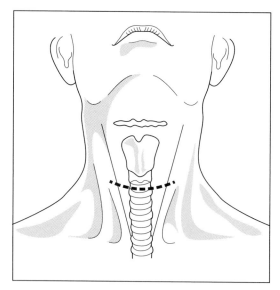

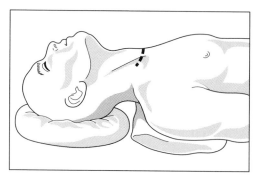

Figure 13–24. An inflatable bag should be placed beneath the shoulders to provide maximal cervical hyperextension. (Redrawn from Urschel HC Jr, Cooper JD: *Atlas of thoracic surgery.* New York, Churchill Livingstone, 1995, p 113.)

Figure 13–23. Subglottic resection. Resection of the subglottic airway is indicated for tumors extending to the cricoid cartilage; traumatic injuries, including cricoid fracture and laryngotracheal separation; idiopathic subglottic stenosis; postintubation injury; and inhalation injuries involving the upper airway. For this procedure, the anastomosis may be carried up to the level of the vocal cords. The head is to the right. An endotracheal tube has been placed through a tracheostomy stoma below the site of the injury (not shown). The anterior perichondrium is incised transversely at the inferior border of the anterior portion of the cricoid ring. A subperichondral plane of dissection is established anterior and posterior to the front of the cricoid ring. (Redrawn from Urschel HC Jr, Cooper JD. *Atlas of thoracic surgery.* New York: Churchill Livingstone, 1995:105.)

thoracotomy incision in the fourth intercostal space. The neck should always be prepared in case a cervical incision needs to be used.

Key Readings

Armstrong WB, Netterville JL. Anatomy of the larynx, trachea, and bronchi. *Otolaryngol Clin North Am* 1995;28:685–699.

Grillo HC. Pediatric tracheal problems. *Chest Surg Clin North Am* 1996;6:693–700. *Review of pediatric diseases of the trachea written by a leader in tracheal surgery.*

Mathisen DJ. Tracheal tumors. *Chest Surg Clin North Am* 1996;6:875–898. *Review of rare tumors that may invade the tracheobronchial tree.*

Selected Readings

Chen HC, Tang YB, Chang MH. Reconstruction of the voice after laryngectomy. *Clin Plast Surg* 2001;28:389–402.

Filler RM, de Fraga JC. Tracheomalacia. *Semin Thorac Cardiovasc Surg* 1994;6:211–215.

Mathisen DJ. Surgical management of tracheobronchial disease. *Clin Chest Med* 1992;.

Messineo A, Filler RM. Tracheomalacia. *Semin Pediatr Surg* 1994;3:253–258.

Rimell FL, Stool SE. Diagnosis and management of pediatric tracheal stenosis. *Otolaryngol Clin North Am* 1995;28:809–827.

Spitz L. Esophageal atresia and tracheoesophageal fistula in children. *Curr Opin Pediatr* 1993;5:347–352.

Weber AL. Radiologic evaluation of the trachea. *Chest Surg Clin North Am* 1996;6:637–673.

Worrell JA. Radiology of the central airways. *Otolaryngol Clin North Am* 1995;28:701–720.

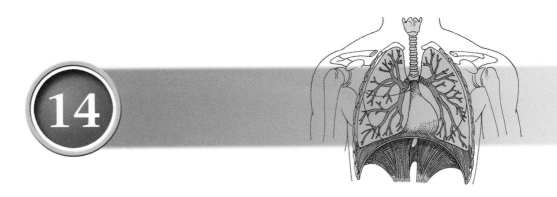

14

Diaphragm

DIAPHRAGMATIC HERNIAS
CONGENITAL HERNIAS
HIATAL HERNIAS
PARALYSIS OF THE DIAPHRAGM

PACING OF THE DIAPHRAGM
EVENTRATION OF THE DIAPHRAGM
DIAPHRAGMATIC TUMORS

Diaphragm: Key Topics

- Understand the following developmental anomalies of the diaphragm: congenital diaphragmatic hernias (Bochdalek and Morgagni) and diaphragmatic eventration
- Describe the pathophysiology of developing acquired diaphragmatic hernias and determining indications for medical versus surgical therapy
- Understand the etiology, diagnosis, and treatment of diaphragmatic paralysis
- Describe what two situations warrant diaphragmatic pacing
- Understand the primary and secondary tumors of the diaphragm

The diaphragm serves two major roles, fulfilling both an anatomical and a functional need. The major anatomical action is separation of the torso into the thoracic and abdominal cavities. Diaphragm comes from the Greek word *dia* ('in between') and *phragma* ('fence'). Functionally, the diaphragm is the principal muscle of respiration, as discussed in Chapter 1.

To review, the diaphragm is anatomically composed of two distinct parts – the costal and crural aspects. The costal muscle is thin and causes some downward displacement of the diaphragm. The costal part of the diaphragm allows the diaphragm to flatten and the lower ribs to lift. The crural aspect of the diaphragm is thicker, supports the heart, and plays less of a role in respiration. Both groups are innervated by the phrenic nerve (Figure 14–1). The pericardiacophrenic artery, musculophrenic artery, and superior phrenic arteries extend to the cranial side of the diaphragm. Small, direct branches of the aorta vascularize the dorsal part of the diaphragm. The caudal area is supplied by the inferior phrenic arteries.

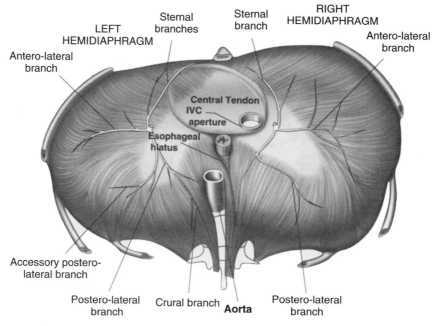

Figure 14–1. Branches of the phrenic nerve at the diaphragm. (Adapted from Meredino KA, Johnson RS, Skinner HH, *et al.* The intradiaphragmatic distribution of the phrenic nerve with particular reference to the placement of diaphragmatic incisions and controlled segmental paralysis. *Surgery* 1956;39:189.)

They branch off the aortal hiatus directly from the aorta or from the celiac trunk.

The diaphragm is a muscle of inspiration and the downward descent of the central tendon is responsible for 75–80% of the air brought into the lungs during quiet breathing. During light inspiration, the two domes of the diaphragm flatten to some extent, whereas the central tendon remains almost stationary. The diaphragm typically moves 1–2 cm during quiet breathing but may lower as much as 6–7 cm with forced inspiration. The peripheral parts of the diaphragm unwrap from the lateral walls of the chest by contraction during deep breathing. This widens the costodiaphragmatic recesses, and the lungs enter that additional volume but do not fill the recess completely.

The development of the diaphragm is a complex process that takes place between the fourth and eighth week of fetal life (Figure 14–2). The large central portion of the diaphragm is formed from the septum transversum. This mesodermal tissue between the developing heart and liver fuses ventrally, leaving behind spaces (pleuroperitoneal canals) for the development of the lungs. As the lungs develop, they form bilateral folds which fuse with the septum transversum to form bilateral pleuroperitoneal membranes. Myoblasts penetrate the membranes to form the muscular part of

the diaphragm. Finally, the mesentery of the esophagus as it develops contributes to the development of the diaphragmatic crura and the most dorsal part of the diaphragm. A delay or alteration in the embryologic structuring can result in a diaphragmatic hernia or congenital eventration.

Diaphragmatic Hernias

There are four hernias that we will consider (Figure 14–3): two congenital hernias (Bochdalek and Morgagni) and two acquired defects (sliding and paraesophageal).

Congenital Hernias

Bochdalek Hernia

Infants with congenital diaphragmatic hernias diagnosed at birth (1/4000 live births) have a poor prognosis despite major advances in prenatal diagnosis and management. Bochdalek hernia is a posterolateral defect in the diaphragm caused by a failure of the pleuroperitoneal canal to close at 8 weeks gestation (Figure 14–4). Eighty-five percent occur on the left side and are typically through a small circular hole;

Figure 14-2. The embryonic relationship of the liver (stippled area) and diaphragm (solid black line). Initially (2 mm embryo), the liver is at the level of the cervical somites. With differential growth of the embryo, the diaphragm assumes a more caudal position. The dashed line represents the contribution of the pleuroperitoneal folds and mediastinal mesenchyme. (From Ashcraft KW, Holder TM. *Pediatric surgery*, 2nd ed. Philadelphia: WB Saunders, 1993:206.)

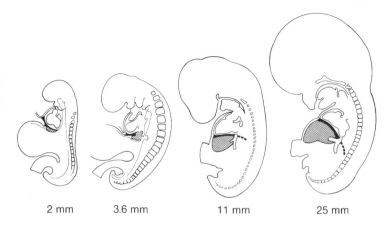

2 mm   3.6 mm   11 mm   25 mm

Figure 14-3. Classification of diaphragmatic hernias.

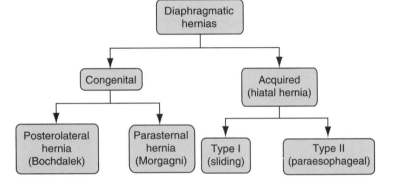

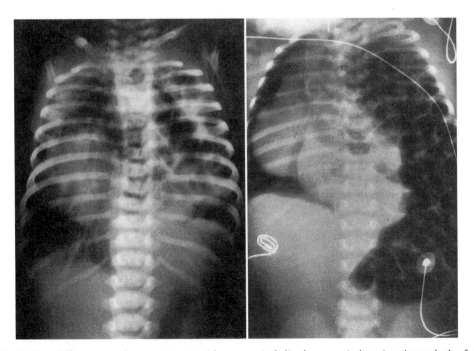

Figure 14-4. Two different newborn patients with congenital diaphragmatic hernias through the foramen of Bochdalek. Preoperative chest radiographs show intestinal organs mostly within the left hemithorax and herniation of the mediastinal structures into the right side. There is absence of most gas shadows from the abdomen, except for a small amount in the stomach and descending colon. (From Kaplan JA, Slinger PD. *Thoracic anesthesia*, 3rd ed. Philadelphia: Churchill Livingstone, 2003:355.)

only 10% have a true hernia sac. When the intestines return to the abdomen from the yolk sac at 10 weeks gestation, the intestines and the other abdominal viscera may herniate into the chest and alter the growth of the ipsilateral lung. If the mediastinum is pushed to the contralateral side of the chest by the abdominal viscera, the contralateral lung can also be affected. Herniation of the viscera through the defect usually occurs during the pseudoglandular stage of lung development. The pressure of abdominal viscera in the thoracic cavity results in a decrease in the number of bronchial branches, total number of acini, and number of vessels.

The cause of congenital diaphragmatic hernias is unknown. They are commonly associated with additional anomalies including congenital heart defects, hydronephrosis, renal agenesis, intestinal atresia, extralobular sequestration, hydrocephalus, anencephaly, and spina bifida (Table 14–1).

Typically, congenital diaphragmatic hernia can cause life-threatening respiratory compromise within the first hours or days of life, depending on the degree of pulmonary hypoplasia, which is the main cause of morbidity and mortality. The defect can occasionally cause respiratory distress or feeding intolerance in later infancy or childhood or may be identified on a radiograph obtained for unrelated reasons. The other element that contributes to the pathophysiology of this disease is pulmonary hypertension. This condition mimics normal fetal circulation and is termed persistent fetal circulation. This can result in hypoxemia and acidosis (Figure 14–5). Severe pulmonary hypertension is manifest by right-to-left shunting through the persistent foramen ovale and the patent ductus arteriosus. The morbidity and mortality associated with a congenital

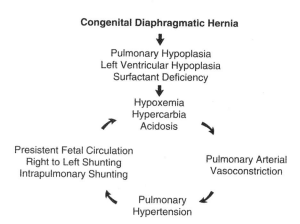

Figure 14–5. The pathophysiology of acute respiratory failure in neonates with congenital diaphragmatic hernia. (From Ashcraft KW, ed. *Pediatric surgery*, 3rd ed. Philadelphia: WB Saunders, 2000:302.)

diaphragmatic hernia is directly related to the age of the patient at presentation.

Half of all congenital diaphragmatic hernias are diagnosed during prenatal ultrasound examination. The diagnosis is generally confirmed by a chest radiograph, which characteristically demonstrates abdominal contents in the chest with mediastinal deviation away from the affected side (Figures 14–6, 14–7). The differential diagnosis includes congenital cystic adenomatoid malformation, other cystic diseases of the lung, and eventration of the diaphragm. Simple passage of an orogastric tube can confirm the diagnosis. The prenatal diagnosis of right-sided defects is extremely difficult because of the similar echogenicity of the liver and lung.

If a patient presents with respiratory distress at birth, the baby is quickly intubated and nasogastric decompression is initiated. Mechanical ventilation with 100% F_iO_2 and

TABLE 14–1 • *Associated Anomalies in Patients with Congenital Diaphragmatic Hernia*	
Organ System	**Malformation**
Cardiovascular	Any form of cyanotic or acyanotic defect
Gastrointestinal	Tracheoesophageal fistula, malrotation, various atresias, omphalocele
Genitourinary	Hypospadias, hydronephrosis, renal dysplasia
Central nervous system	Spina bifida defects, hydrocephalus, cerebral dysgenesis
Musculoskeletal	Syndactyly, amelias
Chromosomal	Trisomy 18, trisomy 21

From Kaplan JA, Slinger PD. *Thoracic anesthesia*, 3rd ed. Philadelphia: Churchill Livingstone, 2003:356.

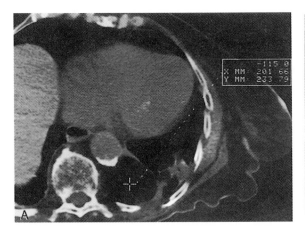
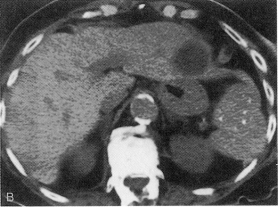

Figure 14–6. Left Bochdalek's hernia. **A,** Computed tomography scan of the left lower thorax demonstrates a large fat-containing structure in the posterior costal phrenic angle. The left crus of the diaphragm is absent. **B,** 2 cm inferiorly, the top of the left kidney is visible, protruding into the hernia. Both adrenal glands are visible. Splenic calcifications are from prior histoplasmosis. A metastasis is present in the left lobe of the liver. (From Moss AA, Gamsu G, Genant HK. *Computed tomography of the body with magnetic resonance imaging,* 2nd ed. Philadelphia: WB Saunders, 1992:278.)

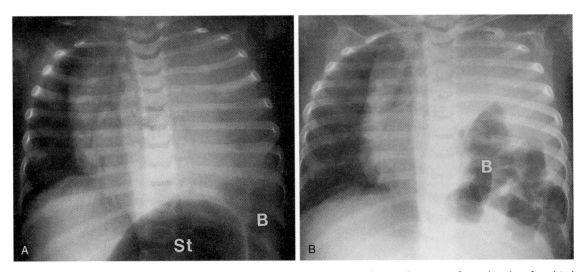

Figure 14–7. Congenital diaphragmatic hernia. **A,** A radiograph obtained in an infant shortly after birth reveals partial opacification of the left hemithorax, a dilated, air-filled stomach (St), and upper abdominal bowel gas (B). **B,** Hours later, air has passed into bowel loops (B) in the left hemithorax, confirming a large congenital hernia. (From Gierada DS, Slone RM, Fleishman MJ. Imaging evaluation of the diaphragm. *Chest Surg Clin North Am* 1998;8:237, courtesy of Marilyn J. Siegel, MD, St Louis, MO.)

low airway pressures (<25 mm Hg) and low positive end-expiratory pressure (PEEP 5 mm Hg) should be used. The patient should then be transported to a facility capable of extracorporeal membrane oxygenation (ECMO; Figure 14–8). Indication to place a baby on ECMO includes an alveolar–arterial oxygen gradient greater than 600 for 8 hours, oxygen index greater than 40, pH less than 7.15, P_aO_2 less than 55, and progressive barotrauma (Box 14–1). ECMO is contraindicated if the patient has pre-existing intraventricular hemorrhage,

weighs less than 2 kg, or has other abnormalities incompatible with life.

In the past, repair of a congenital diaphragmatic hernia was considered to be a surgical emergency. The traditional treatment scheme of emergency operative repair immediately after birth resulted in mortality rates greater than 50% and has recently given way to other forms of management, such as delayed operation, ECMO, inhaled nitric oxide, and partial liquid ventilation, all with improved results (Figure 14–9). Recent studies have

ECMO Circuit

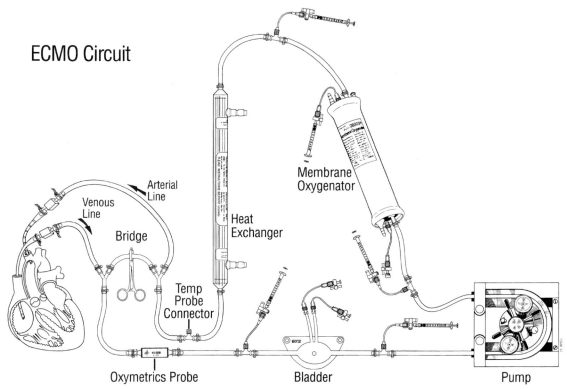

Figure 14–8. Diagram of the extracorporeal membrane oxygenation circuit. (From Ashcraft KW, ed. *Pediatric surgery*, 3rd ed. Philadelphia: WB Saunders, 2000:100.)

demonstrated that preoperative stabilization results in improvement in pulmonary compliance prior to repair. Once the child is stable, the repair can be performed through a para-

median incision or subcostal incision, although a transthoracic approach has been advocated by some for right-sided hernias. From the abdominal approach, the viscera can

BOX 14–1 SELECTION CRITERIA FOR EXTRACORPOREAL MEMBRANE OXYGENATION IN CONGENITAL DIAPHRAGMATIC HERNIA

Respiratory failure refractory to maximal 'conventional' therapy
- With oxygenation index* >40
- With acute deterioration (pH <7.15 and/or P_{O_2} <40 mm Hg for 2 h)
- Inability to hyperventilate (P_{CO_2} <40 mm Hg) despite maximal ventilation effort
- Ventilation index[†] >1000
- A–a gradient >600 mm Hg for >8 h (>4 h if PIP >38)
- Birth weight >2000 g
- Gestational age >34 weeks
- Absence of intracranial hemorrhage > grade I
- Absence of other congenital malformations or chromosomal anomalies
- Preductal P_{O_2} <50 mm Hg for 2 h
- Signs of barotrauma

* Oxygenation index = (MAP×F_iO_2×100/postductal P_{O_2}). † Ventilation index = (MAP×RR).
A–a, alveolar–arterial; F_iO_2, fraction of inspired oxygen; MAP, mean airway pressure; P_{CO_2}, partial pressure of carbon dioxide; PIP, peak inspiratory pressure; P_{O_2}, partial pressure of oxygen; RR, respiratory rate.
From Arensman RM, Bambini DA. Congenital diaphragmatic hernia and eventration. In: Ashcraft KW, ed. *Pediatric surgery*, 3rd ed. Philadelphia: WB Saunders, 2000.

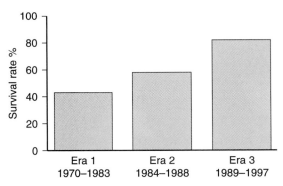

Figure 14–9. Survival rate for 203 patients with congenital diaphragmatic hernia in three therapeutic eras as assessed at Cardinal Glennon Children's Hospital, St Louis University Health Sciences Center, St Louis, MO. The survival rate for the third era was significantly higher than that for the first and second eras because of the institution of novel forms of management (extracorporeal membrane oxygenation, inhaled NO, partial liquid ventilation, rapid transit). (From Weber TR, Kountzman B, Dillon PA, Silen ML. Improved survival in congenital diaphragmatic hernia with evolving therapeutic strategies. *Arch Surg* 1998; 133:498–502.)

be returned from the chest and the hernia sac may need to be excised. Extralobar pulmonary sequestrations are resected at the time of hernia repair. A small diaphragmatic defect is closed with permanent suture and Teflon pledgets. Larger defects can be closed with polytetrafluoroethylene (PTFE) sheets. Typically, bilateral chest tubes are left in place. Intra-abdominal anomalies should be corrected at the time of hernia repair if the patient's condition is stable, although there is some controversy about whether this step should be left for another time.

The goal of postoperative management is to reduce pulmonary vascular resistance, improve oxygenation and treat persistent fetal circulation. Frequent arterial blood gas determinations coupled with continuous pulse oximetry or transcutaneous partial pressure of oxygen and carbon dioxide monitoring provide a constant assessment of ventilatory status. The lungs are at risk of barotrauma. A variety of vasodilators have been used to prevent and reverse pulmonary hypertension. Minor changes in ventilation can precipitate intense pulmonary vasoconstriction. Again, at last resort, ECMO may need to be initiated to reverse pulmonary hypertension if conventional methods fail.

In the absence of lethal anomalies, fetal mortality is directly related to the degree of pulmonary hypoplasia. Poor prognostic indications include additional anomalies, polyhydramnios, presence of an intrathoracic stomach bubble, and underdevelopment of the left heart region. It should be noted that some patients present later in life. These patients may present with a variety of respiratory symptoms or sometimes bowel obstruction.

Morgagni Hernia

Retrosternal anterior diaphragmatic hernia was described by Morgagni in 1769. Morgagni hernias are rare, accounting for only 5% of all diaphragmatic hernias. On each side of the sternum is a potential space, known as the foramen of Morgagni, through which the internal mammary artery becomes the superior epigastric artery. Usually these hernias are true hernias. Commonly, the diaphragmatic defect contains only a piece of omentum that enlarges as the person grows and produces the mass within the hernia sac. However, colon and small intestine are capable of passing through larger defects. A right-sided defect occurs in 90% of the cases because the left side is protected by the pericardium.

A small foramen of Morgagni hernia remains unrecognized and asymptomatic in young children. Larger ones can produce severe respiratory symptoms. Women are affected more commonly than men. Dyspnea is only occasionally observed in patients past early childhood. Plain chest radiographs demonstrate a density, either solid or containing air, adjacent to the right or left side of the heart. A computed tomography (CT) or contrast study is occasionally indicated to confirm the diagnosis (Figure 14–10).

A contrast study can identify whether the stomach, small bowel, or colon is above the diaphragm in the peristernal position. The abdominal approach for surgical repair is preferred for this hernia. A subcostal or right epigastric paramedian incision may be used. The contents of the hernia are reduced into the peritoneal cavity by gentle retraction and the margins of the hernia sac are identified. The sac is removed when possible. The repair of the muscular defect is made with interrupted mattress sutures. Occasionally it is necessary to pull the diaphragm up to the posterior part of the sternum and to the posterior rectus sheath.

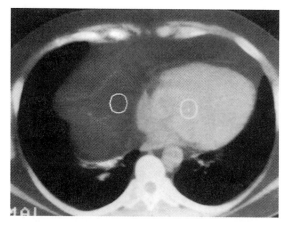

Figure 14–10. Morgagni's hernia. Computed tomography scan through the lower thorax demonstrates a large right pericardial mass consisting of the liver herniating through a large defect in the foramen of Morgagni. Vessels are seen within the liver after inspection of intravascular contrast material. (From Moss AA, Gamsu G, Genant HK. *Computed tomography of the body with magnetic resonance imaging*, 2nd ed. Philadelphia: WB Saunders, 1992:279.)

Hiatal Hernias

Sliding Hernia

Hiatal hernias are classified according to their anatomic characteristics. Sliding hernias (type I) are characterized by a dome-shaped upward migration of the gastroesophageal junction into the posterior mediastinum. Paraesophageal hernias (type II) are characterized by an upward dislocation of the gastric fundus alongside a normally positioned gastroesophageal junction.

Most sliding hernias are acquired defects. The esophagogastric junction moves through the hiatus into the visceral mediastinum so that it occupies an intrathoracic position (Figure 14–11). This occurs because of a weakening or attenuation of the phrenoesophageal ligament. The esophageal hiatus is formed by muscle fibers of the right crus of the diaphragm with little or no contribution from the left crus. These fibers overlap inferiorly where they attach over and along the right side of the median arcuate ligament. Enlargement of the hiatus occurs by separation of the crura, posteriorly and laterally, in proportion to the amount of stomach protruding through it (Figure 14–12). In the beginning, the esophagogastric junction may be located below the diaphragm, but with straining, coughing or recumbency may be above it. As the hernia

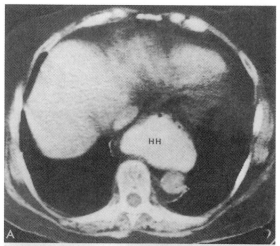

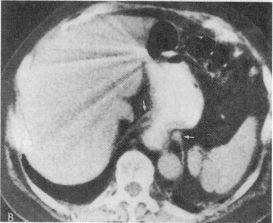

Figure 14–11. Hiatal hernia. **A**, Computed tomography scan after oral administration of contrast material shows a large opacified hiatal hernia (HH) in the lower mediastinum. **B**, At a lower level, the hernia is shown passing through the esophageal hiatus (arrows) to connect with the remainder of the stomach. (From Moss AA, Gamsu G, Genant HK. *Computed tomography of the body with magnetic resonance imaging*, 2nd ed. Philadelphia: WB Saunders, 1992:279.)

enlarges, this sliding component no longer occurs. The phrenoesophageal ligament is stretched especially anteriorly and laterally.

Over time the intrinsic sphincteric component of the diaphragm is lost. The resulting symptoms or damage are directly related to the reflux of gastric contents into the lower third of the esophagus (Figure 14–13). Whether or not esophagitis develops is determined by many factors that remain poorly understood. Despite significant reflux, symptoms may not be apparent. The presence of the sliding hiatal hernia is in itself of little consequence and is a common finding. As the reflux process continues, loss of surface

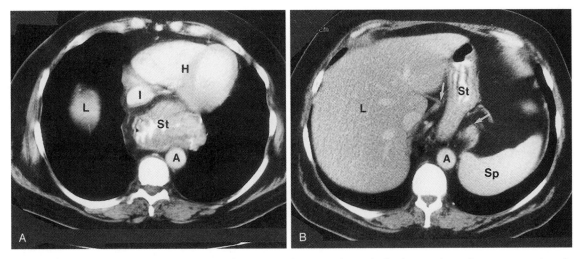

Figure 14–12. Hiatal hernia. **A,** Computed tomography scan through the lower chest demonstrates herniation of a portion of the stomach (St) into the lower mediastinum. **B,** Image obtained several centimeters caudad demonstrates widening of the esophageal hiatus (arrows) and herniation of the stomach (St). A, aorta; H, heart; I, inferior vena cava; L, liver; Sp, spleen. (**A,** from Gierada DS, Slone RM, Fleishman MJ. Imaging evaluation of the diaphragm. *Chest Surg Clin North Am* 1998;8:237; **B,** from Pearson FG, Cooper JD, Deslauriers J, *et al.*, ed. *Thoracic surgery*, 2nd ed. New York: Churchill Livingstone, 2002:1520.)

epithelium in the esophagus leads to superficial ulcerations. These ulcerations can cause scarring during periods of healing and contracture may lead to strictures (Figure 14–14).

Sliding hernias may be due to factors that cause increased intra-abdominal pressure such as pregnancy, obesity, vomiting, and vigorous esophageal contractions. The typical symptoms of retrosternal or epigastric heartburn, postural regurgitation, especially when lying on the right side, and intermittent dysphagia, are results of incompetence of the cardia and varying degrees of esophagitis. Symptoms are typically worse after meals and aggravated by position, as when lying down, stooping, bending over, or straining. Relief may come with sitting or standing.

Figure 14–13. Mechanism of reflux due to hiatal hernia. **A,** A hiatal hernia is an acquired herniation of part of the stomach through the diaphragm. After an episode of reflux (**B**), an esophageal peristaltic contraction (**C**) clears the bolus of acid from the esophagus into the hiatal hernia (**D**). **E,** Subsequently, swallowing-induced relaxation of the lower esophageal sphincter results in reflux of acid from the hernial sac into the esophagus. This sequence can be repeated several times and results in markedly prolonged clearance of acid. (Redrawn from Mittal RK, Balaban DH. The esophagogastric junction. *N Engl J Med* 1997;336:924–932.)

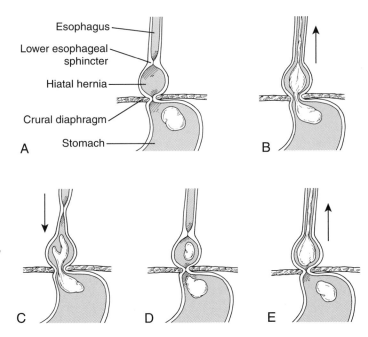

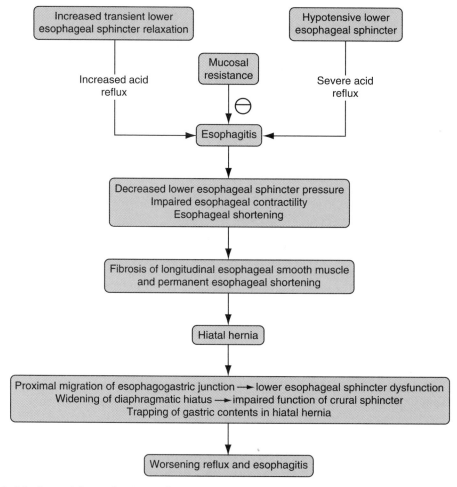

Figure 14–14. Potential mechanism of gastroesophageal reflux disease. Increased transient lower esophageal sphincter relaxation is the predominant mechanism of gastroesophageal reflux disease. A subset of patients with gastroesophageal reflux disease have hypotensive lower esophageal sphincter and usually have severe reflux disease. (Redrawn from Buttar NS, Falk GW. Pathogenesis of gastroesophageal reflux and Barrett esophagus. *Mayo Clin Proc* 2001;76:226–234.)

The diagnosis is commonly made by a barium swallow but a 24 hour pH study is the definitive diagnostic test. Cinefluorography can help assess the degree of reflux. An esophageal motility study may be necessary to evaluate the function of the lower esophageal sphincter as well as any intrinsic abnormalities of peristalsis that may be the result or cause of reflux.

Esophagoscopy should be carried out on all patients with symptoms of gastroesophageal reflux in order to assess esophagitis. The pliability of the esophageal wall can be assessed, as well as the fixation of the esophagogastric junction above the diaphragm, the status of the fundus of the stomach, and the possibility of coincidental malignancy. Biopsy of the mucosa should be performed at the same time to evaluate for Barrett's esophagus. Barrett's esophagus is a disease of the distal esophagus due to metaplastic replacement of the stratified squamous epithelium of the esophagus with columnar epithelium. Esophagogastroscopy should be used to rule out specialized intestinal columnar epithelium within 3 cm of the gastroesophageal junction. The presence of Barrett's esophagus increases the risk of esophageal adenocarcinoma 50–100-fold. Gastroesophageal reflux disease (GERD) plays an important role in the development of Barrett's esophagus. The more frequent and severe the symptoms of reflux, the greater the risk of developing adenocarcinoma.

In the absence of symptoms, no treatment is indicated for an uncomplicated sliding esophageal hernia. Medical treatment is necessary for patients with mild or transient symptoms in whom esophagitis is absent or mild. The goal of medical treatment is reducing reflux and minimizing the irritative effects of gastric secretions. This entails behavior modification such as a change in eating habits. A patient should have smaller meals and should not go to bed within 3 hours of a large meal. Alcohol, caffeine, and chocolate should be eliminated from the diet. A patient should avoid tight-fitting clothing, lose weight, and elevate the head of the bed. Pharmacologically, antacids should be prescribed before meals and bedtime to minimize the acidity of fluid in the esophagus. H_2-receptor antagonists and proton pump inhibitors (PPIs) can minimize acid secretions in the stomach. The introduction of PPIs has significantly advanced the medical management of GERD. These drugs block the H^+–K^+–adenosine triphosphate (ATPase) pump. PPIs can decrease acid secretion by 75–90% of basal and postprandial status.

Several indications for surgery exist. Patients who continue to have severe symptoms affecting their lifestyle despite optimal medical management should be considered for a definitive procedure. Patients who also develop complications from reflux esophagitis such as recurrent aspiration pneumonitis or peptic strictures are candidates. Signs of high-grade dysplasia in Barrett's esophagus should warrant repair of the hernia and resolution of the reflux. The mere presence of a sliding hiatal hernia is not an indication for an operation. However, ongoing damage of the distal esophagus due to GERD and development of Barrett's esophagus can have serious consequences and requires a definitive procedure.

Surgical goals are twofold: to prevent reflux and treat the esophagitis. The solution has been to attempt to reproduce a valve-like mechanism of the distal esophagus by wrapping the fundus of the stomach and the gastroesophageal junction. The wrap must be functional in that it must control reflux yet not interfere with passage of food into the stomach. The most commonly employed procedure is the Nissen fundoplication, a 360° wrap performed via either laparotomy or laparoscopy.

The operation of choice depends on the individual needs of the patient and expertise of the surgeon. Factors that influence the choice include whether a thoracic or abdominal approach is advantageous, whether the patient has already had a previous antireflux repair, whether a resection or esophagomyotomy is necessary, and the patient's body habitus. The principle of these procedures (Nissen, Belsey, Toupe) is the same. The surgeon restores the gastroesophageal junction to the abdomen and reduces the hiatal hernia, also approximating the diaphragmatic crurae and wrapping the gastric fundus around the distal esophagus (fundoplication). Restoration of the distal esophagus to the positive-pressure environment of the abdomen can prevent reflux.

Antireflux procedures can be performed a number of ways. Laparoscopic Nissen fundoplication and open laparotomy accomplish the same operation (Figure 14–15). Although the laparoscopic approach has less perioperative discomfort, long-term outcome depends on the success of the primary operation; therefore, the patient should be given the best

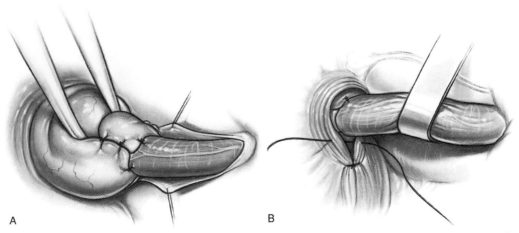

Figure 14–15. (**A**) Completed fundoplication. (**B**) Wrapped distal esophagus placed intra-abdominally and hiatal crura approximated posteriorly with nonabsorbable sutures. (From Ellis FH Jr: The Nissen fundoplication. In Cox JL, Sundt TS III, eds. *Operative Techniques in Cardiac & Thoracic Surgery*, Vol 2. Philadelphia, WB Saunders, 1997:37.)

operation at the disposal of the surgeon. While the Nissen fundoplication is the most popular complete fundoplication, the Toupet is one of the most commonly performed partial wraps. Originally performed for the prevention of reflux following Heller myotomy for achalasia, the partial wrap purports to result in fewer problems with dysphagia (Figure 14–16).

Paraesophageal Hernia

Paraesophageal hiatal hernias are much less common than sliding hernias. The phrenoesophageal membrane is focally weakened anteriorly and laterally to the esophagus. The gastric cardia and lower esophagus remain below the diaphragm in the normal anatomic location. The gastric fundus and abdominal viscera can protrude or roll through the defect into the mediastinum (Figure 14–17). The protruding organs are circumferentially covered by a layer of peritoneum that forms a true hernia sac, unlike the sliding hernia, in which the stomach forms the posterior wall of the hernia sac (Figure 14–18).

Most paraesophageal hernias cause no symptoms and remain undiagnosed for years. Possible complications include bleeding, incarceration, volvulus, obstruction, strangulation, and perforation. Gastritis and ulceration have been visualized in as many as one third of patients with paraesophageal hernias. It is suspected that these ulcers are the result of poor gastric emptying and torsion of the gastric wall, particularly after repeat incarcerations, which may impair the blood supply. Chronic bleeding from gastritis or ulceration may lead to iron-deficiency anemia with

resultant fatigue and exertional dyspnea. Respiratory complications may be associated with a paraesophageal hernia and consist of dyspnea from mechanical compression and recurrent pneumonia from aspiration.

The diagnosis of paraesophageal hiatal hernia is usually first suspected because of an abnormal radiograph of the chest. The most frequent finding is a retrocardiac air bubble with or without an air–fluid level. The sac and its contents occasionally protrude into the right thoracic cavity. A barium study of the upper gastrointestinal tract is the diagnostic study of choice. Once the diagnosis is established, the functional effect on the competence of the lower esophageal sphincter must be determined. This is best accomplished by endoscopy and esophageal function testing.

No acceptable medical treatment regimen exists for patients with paraesophageal hiatal hernia. Because of the serious and life-threatening nature of complications in this disorder, specifically gastric necrosis, the presence of the defect has been considered an indication for operation. When a patient presents with gastric volvulus and obstruction, decompression with a nasogastric tube must be promptly performed. The inability to decompress a gastric volvulus constitutes a surgical emergency and mandates immediate operative intervention, whether or not signs of toxicity exist.

Some controversy exists over how to approach these lesions. The thoracic approach emphasizes the ease of dissection of the hernia sac contents and resection of the sac. The abdominal approach is easily performed and permits the simultaneous placement of a gastrostomy tube. If the patient has objective

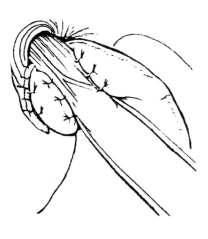

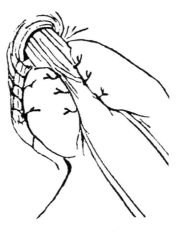

Figure 14–16. Toupet repair according to Ténière. (**A**) Separate closure of the diaphragmatic hiatus and 180-degree gastric wrap around the esophagus. (**B**) Separate closure of the diaphragmatic hiatus and 270-degree gastric wrap around the esophagus.

A   B

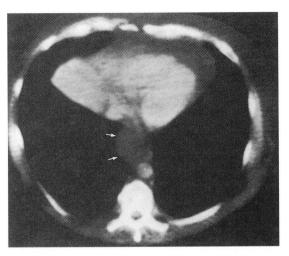

Figure 14–17. Paraesophageal hernia. Computed tomography scan near the diaphragm shows a fatty mass in the mediastinum (arrows), displacing the esophagus to the left. At surgery, a paraesophageal hernia consisting of omentum was found. (From Moss AA, Gamsu G, Genant HK. *Computed tomography of the body with magnetic resonance imaging*, 2nd ed. Philadelphia: WB Saunders, 1992:280.)

evidence of significant reflux esophagitis preoperatively, an antireflux procedure is performed. The stomach is secured within the peritoneal cavity. The crural defect is repaired. Recently this procedure has been accomplished laparoscopically. Controversy remains as to whether a concomitant fundoplication should be performed.

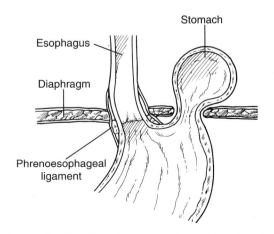

Figure 14–18. Type II paraesophageal hernia with complete herniation of the stomach into the chest. (Redrawn from Rogers MA, Cox JA. Laparoscopic paraesophageal hernia repair with Nissen fundoplication. *AORN J* 1998;67:536–540.)

Paralysis of the Diaphragm

In adults, the most common cause of hemidiaphragm paralysis is phrenic nerve injury, particularly from cardiac operations where topical cold is used. Internal mammary artery takedown is also associated with phrenic nerve injury (Table 14–2). Typically the left nerve is more frequently involved. Now with decreased opening of the pleural space, this has become less of a problem. Inflation of the lung to protect the nerve from contact with ice slush has reduced the incidence to less than 5%. Furthermore, when injury does occur, it is usually temporary. Other traumatic causes of phrenic nerve injury include tumor involvement, surgical injury following mediastinotomy, thoracic and neck resections, injury from subclavian and jugular vein catheter placement, and high cervical spinal cord injuries. Occasionally, idiopathic diaphragmatic paralysis is also seen in adults, but it is thought to be caused by subclinical viral infections (Figure 14–19). Again, this is usually unilateral, though bilateral injury has been reported.

Similarly, in infants, the most common cause of unilateral hemidiaphragmatic paralysis is injury to one of the phrenic nerves during a cardiac surgery procedure. Redo operations have almost twice the incidence of phrenic nerve injury (Figure 14–20). Birth trauma and removal of a mediastinal tumor are occasional causes of nerve injury. Prior to methods of modern management, mortality was 20–25%.

In adults, paralysis of either the left or right hemidiaphragm can occur without significant respiratory compromise. Studies have demonstrated a reduction of 20–30% in the vital capacity and the total lung capacity with isolated hemidiaphragm paralysis. Perfusion is also diminished to a lesser extent. Bilateral diaphragmatic paralysis is compatible with life in adults, however, is associated with excessive movement of the accessory muscles of respiration. In infants and young adults, however, this can be life-threatening. Pulmonary function tests have shown vital capacity to be half the predicted value in the erect position and further decreased by 50% supine. Lung compliance is reduced as a result of widespread atelectasis. During inspiration, the intercostal–accessory muscles contract, expanding the rib cage and producing negative pleural pressure, which draws the diaphragm and the abdominal viscera upward into the thoracic cavity. When upright, gravitational

TABLE 14–2 • *Causes of Phrenic Nerve Paralysis*	
Traumatic	Surgical, obstetric, chest tube
Infectious diseases	Poliomyelitis, herpes zoster, diphtheria, influenza, syphilis, tuberculosis, *Echinococcus* infections
Neoplastic diseases	Mediastinal tumors, N2 diseases
Others	Dystrophia myotonica, pericarditis, subphrenic abscess, lead poisoning
Idiopathic	

From Pearson FG, Cooper JD, Deslauriers J, *et al.*, ed. *Thoracic surgery*, 2nd ed. New York: Churchill Livingstone, 2002:1543.

forces tend to pull down the abdominal contents and the diaphragm, limiting their passive upward movement during inspiration. Therefore, in the erect posture, the intercostal–accessory muscle complex works more efficiently.

Paralysis of the diaphragm can be suggested by basilar atelectasis on a plain chest radiograph. Fluoroscopic observation of paradoxic diaphragmatic motion with a sniff test, however, remains the gold standard. Unilateral diaphragmatic paralysis can be distinguished by the upward movement of the hemidiaphragm with sniffing. The paralysis may escape detection if viewed with normal respiration as the motion of the contralateral diaphragm results in some passive motion of the paralyzed diaphragm (Table 14–3). Percutaneous electrical stimulation of a suspected phrenic nerve can give direct information about function of the nerve and the diaphragm.

Conservative therapy is the treatment of choice for adults. In general, direct repair of severed nerves is rarely successful. Diaphragm plication works well for the symptomatic patient. In infants, the initial therapy is mechanical ventilation. Patients are typically placed with the involved side down and treated with

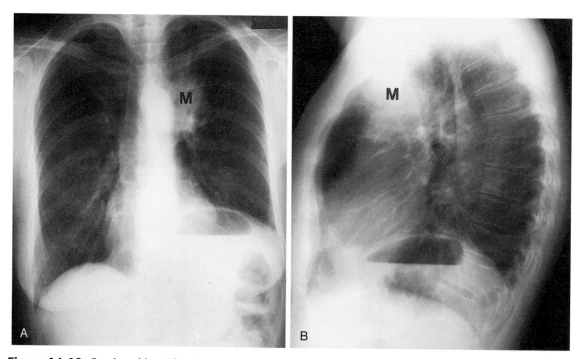

Figure 14–19. Paralyzed hemidiaphragm. Radiography demonstrates an elevated left hemidiaphragm and a large left paramediastinal mass (M) representing bronchogenic carcinoma involving the expected location of the phrenic nerve. Fluoroscopic examination confirmed hemidiaphragm paralysis, consistent with phrenic nerve invasion. (From Gierada DS, Slone RM, Fleishman MJ. Imaging evaluation of the diaphragm. *Chest Surg Clin North Am* 1998;8:237.)

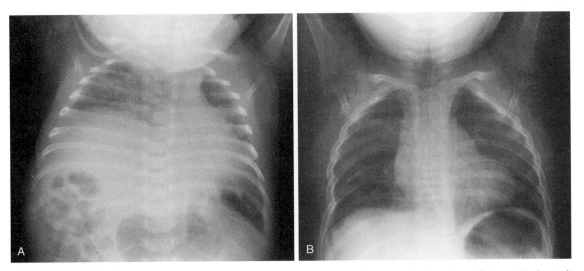

Figure 14–20. A, Preoperative chest radiograph of a neonate with acquired elevation of the right hemidiaphragm secondary to transection of the phrenic nerve, which occurred during chest tube insertion for pneumothorax. **B,** Chest radiograph 12 months after plication and primary repair of the phrenic nerve. (From Pearson FG, Cooper JD, Deslauriers J, *et al.*, ed. *Thoracic surgery*, 2nd ed. New York: Churchill Livingstone, 2002:1547.)

continuous positive airway pressure. If no resolution occurs within 2 weeks, operative intervention is undertaken by plication of the paralyzed diaphragm. Interestingly, plication does not prevent return of diaphragmatic function.

The goal of plicating the diaphragm is to lower the muscle into a flat position to reduce

TABLE 14–3 • *Hemidiaphragm Elevation*	
Unilateral	Lung volume loss (atelectasis, lobar collapse, partial lung resection, radiation fibrosis, congenital pulmonary hypoplasia, encasement by tumor)
	Eventration
	Abdominal disease (dilated stomach or colon, hepatomegaly, splenomegaly, subphrenic abscess)
	Phrenic nerve paralysis
	Splinting (rib fracture, pneumonia, infarction, abscess, peritonitis)
	Mimics (subpulmonic pleural effusion, large pleural mass, diaphragmatic hernia)
	After single lung transplant for pulmonary fibrosis
	Phrenoplasty
Bilateral	Lung volume loss (suboptimal inspiration, supine positioning, atelectasis, lung resection, pulmonary fibrosis)
	Abdominal mass effect (obesity, pregnancy, marked bowel dilation, ascites, hepatosplenomegaly, large abdominal tumors)
	Eventration
	Subpulmonic pleural effusions
	Neuromuscular disease (quadriplegia, multiple sclerosis, amyotrophic lateral sclerosis, Guillain–Barré syndrome, myasthenia gravis, Eaton–Lambert syndrome, muscular dystrophy, steroid or alcohol myopathy, rhabdomyolysis)
	Connective tissue disease (fibrosis in rheumatoid arthritis, scleroderma, and ankylosing spondylitis; weakness in systemic lupus erythematosus, polymyositis)
	Endocrine and metabolic disorders (hypothyroidism, hyperthyroidism, Cushing's disease, hypokalemia, hypophosphatemia, hypomagnesemia, metabolic alkalosis)
	Phrenic nerve paralysis

From Pearson FG, Cooper JD, Deslauriers J, *et al.*, ed. *Thoracic surgery*, 2nd ed. New York: Churchill Livingstone, 2002:1511.

the paradoxical motion and associated shift of the mobile mediastinum to the contralateral side on inspiration. Ventilatory movements become more efficient. We tend to use a thoracic approach – both open and laparoscopically. Either the excess diaphragmatic tissue can be stapled across each other or a portion of the muscle can be removed and then a primary closure performed.

Pacing of the Diaphragm

Electric stimulation of the phrenic nerve to produce artificial respiration emerged as a concept in the 18th century and became an accepted technique in the 19th century. Although pacing of the diaphragm appears to be an attractive treatment for respiratory failure due to a disorder of the respiratory pump, its use is truly indicated for the management of two diseases: central alveolar hypoventilation associated with apnea and high cervical spinal cord injury (Box 14–2). Diaphragmatic pacing has been used with limited success for intractable hiccups and suppressed respiratory drive during oxygen administration for patients with chronic obstructive pulmonary disease. Pacing is not indicated for phrenic nerve dysfunction, whether it is caused by traumatic injury or iatrogenic injury, neuropathy, myasthenia gravis, or obstructive sleep apnea. Central sleep apnea is usually due to medullary injury, either due to stroke, encephalitis, trauma, iatrogenic, or idiopathic (Ondine's curse). Spinal cord injury involving C3, C4, and C5 can disrupt respiration (Figure 14–21). Typically with quadriplegia in this situation, most accessory muscles are also affected. However, the sternocleidomastoid and trapezius, which are innervated by cranial nerve 11, remain functional.

The central principle is that pacing of the diaphragm requires an intact phrenic nerve. Candidates must be severely incapacitated by chronic ventilatory insufficiency and are usually receiving ventilator support before diaphragmatic pacing is instituted.

In evaluating candidates for diaphragm pacing, multiple factors need to be considered (Box 14–3). The lungs must have preserved ability to oxygenate and ventilate. Pacing cannot compensate for severe restrictive or obstructive lung disease. Measured pulmonary function tests should be normal. It is of paramount importance to verify the integrity of peripheral phrenic nerve conduction and diaphragmatic contractile function. A diaphragm that has been affected by a primary muscular disorder is not appropriate for pacing. The medullary respiratory center should be evaluated by measuring arterial blood gas levels at rest and during sleep.

Multiple methods exist for diaphragmatic pacing. For implantation of a pacer, both the neck and thoracic approaches offer certain advantages. The neck approach avoids the need for a thoracotomy; however, stimulation before all spinal contributions to the nerve have arrived can result in a suboptimal response. Activation of other nerves in the vicinity can cause painful contractions in the arm. In patients with a tracheostomy, contamination of a nearby surgical site can be difficult to avoid. Therefore, we prefer a thoracic approach.

Eventration of the Diaphragm

Eventration of the diaphragm is a rare anomaly usually associated with newborn infants and acquired during the fetal period. It refers to elevation of part or all of the hemidiaphragm, usually on the left side, although bilateral disease is possible. Congenital eventration of the diaphragm exhibits marked diaphragm thinning with an abnormal elevation of the diaphragm with poor or absent muscle development between the pleura and peritoneum. Although the pathophysiology of true eventrations in unknown, it is suspected to be caused by a premature return of the viscera to the peritoneal cavity after their rotation and the absence of ingrowth of striated muscles to the pleuroperitoneal membrane from the septum transversum. By returning prematurely, the viscera prevents complete development of the diaphragm. Like Bochdalek hernias, these occur more frequently on the left side. Based on their location, eventrations can be divided into three types: anterior, posterior, and median (Table 14–4). Microscopically the

BOX 14–2 INDICATIONS FOR DIAPHRAGMATIC PACING

- Central alveolar hypoventilation associated with central apneas
- Ventilator-dependent patient after high cervical cord injury

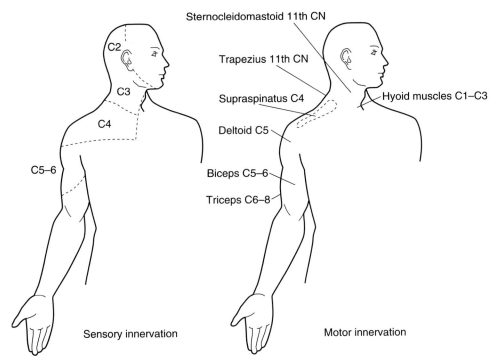

Sternocleidomastoid 11th CN

Trapezius 11th CN

Supraspinatus C4

Deltoid C5

Hyoid muscles C1–C3

Biceps C5–6

Triceps C6–8

C2

C3

C4

C5–6

Sensory innervation

Motor innervation

Figure 14–21. Sensory and motor findings that distinguish 'high' quadriplegia. Quadriplegia at C2–3 is amenable to diaphragm pacing. CN, cranial nerve. (Redrawn from Shields TW. *General thoracic surgery*, 4th ed. Baltimore: Williams & Wilkins, 1994.)

muscle fibers in the defective diaphragmatic region are fewer in number and unorganized in direction. Often the tissue is scarred, has a high collagen content, and is infiltrated with leukocytes.

Most small eventrations are asymptomatic, or they can result in a paradoxical motion of the affected hemidiaphragm during inspiration and expiration (Figure 14–22). The diagnosis of eventration of the diaphragm can usually be made by examining the posteroanterior and lateral chest x-rays (Figure 14–23). Chest radiographs typically demonstrate an elevated hemidiaphragm, sometimes with loss of volume of the lower lobe and mediastinal

shift to the contralateral side (Figure 14–24). Fluoroscopy and ultrasound can provide additional information about the location of solid organs such as the liver and demonstrates paradoxical motion of the diaphragm and mediastinal shift with inspiration and expiration. These findings help differentiate the eventration from subpulmonic pleural conditions, phrenic nerve paralysis and primary hepatic abnormalities (Table 14–5).

Management of diaphragmatic eventration varies greatly depending on whether the diagnosis is made in infants or adults. Initial treatment of eventration includes upright positioning, supplemental oxygen, and nutritional

BOX 14–3 CLINICAL REQUIREMENTS FOR DIAPHRAGMATIC PACING

- Stable clinical condition
- Good lung function
- Good phrenic nerve and diaphragmatic function
- Evaluation of medullary respiratory center

TABLE 14-4 • *Anatomic Classification of Eventration*		
Total		
Partial (localized)	Anterior	
	Posterolateral	
	Medial	
Bilateral	Partial	
	Complete	

From Thomas TV. Non-paralytic eventration of the diaphragm. *J Thorac Cardiovasc Surg* 1968;55:586.

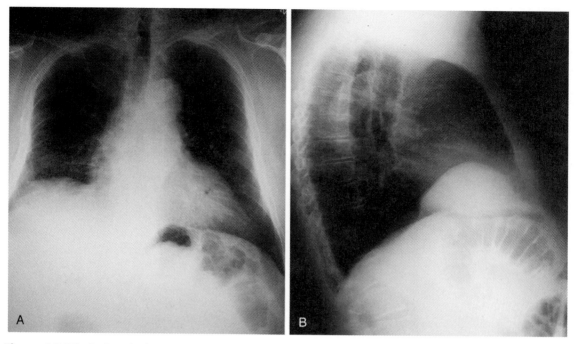

Figure 14–22. A, Standard posteroanterior chest radiograph showing an asymptomatic congenital eventration of the right hemidiaphragm diagnosed in an adult moderate right diaphragm eventration. **B,** Lateral view showing the incomplete anterior nature of the eventration. (From Pearson FG, Cooper JD, Deslauriers J, *et al.,* ed. *Thoracic surgery,* 2nd ed. New York: Churchill Livingstone, 2002:1538.)

support. Mechanical ventilation may be necessary. Once the patient is stabilized from a cardiopulmonary point of view, surgical correction of the eventration is indicated for all symptomatic disease (Table 14–6). Small asymptomatic eventrations may not require any treatment. Simple plication is recommended in children because it is fast, can be done with minimal blood loss, and involves no entry into the peritoneal cavity.

When eventration occurs in older children and adults, it is usually the result of an acquired paralysis of the diaphragm due to phrenic nerve dysfunction (Table 14–7). This

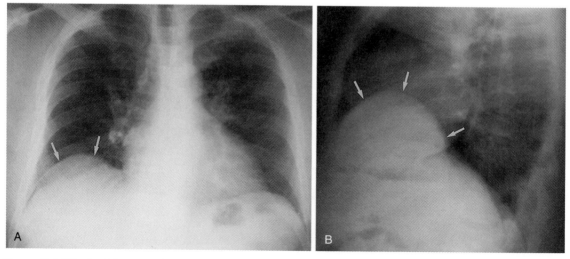

Figure 14–23. Partial eventration. Posteroanterior (**A**) and lateral (**B**) radiographs in a 42-year-old man reveal a broad, upwardly bulging segment (arrows) of the anteromedial right hemidiaphragm. (From Pearson FG, Cooper JD, Deslauriers J, *et al.,* ed. *Thoracic surgery,* 2nd ed. New York: Churchill Livingstone, 2002:1512.)

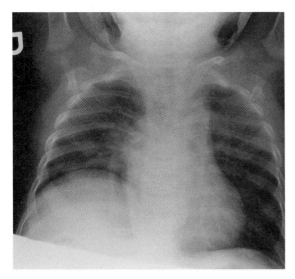

Figure 14–24. Standard posteroanterior chest radiograph of a 10-month-old child with complete eventration of the right hemidiaphragm. (From Pearson FG, Cooper JD, Deslauriers J, *et al.*, ed. *Thoracic surgery*, 2nd ed. New York: Churchill Livingstone, 2002:1539.)

can occur due to birth trauma, injury during cervical or thoracic operations, invasion by tumors, and some pleural or pulmonary infections. At birth, breach delivery or difficult and prolonged forceps delivery can result in phrenic nerve injury, often associated with vocal cord paralysis or brachial plexus injuries. Neoplastic involvement of the phrenic nerve is often the cause of diaphrag-

matic elevation and, in patients with bronchogenic carcinomas, phrenic nerve paralysis is usually secondary to mediastinal nodal (N2) disease. Usually occurring on the right, the liver protrudes through the defect but does not require surgical intervention. Most cases of adult eventration can be treated conservatively.

Diaphragmatic Tumors

Primary tumors of the diaphragm are rare (Box 14–4). Most are mesothelial in origin, although neurogenic tumors do occur to a lesser extent, and are discovered in the fifth to seventh decade of life. Most benign tumors are asymptomatic and are usually noted on routine radiographs of the chest or found incidentally at time of surgical operation. Simple cysts have been described, as well as lipomas, fibromas, and benign neurogenic tumors. Symptomatic diaphragmatic hernias are usually malignant and present with pain with respiration. These tumors are usually fibrosarcomas or rarely vascular or muscular sarcomas. Most commonly, the diaphragm is invaded secondarily by a malignant tumor from surrounding structures.

Computed tomography and magnetic resonance imaging are usually necessary for full visualization of diaphragmatic tumors. The differential for a suspected diaphragmatic mass includes an infectious collection (including

	Eventration	**Phrenic Nerve Palsy**
Incidence	Rare	Common
Etiology	Congenital anomaly in formation of the diaphragm	Acquired lesion (at birth or during adult life) of the phrenic nerve
Gross appearance	Normal muscle rim at the periphery and thin membranous eventrated portion	Atrophic muscle throughout the diaphragm
Microscopy	Attenuated portion composed of fibroelastic tissue	Muscle fibers and nerve bundles seen throughout the diaphragm
	Phrenic nerve normal	
Clinical presentation	Newborn: can present with respiratory failure; no history of obstetrical trauma	Newborn: history of obstetrical trauma nearly always present
	Adult: respiratory or gastrointestinal symptoms	Adult: respiratory or gastrointestinal symptoms
Diagnosis	No paradoxical movement on fluoroscopy	Paradoxical motion
	Response positive to faradic intraoperative stimulation	No response to faradic stimulation
	Restrictive pattern on spirometry	Restrictive pattern on spirometry

TABLE 14–5 • *Differences Between Eventration and Phrenic Nerve Palsy*

From Deslauriers J. Eventration of the diaphragm. *Chest Surg Clin North Am* 1998;8:324.

TABLE 14–6 • *Surgical Techniques for Repair of Congenital Eventration*

Technique	Advantages
Plication	Easier and faster operation
	Minimal blood loss
	No entry in peritoneal cavity
Excision and plication	Possible reapproximation of normal muscle with recovery of functions
	Avoids inadvertent injury to abdominal organs

From Pearson FG, Cooper JD, Deslauriers J, *et al.*, ed. *Thoracic surgery*, 2nd ed. New York: Churchill Livingstone, 2002:1542.

TABLE 14–7 • *Acquired Elevation of the Diaphragm*

Intact phrenic nerve	Mechanical factors or blunt trauma
	Idiopathic
Abnormal phrenic nerve	Post-traumatic or postoperative
	Sequela of neuromuscular or infectious disorders
	Malignancies of lung or mediastinum
	Idiopathic

From Pearson FG, Cooper JD, Deslauriers J, *et al.*, ed. *Thoracic surgery*, 2nd ed. New York: Churchill Livingstone, 2002:1539.

Mycobacterium tuberculosis), hematoma, congenital abnormality and hernia. On CT scans, lipomas typically appear large, sharp-bordered, and smooth.

Surgical removal is indicated for all tumors of the diaphragm. Resection and reconstruction of the diaphragm usually does not represent a technical challenge. The pleural and peritoneal layers are excised *en bloc* with the diaphragm. The remaining defect is closed primarily either using nonabsorbable mattress sutures or with a prosthetic soft tissue patch of Gore-Tex or

BOX 14–4 DIAPHRAGMATIC TUMORS

Benign
- Lipoma
- Cystic masses
- Bronchogenic
- Mesothelial
- Teratoid

Malignant
- Sarcoma
- Schwannoma
- Chondroma
- Pheochromocytoma
- Endometriosis

polypropylene mesh. Morbidity and mortality from these procedures is low and there is usually minimal respiratory compromise. For benign tumors, the overall prognosis is quite good. However, for malignant tumors, recurrence is common and patients tend to do poorly.

Suggested Readings

Deslauriers J. Eventration of the diaphragm. *Chest Surg Clin North Am* 1998;8:315–330.

Horgan S, Pellegrini CA. Surgical treatment of gastroesophageal reflux disease. *Surg Clin North Am* 1997; 77:1063–1082.

Moxham J, Shneerson JM. Diaphragmatic pacing. *Am Rev Respir Dis* 1993;148:533–536.

Naunheim K, Baue A. Paraesophageal hiatal hernia. In: Shields T, ed. *General thoracic surgery*, vol. 1. Philadelphia: Williams & Wilkins, 1994:644–651.

Reynolds M. Congenital posterolateral diaphragmatic hernias. In: Shields T, ed. *General thoracic surgery*, vol. 1. Philadelphia: Williams & Wilkins, 1994:628–634.

Schumpelick V, Steinau G, Schluper I, Prescher A. Surgical embryology and anatomy of the diaphragm with surgical applications. *Surg Clin North Am* 2000;80: 213–239.

Shields T. Tumors of the diaphragm. In: Shields T, ed. *General thoracic surgery*, vol. 1. Philadelphia: Williams & Wilkins, 1994:652–656.

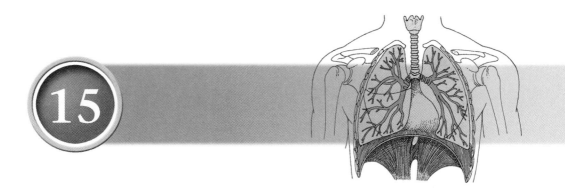

The Pleura

ANATOMY AND PHYSIOLOGY	PLEURAL EFFUSIONS
PNEUMOTHORAX	EMPYEMA
HEMOTHORAX	BRONCHOPLEURAL FISTULA
CHYLOTHORAX	PLEURAL TUMORS

The Pleura: Key Points

- Understand the pathophysiology of a pneumothorax and its management
- Know the differential diagnosis for fluid in the pleural space
- Understand how patients develop a hemothorax and chylothorax and the appropriate treatment options
- Understand the stages of the development of an empyema
- Describe the typical characteristics of pleural tumors

Anatomy and Physiology

The lungs are ensheathed by a thin serous membrane in the form of a closed invaginated sac. A portion of the serous membrane called the visceral pleura covers the surface of the lung and extends into the fissures between its lobes. The rest of the membrane, called the parietal pleura, lines the inner surface of the chest wall, covers the diaphragm, and reflects over the structures occupying the middle of the thorax. The two layers are continuous with one another around and below the lung root (Figure 15–1). The potential space between them is known as the pleural cavity. When the lung collapses or

when air or fluid collects between the two layers, the cavity becomes apparent. The right and left pleural sacs do not communicate.

Like other serous membranes, the pleura is covered by a single layer of flattened, nucleated cells, sealed at their edges by cement substance. These cells are modified connective-tissue corpuscles and rest on a basement membrane. Beneath the basement membrane there are networks of yellow elastic and white fibers, imbedded in ground substance, which contain connective-tissue cells. Blood vessels, lymphatics, and nerves are distributed in the substance of the pleura. The arteries supplying the pleura are derived from the intercostal, internal

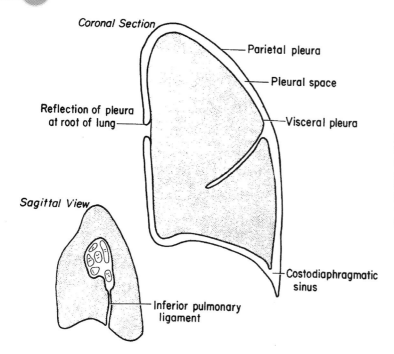

Figure 15–1. Schematic coronal section of a hemithorax and sagittal view of the root of the lung showing the pleural coverings. Note the location of the costodiaphragmatic sinus. (From Sabiston DC Jr, Spencer FC. *Surgery of the chest*, 6th ed. Philadelphia: WB Saunders, 1995:524.)

mammary, musculophrenic, thymic, pericardiac, and bronchial vessels.

Pleural pressure is maintained by the opposite pull on the pleural space by the transthoracic pressure developed by the chest wall and the transpulmonary pressure created by the lungs. The pleural pressure is typically negative, and at functional residual capacity, reaches -2 to -8 cm H_2O in the sitting position (Figure 15–2). As lung volume increases during inspiration, the pleural pressure becomes more negative, reaching -25 to -35 cm H_2O at full inspiration.

Pleural fluid is continuously produced and reabsorbed, essentially maintaining an equilibrium (Box 15–1). Pleural fluid moves into the

BOX 15–1 COMPOSITION OF NORMAL PLEURAL FLUID

- Volume: 10 mL
- pH >7.6
- Protein: 10–20 g/L
- Albumin: 60%
- $[LDH]_{pleural fluid}$ <50% $[LDH]_{plasma}$
- $[Glucose]_{pleural fluid}$ = $[Glucose]_{plasma}$
- Cellular composition
  - Mesothelial cells: 10–70%
  - Monocytes 30–70%
  - Lymphocytes: 5–30%
  - Granulocytes: 10%

pleural space due to oncotic and hydrostatic pressure of the systemic circulation. Although the resorption rate ranges from 20 to 1000 mL/24 h, at any given time there is only less than 10 mL fluid in the pleural space. The lymphatic system, particularly that of the parietal pleura, plays an important role in the reabsorption of excess fluid and proteins.

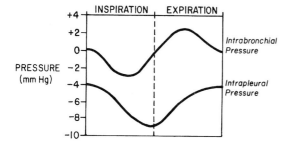

Figure 15–2. Pressure tracing of the intrabronchial and intrapleural pressures during inspiration and expiration, showing the constant pressure gradient between the bronchus and the pleural space. (From Sabiston DC Jr, Spencer FC. *Surgery of the chest*, 6th ed. Philadelphia: WB Saunders, 1995:525.)

Pneumothorax

A pneumothorax occurs when air from an injured lung or airway is trapped within the pleural cavity, increasing or obliterating the normal negative intrapleural pressure (Figure 15–3). It may be spontaneous, traumatic, or iatrogenic (Table 15–1). Under normal conditions, the pleural space is under negative pressure, fluctuating between −10 mm Hg during inspiration and −5 mm Hg during expiration. This negative pressure is maintained by continual reabsorption of lymphatic fluid from the pleural space by the pleural capillaries. In a spontaneous pneumothorax, whether due to a bleb or bullae or ruptured cyst, air escapes into the pleural space via the bronchoalveolar tree (Figure 15–4). Often, a valve effect prevents return of air from the pleural space. Accumulation of air in the pleural space can cause intrapleural pressure to rise to 20 cm H_2O, preventing effective venous return to the right atrium (Figure 15–5). This scenario describes a tension pneumothorax, a rare but life-threatening situation.

Primary spontaneous pneumothorax occurs in patients without clinically apparent lung disease. Secondary spontaneous pneumothorax is a complication of pre-existing lung disease. Most patients who develop a primary

TABLE 15–1 • *Categories of Pneumothorax*	
Spontaneous	
Primary	
Secondary	Chronic obstructive pulmonary disease
	Bullous disease
	Cystic fibrosis
	Pneumocystis-related congenital cysts
	Idiopathic pulmonary fibrosis (IPF)
	Pulmonary embolism
Catamenial	
Neonatal	
Traumatic	
Penetrating	
Blunt	
Iatrogenic	
Mechanical ventilation	
Thoracentesis	
Lung biopsy	
Venous catheterization	
Postsurgical	
Other	
Esophageal perforation	

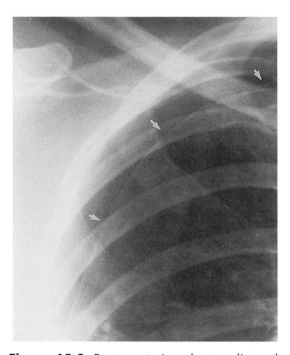

Figure 15–3. Posteroanterior chest radiograph showing pneumothorax. Close-up demonstrates well the visceral pleural line (arrows) and also the lack of pulmonary vascular markings lateral to the pleural line. Also see Figure 15–6. (From Meholic A, Ketai L, Lofgren R. *Fundamentals of chest radiology.* Philadelphia: WB Saunders, 1996:146.)

spontaneous pneumothorax are less than 40 years of age. Typically, patients are tall, thin men with a history of smoking. Pneumothorax results from rupture of a pulmonary bleb, which is a small air-filled sac between the lung parenchyma and the visceral pleural. Blebs tend to occur in the apices of the upper lobes and fissures. Of note, spontaneous pneumothoraces tend to recur. After a primary spontaneous pneumothorax, the incidence of a repeat episode on the ipsilateral side is 30% (Box 15–2). After a recurrence, the chance of another pneumothorax exceeds 50%.

Secondary causes of pneumothorax include airway disease, infectious lung disease, interstitial lung disease, connective tissue disease, and cancer. Underlying airway disease such as asthma, bullous disease, and chronic obstructive pulmonary disease (COPD) can predispose to pneumothorax. COPD patients are typically older, have limited pulmonary reserve and have lost the intrinsic elastic recoil of the lung, causing the lung to collapse slowly. Interstitial diseases such as idiopathic pulmonary fibrosis, sarcoidosis, and collagen-vascular diseases can also lead to pneumothorax. Infections can

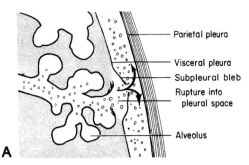

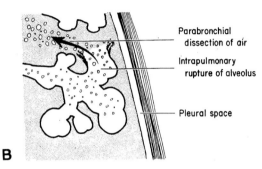

Figure 15–4. Schematic drawing of the distended apical alveoli caused by mechanical stress from the weight of the upright lung. Alveolar rupture allows alveolar gas to dissect peripherally and form blebs that eventually rupture into the pleural space and cause a pneumothorax (**A**) or dissect centrally along lobular septa and produce a pneumomediastinum (**B**). (From Sabiston DC Jr, Spencer FC. *Surgery of the chest*, 6th ed. Philadelphia: WB Saunders, 1995:529.)

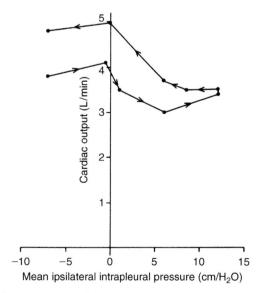

Figure 15–5. Reduction in cardiac output caused by increasing intrapleural pressure. A positive pleural pressure interferes with venous return to the heart. (From Sabiston DC Jr, Spencer FC. *Surgery of the chest*, 6th ed. Philadelphia: WB Saunders, 1995:525.)

BOX 15–2 RISK FACTORS FOR RECURRENCE OF SPONTANEOUS PNEUMOTHORAX

- More than one prior episode
- Chronic obstructive lung disease
- Bullae and cysts visible on chest radiographs
- Air leak for more than 48 h during first episode

cause inflammatory processes of the pleura that can disrupt the mesothelial lining of the lung and cause a pneumothorax. An iatrogenic pneumothorax can be the result of thoracentesis, mechanical ventilation, central vein catheterization, or postoperative in nature. Tumors can also disrupt pulmonary anatomy, causing accumulation of air in the pleural space. Growth of the tumor can cause obstruction of the airway. Increased alveolar pressure can rupture into the pleural space. Similarly, tumors can grow in the peripheral lung tissue, creating an ischemic path from alveoli to the pleural cavity.

Pneumothoraces are classified according to the volume of lung loss or collapse identified on chest x-ray or by respiratory and systemic signs. Arterial hypoxemia occurs with the collapse of 50% or more of the lung and is due to significant ventilation-perfusion mismatch.

In a small pneumothorax, the volume loss is one third of the normal lung volume (Figure 15–6). In a large pneumothorax, the lung is completely collapsed but there is no mediastinal shift or associated hypotension. Patients usually have symptoms, most commonly complaining of pain and shortness of breath. Clinical findings suggestive of a pneumothorax include decreased breath sounds, hyperresonance to percussion, and decreased expansion of the affected lung during inspiration. The presence of subcutaneous emphysema is alarming in appearance but is relatively harmless (Figure 15–7). This is not an indication for chest-tube insertion if the lung remains inflated. However, most traumatic pneumothoraces should be managed with a chest tube. Delayed increase in the volume of a pneumothorax may occur at any time and may become life-threatening.

A tension pneumothorax is characterized by complete lung collapse, tracheal deviation, mediastinal shift leading to decreased venous return to the heart, hypotension, and respiratory distress (Figure 15–8). It usually occurs in

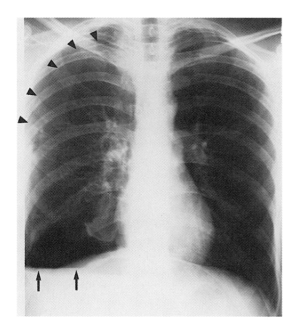

Figure 15–6. Posteroanterior upright chest view: small pneumothorax with air–fluid level in the costophrenic angle. Full radiograph of the same patient shown in Figure 15–3 demonstrates an air–fluid level (arrows) that is well-defined at the right costophrenic angle. In some instances, the air–fluid level is very small and the only indication of free air within the pleural space. The visceral pleural line (arrowheads) is better seen in the close-up (Fig. 15–3). (From Meholic A, Ketai L, Lofgren R. *Fundamentals of chest radiology*. Philadelphia: WB Saunders, 1996:147.)

patients with parenchymal lung injury in the presence of positive pressure ventilation. Clinical signs and symptoms include dyspnea, tachypnea, hypotension, diaphoresis, and dis-

tended neck veins and a notable increase in peak airway pressure of the ventilated patient. It is diagnosed clinically, and constitutes a life-threatening emergency. Chest x-rays are not necessary to confirm the diagnosis and may delay definitive treatment, thus significantly increasing the risk of circulatory collapse and cardiorespiratory arrest.

This is a true surgical emergency and treatment includes chest decompression initially with a large-bore needle inserted in the second intercostal space on the midclavicular line, and subsequent tube thoracostomy. Re-expansion of the lung and re-approximation of the pleural surfaces usually seals the lung defect. All patients with a pneumothorax, regardless of its size, who will undergo positive-pressure ventilation should have a chest tube placed before starting mechanical ventilation.

Surgery is indicated for the definitive management of pneumothoraces on patients with persistent air leak (Box 15–3). Chemical pleurodesis via the chest tube is sometimes an option but the procedure is painful and should usually be done following placement of an epidural catheter. Various agents such as talc, tetracycline and *Corynebacterium* sp. have been used with effective results.

Video-assisted thoracoscopic surgery (VATS) with multiple chest ports allows wide visualization of the pleural space for the resection of bulla and mechanical pleurodesis. The rate of complications associated with VATS is higher among patients with secondary pneumothorax than among those with primary pneumothorax.

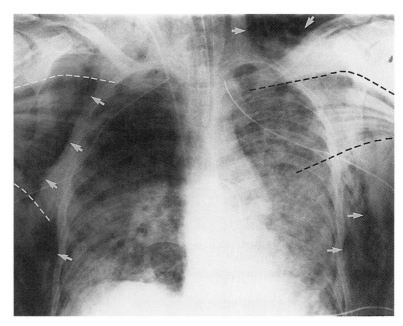

Figure 15–7. Anteroposterior chest radiograph showing subcutaneous emphysema. Subcutaneous air extends throughout the soft tissues of the thorax, defining the major pectoral muscles bilaterally (radial lucencies inside dotted lines). The emphysema also extends inferolaterally into the soft tissues external to the ribs and into the supraclavicular regions (arrows). (Diffuse air space and interstitial infiltrates of adult respiratory distress syndrome are evident. Also note bilateral chest tubes.) (From Meholic A, Ketai L, Lofgren R. *Fundamentals of chest radiology*. Philadelphia: WB Saunders, 1996:149.)

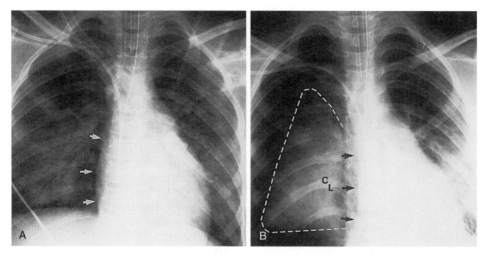

Figure 15–8. Serial posteroanterior chest radiographs showing tension pneumothorax. **A,** Initial frontal radiograph demonstrates normal appearance of the chest following central venous pressure catheter placement. The right cardiac border shows on mediastinal shift (arrows). **B,** Follow-up chest radiograph obtained for acute onset of dyspnea shows a large pneumothorax with the mediastinal structures and right cardiac border shifted to the left (arrows). The dome of the right diaphragm is depressed, and the compressed lung (CL) is now airless and collapsed inferomedially (dotted lines). (From Meholic A, Ketai L, Lofgren R. *Fundamentals of chest radiology.* Philadelphia: WB Saunders, 1996:149.)

For young patients with spontaneous pneumothorax, indications for VATS procedure include air leak for more than 48 hours, recurrent pneumothorax, or a history of pneumothorax on both sides.

Hemothorax

Blood may accumulate in the pleural cavity after blunt or penetrating injuries, after open heart surgery, and because of spread of malignant disease. Bleeding can result from nontraumatic causes (Box 15–4). It may vary from minor to massive. The pleural space can accumulate up to 3 L of blood. Most often, hemothorax occurs because of injury to an intercostal artery or the internal mammary artery. Massive hemothorax is the result of major pulmonary vascular or parenchymal injury or major arterial wounds, while minor lung injuries would only cause a small hemothorax.

Symptoms depend on the amount of blood that accumulates in the pleural space. On physical examination, breath sounds may be decreased on the side of the injury. A chest x-ray obtained in the upright position may reveal accumulations of blood greater than 200 mL; however, a supine film may demonstrate a diffuse haziness or none at all.

Management is directed at correcting the hypovolemia and at evacuating the blood from the pleural cavity. Hemothoraces are

BOX 15–3 INDICATIONS FOR THORACOTOMY IN PATIENTS WITH SPONTANEOUS PNEUMOTHORAX

- Massive air leak that prevents lung re-expansion
- Persistent air leak for more than 5 days
- Recurrent pneumothorax (second episode)
- Complications of pneumothorax:
  - Hemothorax
  - Empyema
- Chronic pneumothorax
- Specific surgical indications for conditions causing secondary spontaneous pneumothorax
- Occupational indications after first episode:
  - Airline pilots
  - Scuba divers
  - Individuals living in remote areas
- Previous contralateral pneumothorax
- Bilateral simultaneous pneumothorax
- Presence of large cysts visible on chest x-ray

From Sabiston DC Jr, Spencer FC. *Surgery of the chest*, 6th ed. Philadelphia: WB Saunders, 1995:531.

BOX 15–4 ETIOLOGY OF SPONTANEOUS HEMOTHORAX

Pulmonary
- Bullous emphysema
- Necrotizing infections
- Pulmonary embolus with infarction
- Tuberculosis
- Arteriovenous malformation
- Hereditary hemorrhagic telangiectasia

Pleural
- Torn pleural adhesions secondary to spontaneous pneumothorax
- Neoplasms
- Endometriosis

Pulmonary Neoplasms
- Primary
- Metastases
  - Melanoma
  - Trophoblastic tumors

Blood Dyscrasias
- Thrombocytopenia
- Hemophilia
- Complication of systemic anticoagulation
- Von Willebrand's disease

Abdominal Pathology
- Pancreatic pseudocyst
- Splenic artery aneurysm
- Hemoperitoneum

Thoracic Pathology
- Ruptured thoracic aortic aneurysm

From Sabiston DC Jr, Spencer FC. *Surgery of the chest*, 6th ed. Philadelphia: WB Saunders, 1995:534.

initially treated by large-bore (36 French) chest tube placement and, in approximately 85% of the cases, the bleeding will stop as the lung is re-expanded because of the low pressure in the systemic circulation. Clotted hemothorax when not completely evacuated may result in organized fibrin deposition on the pleural surfaces and lung entrapment. This may require formal decortication in order to allow the lung to fully re-expand.

A small number of patients will have continued bleeding and require a thoracotomy. Most commonly, injuries in systemic arteries (intercostal arteries or internal mammary artery) or the lung parenchyma are found as the cause. Major pulmonary vessel injury is usually rap-idly fatal and these patients rarely survive. As previously described, indications for emergent thoracotomy are initial chest tube output of 1500 mL of blood or persistent drainage of 200–300 mL per hour.

Chylothorax

Chylothorax is defined by the presence of chyle in the pleural space. Chyle is the lymphatic drainage from the abdomen. This problem has become more common with the increased incidence of chest trauma and surgical procedures on mediastinal structures. The thoracic duct starts at the cisterna chili, transverses the thoracic cavity along the spine with multiple small rami and ends at the left jugulosubclavian junction. The cisterna chili is a tubular dilatation 3 cm in diameter sitting on the vertebral column between L3 and T10 on the right side of the aorta. The thoracic duct enters the chest through the aortic hiatus at T12–T10. The duct lies on the anterior surface of the vertebral column behind the esophagus and between the aorta and azygous vein. At the level of the fifth thoracic vertebra the duct turns to the left, ascends behind the aortic arch into the left side of the posterior mediastinum, and passes superiorly adjacent to the left side of the esophagus (Figure 15–9). This course explains why damage to it below T5 or T6 results in a right-sided effusion and damage above this level results in a left-sided effusion. In the neck, the duct passes behind the left carotid sheath and jugular vein and empties into the left jugulosubclavian junction.

Flow through the duct varies with meals and particularly the fat content of the meal (Table 15–2). Of the thoracic duct lymph, 95% comes from the liver and intestinal lymphatics. The thoracic duct has valves to ensure unidirectional flow up the chest. Forward flow is assisted by respiration, because on inspiration the increase in intra-abdominal pressure causes compression of the cisterna chili and the negative intrathoracic pressure creates a gradient between the abdomen and thorax.

There are several causes of chylothorax; trauma and neoplasms are the two most common causes (Box 15–5). The most common mechanism of nonpenetrating injury to the thoracic duct is sudden hyperextension of the spine due to blast or blunt trauma with rupture of the duct just above the diaphragm. Vomiting episodes or violent coughing can tear the thoracic duct. Spontaneous rupture of the duct,

THORACIC DUCT

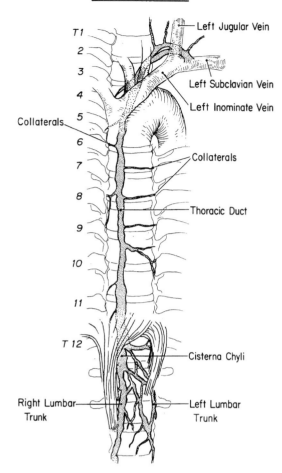

Figure 15–9. Schematic drawing of the most usual pattern and course of the thoracic duct. The single duct that enters the chest through the aortic hiatus between T12 and T10 is a relatively consistent finding and the usual site for surgical ligation. (From Sabiston DC Jr, Spencer FC. *Surgery of the chest*, 6th ed. Philadelphia: WB Saunders, 1995:536.)

TABLE 15–2 • *Characteristics of Chyle*	
Milky appearance with creamy layer on standing; clears when fat is extracted by alkali and ether	
Fat globules stain with Sudan III	
Alkaline, odorless	
Sterile, bacteriostatic	
Specific gravity: 1.012–1.025	
Lymphocytes	400–7000/mm³
Erythrocytes	50–600/mm³
Total fat	0.4–5.0 g/dL
Total cholesterol	65–220 mg/dL
Triglycerides	>110 mg/dL
Cholesterol–triglyceride ratio	<1
Total protein	2–6 g/dL
Albumin	1–4 g/dL
Glucose	50–100 g/dL
Electrolytes	Similar to plasma

such as coughing or stretching after ingestion of a fatty meal.

Symptoms from a chylothorax arise from mechanical compression of the ipsilateral lung from the fluid, which can result in dyspnea and cough. Chyle has bacteriostatic properties and, therefore, rarely becomes infected. Nutritional losses can be high, losing fat and protein, which can rapidly deplete the individual and cause increasing fatigue. The huge loss of white blood cells results in immunosuppression.

Chylothorax is diagnosed from the milky, turbid fluid drained from a pleural tap or thoracostomy tube to relieve the effusion. The triglyceride level of the fluid should be determined and usually is greater than 150 mg/dL. All patients with chylothorax should be managed initially by thoracostomy tube drainage, correction of fluid losses and electrolyte imbalances, hyperalimentation, and bowel rest. One quarter of patients will respond, while others will continue to have a persistent fistula. The most common procedure is ligation of the thoracic duct at the hiatus approached via the right chest, making no attempt to locate the leak. Finding this duct can be assisted by high-fat content feeding through a nasogastric tube to stimulate chylous secretions, however mass ligation of all structures on the spine between the aorta and the esophagus will always include the duct. Pleurectomy and pleurodesis are recommended when the site of the leak is not identified and ligation of the duct at the aortic hiatus is performed.

although rare, is more likely when it is full after a fatty meal. There is a delay of 2–10 days before an effusion develops from a thoracic duct injury. Chyle needs to accumulate in the posterior mediastinum before the mediastinal pleura will rupture and a fistula forms to the pleural space.

Benign tumors of the lymphatic system such as lymphangiomas and mediastinal hygromas can cause a chylothorax. Abdominal and thoracic tumors, particularly lymphomas, can cause a chylothorax by invasion of the thoracic duct, lymphatic permeation of the duct, or tumor embolus into the main duct. Malignant chylous leaks can fill the pericardial sac and cause tamponade. In adults, most cases of idiopathic chylothorax are due to minor trauma

BOX 15–5 ETIOLOGY OF CHYLOTHORAX

Traumatic (Chest and Neck)
- Blunt
- Penetrating

Iatrogenic
- Catheterization, particularly subclavian venous
- Postsurgical
- Excision of cervical/supraclavicular lymph nodes
- Radical lymph node dissections of the neck
- Radical lymph node dissections of the chest
- Esophagectomy
- Lobectomy or pneumonectomy
- Mediastinal tumor resection
- Thoracic aneurysm repair
- Sympathectomy
- Congenital cardiovascular surgery

Neoplasms
- Lymphoma
- Lung cancers
- Esophageal cancers
- Mediastinal malignancies
- Metastatic carcinomas

Infectious
- Tuberculous lymphadenosis
- Mediastinitis
- Ascending lymphangitis

Other
- Lymphangioleiomyomatosis
- Venous thrombosis

Congenital

Pleural Effusions

Pleural effusions are due to a transudation or exudation of interstitial fluid from the pleural surface. Symptoms include pleuritic chest pain and dyspnea. Pleuritic pain is sharp and stabbing in nature and intensifies during deep inspiration when the patient perceives a 'catch.' Excessive pleural fluid can alter pulmonary function by impairing lung expansion and causing shortness of breath. This can lead to atelectasis, recurrent infections, and lung trapping.

Pleural effusions are classified as either transudates or exudates. A transudate occurs when systemic factors that influence the formation or absorption of pleural fluid are altered. Changes in plasma colloid osmotic pressure and hydrostatic pressure in the systemic or pulmonary circulation can alter fluid movement. The pleural surface is not involved with the primary pathological process. In an exudate, the disease starts from the pleural surface. Pleural disease causes pleural fluid accumulation by an increase in the permeability of the capillaries for protein similar to that which occurs for pulmonary embolus, bacterial pneumonia, tuberculosis, or tumor implantation. Once a pleural effusion is discovered, its nature must be determined. If it is a transudate, the underling systemic disease must be treated. Congestive heart failure is responsible for the vast majority. Other causes in the differential should include cirrhosis, nephritic syndrome, myxedema, peritoneal dialysis, hypoproteinemia, Meigs syndrome, and sarcoidosis (Box 15–6).

The vast majority of exudative effusions are due to neoplasia, infection, and trauma (Box 15–7). The malignancies that cause pleural effusion most frequently are carcinoma of the lung in men and carcinoma of the breast in women. Less common causes are lymphomas, ovarian carcinoma, and colon tumors. The effusion is usually caused by scattered metastatic tumor implants on the parietal and visceral pleura. Effusion is seen in 10% of patients with viral or mycoplasmal pneumonia and 50% of patients with bacterial pneumonia. A pleural effusion develops in 50% of patients with a pulmonary embolism with or without a pulmonary infarction.

Pleural fluid can be analyzed for composition. If the pleural fluid protein divided by the serum protein is greater than 0.5, the pleural fluid lactate dehydrogenase (LDH) divided by the serum LDH is greater than 0.6, or the pleural fluid LDH is more than two thirds of

BOX 15–6 COMMON ETIOLOGIES OF A TRANSUDATIVE PLEURAL EFFUSION

- Congestive heart failure
- Fluid overload
- Cirrhosis
- Nephrotic syndrome
- Pulmonary embolism
- Hypoalbuminemia
- Lobar collapse

BOX 15–7 ETIOLOGY OF EXUDATIVE PLEURAL EFFUSIONS

Malignant
- Bronchogenic carcinoma
- Metastatic carcinoma
- Lymphoma
- Mesothelioma
- Pleural adenocarcinoma

Infectious
- Bacterial/parapneumonic
- Empyema
- Tuberculosis
- Fungal
- Viral
- Parasitic

Collagen–Vascular-Disease-Related
- Rheumatoid arthritis
- Wegener's granulomatosis
- Systemic lupus erythematosus
- Churg–Strauss syndrome

Abdominal/Gastrointestinal-Disease-Related
- Esophageal perforation
- Subphrenic abscess
- Pancreatitis/pancreatic pseudocyst
- Meigs syndrome

Others
- Chylothorax
- Uremia
- Sarcoidosis
- Post coronary artery bypass grafting
- Post radiation therapy
- Trauma
- Dressler syndrome
- Pulmonary embolism with infarction
- Asbestosis-related

From Lukanich. In: Townsend CM Jr. *Sabiston Textbook of surgery: The biological basis of modern surgical practice*, 16th ed. Philadelphia: WB Saunders, 2001.

the upper limit of normal for serum LDH, the fluid can be assumed to be an exudate. There are many clues to the nature of an effusion. Massive pleural effusions that involve a single pleural space tend to be exudates of malignant origin. Fluid from most transudates is strawcolored, clear, and odorless. Exudates are typically turbid because they contain white blood cells. Neutrophils predominate in effu-

sions associated with pneumonia, pulmonary infarction, and pancreatitis. Lymphocytes are more common in tuberculosis, lymphoma, and malignancy. Eosinophilia is usually noted with parasitic disease and asbestos effusions. All pleural fluid specimens should be sent for Gram stain and culture. Amylase, glucose, and lipid levels can give insight into other disease processes. Elevated amylase can suggest acute pancreatitis or rupture of a pancreatic pseudocyst. Low glucose levels are observed in tuberculosis, rheumatoid arthritis, empyema, and malignant tumor. A low pH (7.2) suggests that an effusion is contaminated with bacteria. Cytopathology should be requested on every specimen.

The presence of fluid in the pleural space is detected on plain chest films. The effusion is noted as a loss of the costophrenic sulcus. At least 250 mL of fluid must be present to obliterate the sulcus. A film taken in the lateral decubitus position allows differentiation between pleural fluid and pleural thickening because fluid gravitates to the dependent part of the pleural space (Figure 15–10). Free pleural fluid may have an atypical distribution. Accumulation of an effusion between the lung and the diaphragm, i.e. a subpulmonic effusion, is suggested by an apparent elevation of one hemidiaphragm, a shallow costophrenic sulcus, or a large distance between the stomach air shadow and the top of the diaphragm on the lateral view (Figure 15–11). Large pleural effusions can be confused with atelectasis of an entire lung (Figure 15–12). Pleural effusion alone seldom fills the entire hemithorax, but leaves some visible lung superiorly. Loculated fluid collections have tapered edges and are best identified in a profile view (Figure 15–13).

Management of pleural effusion depends on the size of the effusion and the symptoms present. Small, asymptomatic effusions do not need to be drained unless diagnostic data is required. Treatment of causative neoplasms with multidrug chemotherapy or radiation therapy may result in resolution of the pleural effusion and improvement of respiratory symptoms. Thoracentesis is useful in evaluating the initial effusion and to relieve acute life-threatening respiratory problems. In 95% of the patients, the effusion recurs within 1 month. Repeated thoracentesis can lead to hypoproteinemia and rapid re-accumulation.

When a malignant pleural effusion is recurrent and systemic therapy is ineffective or not indicated, the most effective treatment is

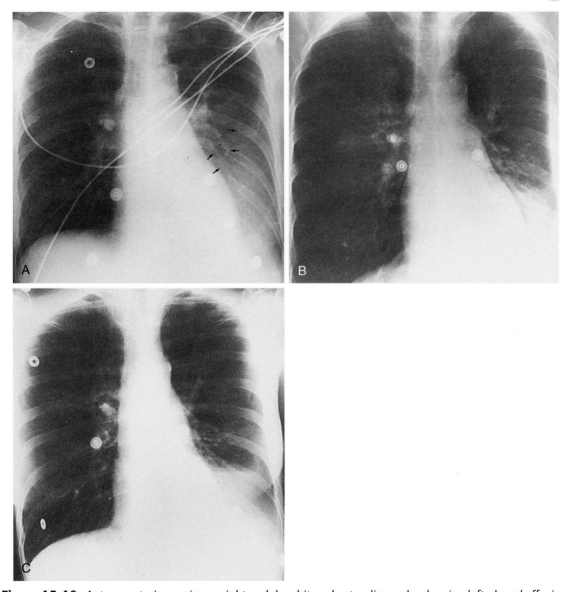

Figure 15–10. Anteroposterior supine upright and decubitus chest radiographs showing left pleural effusion. **A**, Supine chest view demonstrates partial opacification of the left hemithorax inferiorly. Pulmonary vessels are seen throughout this area (arrows), suggesting that the opacity is not due to consolidation. A decubitus study is helpful to detect concomitant air space disease or mass lesions that might otherwise be obscured. **B**, Left lateral decubitus chest radiograph shows the movement of the free-flowing effusion laterally along the left chest wall. **C**, Upright radiograph shows effusion layering in the left base. A meniscus is visible laterally that is not present on the other radiographs. (From Meholic A, Ketai L, Lofgren R. *Fundamentals of chest radiology*. Philadelphia: WB Saunders, 1996:154.)

production of a sterile adhesive pleuritis and obliteration of the potential pleural space. In order to achieve successful pleurodesis, complete evacuation of the fluid must occur so that there is apposition between visceral and parietal pleura. When other methods fail, surgical options include pleurectomy and insertion of a pleuroperitoneal shunt.

Empyema

Pleural empyemas occur chiefly in two settings: infected parapneumonic effusions and postsurgical infections (Box 15–8). A parapneumonic empyema is defined as the presence of a grossly purulent effusion with a positive Gram stain. The white blood cell

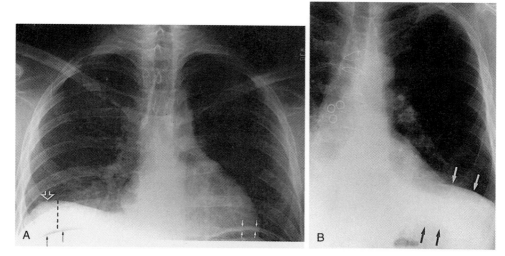

Figure 15–11. Posteroanterior upright chest radiograph demonstrating subpulmonic effusion. **A,** Upright frontal chest radiograph shows a small pneumoperitoneum (black arrows) in a patient with recent abdominal surgery that outlines a large right subpulmonic effusion, not otherwise suspected (dotted lines). Note that the apex of the right diaphragm has shifted laterally (open arrow). Normal width of diaphragm and adjacent stomach wall is seen on the left (white arrows). **B,** Close-up of a left subpulmonic effusion (upright radiograph in a different patient) demonstrates the increased width between the top of the left hemidiaphragm (white arrows) and the top of the stomach bubble (black arrows). Normally this width is less than 2 cm. (From Meholic A, Ketai L, Lofgren R. *Fundamentals of chest radiology.* Philadelphia: WB Saunders, 1996:151.)

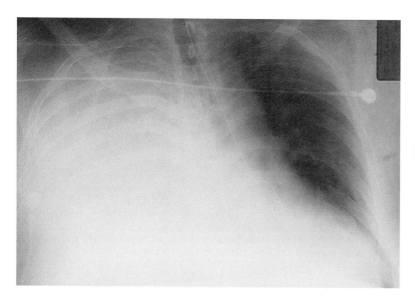

Figure 15–12. Posteroanterior upright chest radiograph demonstrating massive pleural effusion. This examination shows complete opacification of the right hemithorax, which could be caused by a massive effusion or parenchymal disease with an obstructed bronchus. There is tracheal deviation to the left. This indicates that much of the opacity is due to a large pleural effusion (with secondary compressive atelectasis). (From Meholic A, Ketai L, Lofgren R. *Fundamentals of chest radiology.* Philadelphia: WB Saunders, 1996:160.)

count is more than 15 000 cells/mm³, the protein level is greater than 3 g/dL, the pH is less than 7.0, the pleural fluid glucose level is below 50 mg/dL, and the LDH is greater than 1000 IU/L (Box 15–9).

Contamination from any source can lead to a major infection when the host reaction is overwhelmed by the number and virulence of the inoculum. Most empyemas result from bacterial contamination from a source contiguous to the pleural space. The second most frequent cause of empyema is the postsurgical development of infection in the pleural space following surgery of the esophagus, lungs, or mediastinum.

Thoracic empyemas are typically described as developing in three stages: the exudative or acute phase, the fibrinopurulent or transitional phase, and the organizing or chronic phase. The exudative phase is represented by

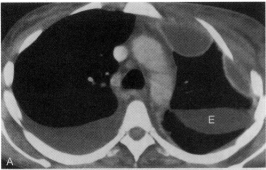

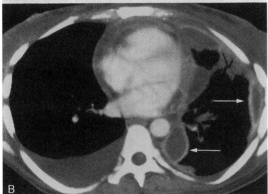

Figure 15–13. Multiple loculated pleural effusions with an empyema. **A,** Computed tomography (CT) scan at the level of the aortic arch demonstrates bilateral pleural effusions. The effusion on the right is free flowing, and the one on the left is loculated at multiple sites. **B,** CT scan at a level of the heart again shows the free-flowing right pleural effusion. On the left side, two empyema cavities (arrows) are visible laterally and paraspinously. Lung consolidation with air bronchograms is seen in the lingula. (From Moss AA, Gamsu G, Genant HK. *Computed tomography of the body*, 2nd ed. Philadelphia: WB Saunders, 1992:270.)

BOX 15–8 ETIOLOGY OF EMPYEMA

- Pneumonia (viral bacterial tuberculosis, mycotic)
- Lung abscess
- Trauma
- Postoperative
- Extension of subphrenic abscess
- Spontaneous pneumothorax
- Generalized sepsis

From Sabiston DC Jr, Spencer FC. *Surgery of the chest*, 6th ed. Philadelphia: WB Saunders, 1995:548.

accumulation of pleural fluid as a result of increased permeability of the visceral pleura contiguous to an underlying parenchymal infection. Alternatively, postsurgical empye-

BOX 15–9 CHARACTERISTICS OF AN EMPYEMA

- Positive Gram stain
- WBC >15 000 cells/mm³
- pH <7.0
- [Glucose]$_{pleural fluid}$ <50 mg/dL
- [LDH]$_{pleural fluid}$ >1000 IU/L

mas can develop from inoculation of a hemothorax, contamination through a chest tube and translocation from the chest wall incision. There is little evidence that hematogenous bacterial seeding of the pleural space occurs.

The sterile fluid can evolve into the fibropurulent stage with infection of the fluid. This collection develops an increased white blood cell count. Fibrin is deposited in layers on both pleural surfaces of the involved area, and loculations of the fluid collection may occur relatively early in the phase.

During the final phase fibroblasts and capillaries grow into the deposited fibrin layers to produce a firm, inelastic membrane termed the pleural peel. The pleural fluid is thick and viscous. The organizing phase may begin as early as 7–10 days after the onset of the parapneumonic effusion. Complications that occur during this stage include dissection of pus through the soft tissues of the chest wall and through the skin. Purulent sputum can be a harbinger of the development of a bronchopleural fistula.

Patients' symptoms may range from no clinical manifestations to severe toxemia. Patients may have chest pain, fever, cough, chest tightness, and dyspnea. Physical findings can include decreased breath sounds and restricted chest wall movements. Diagnosis can be made by chest x-ray or computed tomography (CT) scanning (Figure 15–14). Ultrasound is useful in distinguishing between pleural fluid and parenchymal consolidation or pleural thickening. The diagnosis of an empyema should be established by thoracentesis. A Gram stain should be done immediately and cultures started. The majority of empyemas are composed of multiple aerobic and anaerobic organisms.

The principle of treatment of a parapneumonic effusion include fluid evacuation, pleural space obliteration, nutrition, and antimicrobial support. Prior to loculations in early stages, aspiration and chest tube drainage will suffice. However, organized empyemas can

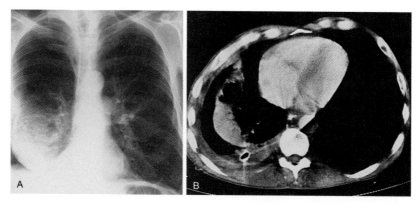

Figure 15–14. Posteroanterior chest radiograph and computed tomography showing trapped lung following empyema. Despite a chest drainage tube well positioned in the pleural space, the right lung is not fully re-expanded. Complete re-expansion is prevented by a thick visceral pleural peel. (From Meholic A, Ketai L, Lofgren R. *Fundamentals of chest radiology*. Philadelphia: WB Saunders, 1996:159.)

require thoracoscope-assisted debridement and irrigation or open thoracotomy for drainage and possible decortication (Figure 15–15).

Acute empyemas can be drained by thoracentesis. Recurrent fluid accumulation may require the placement of a chest tube. The drainage is continued until the space is obliterated or drainage falls to less than 25 mL/day. The tube can be withdrawn from the chest cavity in steady increments over several days. Some success has also been noted with instilling fibrinolytics into the empyema via the chest tube. Chronic empyemas require either rib resection and drainage or decortication depending on the nature of the residual space or presence of a pleural peel (Figure 15–16). Experience has demonstrated that anything less than complete evacuation and removal of the fibrin peel compromises pulmonary recovery.

Bronchopleural Fistula

A bronchopleural fistula is a communication that develops between the bronchus and the pleural space, usually as a result of infection or

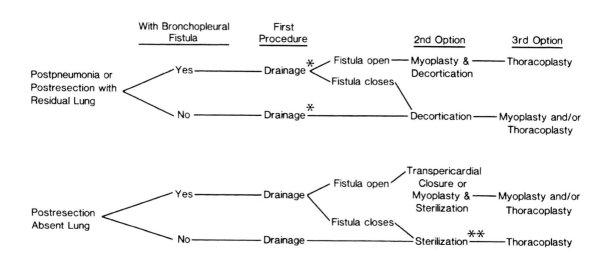

✱ Convert to open drainage if cavity fails to obliterate with tube drainage alone

✱✱ Can be attempted several times

Figure 15–15. Algorithm for the management of an empyema. (From Sabiston DC Jr, Spencer FC. *Surgery of the chest*, 6th ed. Philadelphia: WB Saunders, 1995:550.)

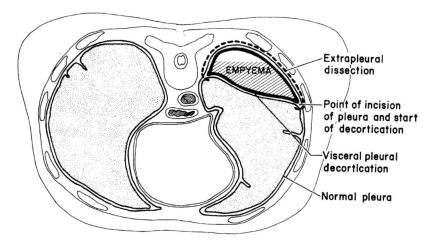

Figure 15–16. Schematic drawing of a cross-section of the thorax showing where an extrapleural dissection and decortication dissection are performed during an empyectomy. (From Sabiston DC Jr, Spencer FC. *Surgery of the chest*, 6th ed. Philadelphia: WB Saunders, 1995:554.)

trauma. Although a pneumothorax by definition implies a connection between the pleural space and the lung parenchyma, clinically this is not considered a fistula tract. A bronchopleural fistula is typically due to a complication of necrotizing pneumonia. Traumatic fistula may also occur postoperatively from the cut surface of lung parenchyma or a failed bronchial closure. Risk factors include malnutrition, diabetes, radiation therapy, inflammatory involvement of the bronchial stump, and residual tumor at the bronchial closure. The most important factor in preventing bronchial leak is meticulous apposition of cartilaginous to membranous bronchus and a good blood supply to the stump.

Typically, bronchopleural fistulas occur within 2 weeks of an operation and manifest with fevers, chills, and continuous cough with productive sputum. Severe complications can include tension pneumothorax and respiratory distress but the major problem is the infected pleural space.

Diagnosis can be made by simple radiograph (Figure 15–17). When an acute bronchopleural fistula occurs, the patient should be turned with the affected side down to prevent aspiration of pleural space contents into the contralateral field. The patient should be taken to the operating room and the bronchus resutured if the leak occurs within several days of the first operation. The bronchial stump should be shortened and reinforced with viable tissue. Additional pulmonary resection must be considered.

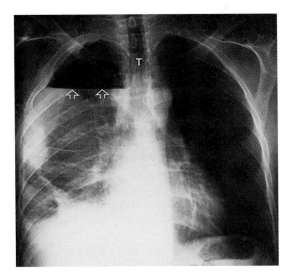

Figure 15–17. Posteroanterior radiographs showing bronchopleural fistula. The upright chest x-ray demonstrates a large air–fluid level in the apical area (arrows) compatible with hydropneumothorax. The air collection follows the contour of the chest wall. T, trachea. (From Meholic A, Ketai L, Lofgren R. *Fundamentals of chest radiology*. Philadelphia: WB Saunders, 1996:159.)

If the fistula develops weeks or months after an operation, drainage should be performed, either open or closed. The chest cavity should be cleaned out and all sources of infection drained. Chronic bronchopleural fistulas are more difficult to care for because the empyema cavity is thick-walled and has extensive fibrosis, but the space must be completely drained. Infected material should be removed and a pedicle muscle flap may be used to seal the bronchial stump and obliterate the space. Options for muscle flaps include the latissimus dorsi, pectoral, and serratus anterior muscles.

Pleural Tumors

Some 95% of all pleural tumors are metastatic in origin. The most common primary tumor of the pleural cavity is malignant mesothelioma, a rare neoplasm. Mesotheliomas are neoplasms of the serosal membranes of the body cavities. Diffuse mesotheliomas account for 90% of mesotheliomas. They are of special interest because of their increasing frequency, dismal prognosis, and medicolegal issues associated with asbestos exposure. So-called 'localized' mesotheliomas may be benign, are not of mesothelial origin, and should be referred to as solitary fibrous tumors. The malignant potential of these lesions is variable.

Asbestos inhalation has been definitely associated with malignant mesotheliomas: 80% of cases are estimated to be caused by asbestos. Hundreds of cohort studies and case reports have established the connection between asbestos and pleural malignancies. Together, these epidemiological studies have analyzed over 50 000 male and female asbestos-related workers and come to the same conclusion: asbestos unequivocally causes mesotheliomas. Some other etiologies that have been thought to cause malignant mesothelioma include zeolite and other organic fibers, Thorostat, prior iatrogenic radiation exposure, and chronic inflammation.

The molecular pathophysiology of malignant mesothelioma can be described by reviewing the chronic inflammatory response. Deposition of asbestos fibers sets off a chain of events involving inflammatory cell activation and mesothelial cell damage. Ordinarily, normal remesothelialization to acute pleural damage involves depositing collagen and serosal fibrosis, which is eventually broken up and cleared. In the case with asbestos, the prolonged presence of asbestos causes a chronic inflammatory response that culminates with malignant transformation of mesothelial cells. Malignant mesothelioma is a rapidly invasive tumor that usually involves the entire pleural space.

Grossly, early malignant mesothelioma appears as many small nodules on the parietal and/or visceral surfaces. Progression of the tumor results in coalescence of the nodules to form plaques that merge to form a sheet tumor. In later stages, malignant mesotheliomas appear with diffuse involvement of the visceral and parietal pleura, involvement of the fissures, and obliteration of the pleural cavity. This hard, white tumor spreads over the entire lung, encasing it with a thickness up to several centimeters (Figures 15–18, 15–19). Large nodular densities are common. Areas of necrosis and hemorrhage are often seen. The neoplasm may invade the chest wall and mediastinum and spread to the opposite pleural cavity or to the peritoneal cavity. Pleural effusions and ascites are common findings. Three basic histological types are described, epithelioid, sarcomatous, and mixed. Pure epithelial mesotheliomas are associated with the best prognosis.

Patients who present with malignant mesothelioma most commonly are in their 60s or 70s, and may look surprisingly good. There is an average 3-month delay before patients seek medical consultation. The most common presenting symptoms are dyspnea (60–70%) and insidious onset of chest pain (50–70%). At later stages, patient will begin experiencing weight loss (25–30%), cough (27%), fever (33%),

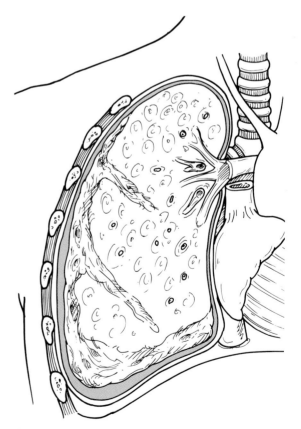

Figure 15–18. Malignant mesothelioma progresses to encase the lung surface with sheets up to several centimeters thick.

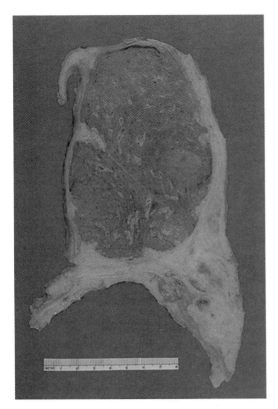

Figure 15–19. Gross picture of malignant mesothelioma encasing a lung. [See color insert, plate 2]

weakness (33%), and anorexia (10%). Other symptoms noted at presentation have included stridor, nausea, headache, and perceived tachycardia. The symptoms of malignant mesothelioma are secondary to the effects of the tumor in the pleural cavity: the enlarging mass, invasion of adjacent structures, and accumulation of fluid within the pleural space.

By the time the patient presents, the tumor often is bulky and encompasses the lung. The patient will experience dyspnea because the tumor encases the lung and restricts ventilation and normal chest wall mechanics. Pleural effusion is usually present and may lend to earlier presentation. A dry pleuritic type of cough may be elicited when the patient is asked to breathe deeply. In later stages, patients develop significant weight loss due to the extensive thoracic involvement and creation of a hypermetabolic state. Median survival from the diagnosis is 12–14 months.

Any patient with pleural thickening should be aggressively evaluated. Radiologic diagnosis of pleural mesothelioma requires a high degree of clinical suspicion. Some 95% of pleural tumors are metastatic, whereas only 5% of malignant pleural tumors are primary. The major pathological features of mesothelioma are well demonstrated by conventional chest radiography and CT (Figure 15–20). CT, however, demonstrates the findings more frequently and in greater detail. Ultrasound and magnetic resonance imaging (MRI) are additional imaging modalities with helpful but limited application in studying malignant mesotheliomas. Positron-emission tomography (PET) scan may also be helpful.

The most common radiological presentation (40–95%) is a large, unilateral pleural effusion. Only 10% of patients present with bilateral effusions. The effusion can be quite large, with near-complete opacification of the hemithorax. Fluid may be loculated, surrounded by areas of thickened or nodular pleura. Because of the loculations, there may only be a small amount of free-flowing pleural fluid. The other most common radiographic finding with

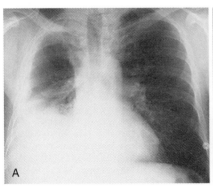
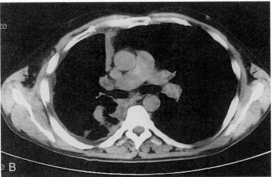

Figure 15–20. Posteroanterior chest radiograph and computed tomography (CT) scan showing malignant mesothelioma. **A,** There is volume loss in the right hemithorax, probably due to decreased chest wall compliance. **B,** CT shows involvement of the mediastinal pleura (a sign that suggests malignancy). (From Meholic A, Ketai L, Lofgren R. *Fundamentals of chest radiology*. Philadelphia: WB Saunders, 1996:162.)

malignant pleural mesothelioma is diffuse, circumferential pleural thickening (60–100%), usually associated with plaques and effusions. The prime importance of CT lies in its ability to define the extent of disease and follow response to treatment. It is also used to look for metastatic disease to the contralateral lung and peritoneal cavity. Serial CT has demonstrated increased accuracy over conventional radiography in determining the extent of pathology and response to treatment.

A CT scan is helpful in differentiating benign from malignant pleural thickening. The most common finding on CT scans with malignant mesothelioma is unilateral thickening with irregular pleuropulmonary contours. The single most important variable in favor of making a correct diagnosis is an appropriate clinical presentation, including a history of asbestos exposure, recurrent pleural effusions, chest pain, and pleural thickening. Thoracoscopic biopsy is the most reliable means of obtaining diagnostic tissue. Pleural fluid cytology often is not definitive. The distinction between adenocarcinoma and mesothelioma may present a significant challenge to the pathologist.

For patients with early disease, stage I, pleurectomy with decortication may be an option. Mesotheliomas tend to spread entirely intrapleurally in their early stages and can remain in confined to the pleural cavity for a long time, making them suitable for radical surgery. Once the tumor has penetrated the parietal pleura, radical surgery will most probably be useless and provide little relief. Chemotherapy or radiotherapy should be considered at this point. For stages III and IV, only palliative treatment is recommended.

Two surgical techniques exist for the management of malignant mesothelioma: pleurectomy with or without decortication, and radical extrapleural pneumonectomy (pleuropneumonectomy). Only 20% of all patients with malignant mesothelioma are candidates for surgery. The indications for surgical management are threefold. First, thoracoscopy for biopsy is necessary if other invasive diagnostic techniques have failed. Second, attempts at cure should be attempted with early, potentially resectable disease if the histology is epithelioid. Third, surgical palliative measures should be considered. Palliation entails controlling effusions and effecting pleurodesis.

Single-modality treatment, whether chemotherapy, radiation, surgery, immunotherapy, or gene therapy, cannot cure or prolong median life more than several months at best. Surgery is rarely used as the exclusive mode of therapy. A small subset of patients with epithelioid histology who cannot undergo complete resection may be long-term survivors when operation is combined with postoperative chemotherapy and radiation therapy.

Key Readings

Lee-Chiong TL Jr, Matthay RA. Current diagnostic methods and medical management of thoracic empyemas. *Chest Surg Clin North Am* 1996;6:419–438. *A look at state-of-the-art care for thoracic empyema.*

Sahn SA, Heffner JE. Spontaneous pneumothorax. *New Engl J Med* 2000;342:868–874. *An excellent review of this disease for surgeons and nonsurgeons.*

Yeam I, Sassoon C. Hemothorax and chylothorax. *Curr Opin Pulm Med* 1997;3:310–314. *A good review of the basis of care for patients with these two diseases.*

Selected Readings

Antony VB, Loddenkemper R, Astoul P, *et al.*, Management of malignant pleural effusions. *Eur Respir J* 2001;18:402–419.

Baumann MH. Treatment of spontaneous pneumothorax. *Curr Opin Pulm Med* 2000;6:275–280.

Baumann MH, Strange C, Heffner JE, *et al.*, Management of spontaneous pneumothorax: an American College of Chest Physicians Delphi consensus statement. *Chest* 2001;119:590–602.

Bryant RE, Salmon CJ. Pleural empyema. *Clin Infect Dis* 1996;22:747–762; quiz 763–744.

Carrillo EH, Richardson JD. Thoracoscopy in the management of hemothorax and retained blood after trauma. *Curr Opin Pulm Med* 1998;4:243–246.

Deschamps C, Pairolero PC, Allen MS, Trastek VF. Management of postpneumonectomy empyema and bronchopleural fistula. *Chest Surg Clin North Am* 1996;6:519–527.

Feliciano DV, Rozycki GS. Advances in the diagnosis and treatment of thoracic trauma. *Surg Clin North Am* 1999;79:1417–1429.

Gallardo X, Castaner E, Mata JM. Benign pleural diseases. *Eur J Radiol* 2000;34:87–97.

Light RW. The management of parapneumonic effusions and empyema. *Curr Opin Pulm Med* 1998;4:227–229.

Lowdermilk GA, Naunheim KS. Thoracoscopic evaluation and treatment of thoracic trauma. *Surg Clin North Am* 2000;80:1535–1542.

Singh M, Singh SK, Chowdhary SK. Management of empyema thoracic in children. *Indian Pediatr* 2002;39:145–157.

Srinivas S, Varadhachary G. Spontaneous pneumothorax in malignancy: a case report and review of the literature. *Ann Oncol* 2000;11:887–889.

Wain JC. Management of late postpneumonectomy empyema and bronchopleural fistula. *Chest Surg Clin North Am* 1996;6:529–541.

Yim AP, Ng CS. Thoracoscopy in the management of pneumothorax. *Curr Opin Pulm Med* 2001;7:210–214.

Zellos LS, Sugarbaker DJ. Multimodality treatment of diffuse malignant pleural mesothelioma. *Semin Oncol* 2002;29:41–50.

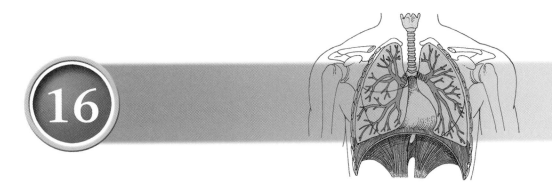

Mediastinal Masses

Mediastinal Masses: Key Points

- Describe the key organs in each mediastinal compartment and the potential pathology that can arise
- Know the general incidence of the most common mediastinal masses
- Develop an understanding of the options to evaluate mediastinal masses and the advantages and disadvantages of both
- Know the differential for lesions that can be confused for primary mediastinal masses
- Name the three most common tumors in each compartment
- Know the differential diagnosis for a germ-cell tumor
- Know the potential diagnostic markers for paraneoplastic, endocrine, and germ-cell tumors

Lesions that originate in the mediastinum are rare compared to the diverse lesions that can involve the mediastinum secondarily (Box 16–1). Although neoplasms of the mediastinum are diverse, they have in common a single clinical manifestation: widening of the mediastinum on the chest radiograph taken in the upright position. This shared feature has not lent itself readily to differential diagnosis. In recent years, however, the advent of computed tomography (CT) and magnetic resonance imaging (MRI) has greatly enhanced the evaluation and subsequent treatment of these lesions.

The mediastinum extends from the thoracic inlet to the diaphragm superoinferiorly and from pleural space to pleural space. Contained within it are heart, aorta, brachiocephalic vein, esophagus, tracheobronchial tree, and elements of the autonomic nervous system and the lymphatic system. Further, various endocrine organs may project into it, distant malignancies may metastasize to it, and infectious processes can manifest themselves within it (Figure 16–1).

BOX 16–1 CLASSIFICATION OF PRIMARY MEDIASTINAL TUMORS AND CYSTS

Neurogenic Tumors
- Neurofibroma
- Neurilemoma
- Neurosarcoma
- Ganglioneuroma
- Neuroblastoma
- Chemodectoma
- Paraganglioma

Thymoma
- Benign
- Malignant

Lymphoma
- Hodgkin's disease
- Lymphoblastic
- Large-cell diffuse growth pattern
  - T-immunoblastic sarcoma
  - B-immunoblastic sarcoma
  - Sclerosing follicular cell

Germ-Cell Tumors
- Teratodermoid
  - Benign
  - Malignant
- Seminoma
- Nonseminomas
  - Embryonal
  - Choriocarcinoma
  - Endodermal

Primary Carcinomas

Mesenchymal Tumors
- Fibroma/fibrosarcoma
- Lipoma/liposarcoma

BOX 16–1 (CONT'D)

- Leiomyoma/leiomyosarcoma
- Rhabdosarcoma
- Xanthogranuloma
- Myxoma
- Mesothelioma
- Hemangioma
- Hemangiopericytoma
- Lymphangioma
- Lymphangiomyoma
- Lymphangiopericytoma

Endocrine Tumors
- Intrathoracic thyroid
- Parathyroid adenoma/carcinoma
- Carcinoid
- Cysts
- Bronchogenic
- Pericardial
- Enteric
- Thymic
- Thoracic duct
- Nonspecific

Giant Lymph Node Hyperplasia
- Castleman's disease

Chondroma

Extramedullary Hematopoiesis

Mediastinal Compartments

The mediastinum has been variably described by different authors. The simplest system divides the mediastinum into three compartments: anterosuperior, visceral (or middle), and paravertebral (or posterior).

Anterosuperior Compartment

This compartment extends from the manubrium and the first ribs to the diaphragm. Its posterior border is defined by the anterior aspect of the pericardium inferiorly and curves posteriorly to include the arch of the aorta and great vessels. Structures contained within it include the ascending aorta, the superior vena cava, the azygous vein, the thymus gland, lymph nodes, fat, connective tissue, transverse aorta, and great vessels. Common major lesions contained within the anterosuperior mediastinal compartment are thymomas, lymphomas, and germ-cell tumors. Less common lesions are tumors of

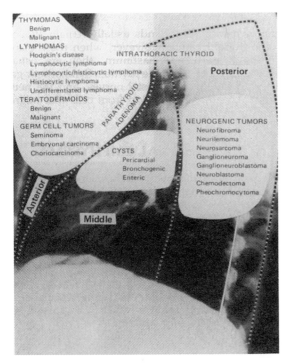

Figure 16–1. Lateral chest film divided into three anatomic subdivisions with the most common location of the tumors and cysts. (From Davis RD Jr, Sabiston DC Jr. Primary mediastinal cysts and neoplasms. In: Sabiston DC Jr, ed. *Essentials of surgery.* Philadelphia: WB Saunders, 1987.)

mesenchymal origin, vascular lesions, and displaced thyroid or parathyroid glands.

Middle Compartment

The middle compartment is also called the visceral compartment. The superior pericardial reflection defines the superior border, while the diaphragm defines the inferior border. The posterior border extends to the spine. Contained within this compartment are the heart and pericardium, trachea and major bronchi, pulmonary vessels, lymph nodes, fat, and connective tissue. Lesions contained within the visceral compartment include cysts of the foregut, primary and secondary tumors of the lymph nodes, and, less commonly, pleural, pericardial, neuroenteric, and gastroenteric cysts.

Posterior Compartment

The posterior compartment is also called the paravertebral compartment. It extends from the superior aspect of the first thoracic vertebral body to the diaphragm anteriorly and then posteriorly to the posterior-most curvature of the ribs. Contained within it are the sympathetic chain, vagus nerves, esophagus, thoracic duct, various lymph nodes, and the descending aorta. Lesions contained within it are primarily tumors of neurogenic origin. Less common is a potpourri of lesions including vascular tumors, mesenchymal tumors, and lymphatic lesions.

Epidemiology and Incidence

Great differences exist between children and adults with respect to the location of mediastinal lesions. In adults, 65% of the lesions arise in the anterosuperior, 10% in the middle, and 25% in the posterior compartments; this distribution is reversed in children, in whom 25% of lesions arise in the anterosuperior, 10% in the middle, and 65% in the posterior compartments. In general, the incidence of posterior lesions is higher in children, whereas anterior lesions predominate in adults.

Signs and Symptoms

Approximately half of mediastinal lesions are asymptomatic and are detected on chest radiographs taken for unrelated reasons. As a rough guideline, the absence of symptoms suggests that a lesion is benign, whereas the presence of symptoms suggests malignancy. The percentage of patients with symptoms from mediastinal masses precisely parallels, or equals, the percentage of malignant lesions. In adults, 50–60% of lesions are symptomatic, whereas the percentage of symptomatic lesions is higher in children – 60–80%. Since the incidence of symptoms parallels the incidence of malignancy, a child with a mediastinal mass is considerably more likely to have a malignancy than is an adult with a mediastinal mass.

The most common symptoms are cardiorespiratory, specifically chest pain and cough. Other manifestations are heaviness in the chest, dysphagia, dyspnea, hemoptysis, signs of superior vena caval obstruction with facial swelling, and cyanosis (Box 16–2). Recurrent respiratory infections are a common complaint. As discussed below, several mediastinal lesions are associated with other clinical syndromes: thymoma with myasthenia gravis, red-cell aplasia, hypogammaglobulinemia, and nonthymic cancers; Hodgkin's disease with recurrent fevers; and von Recklinghausen's disease with neurofibromas.

BOX 16–2 CLINICAL MANIFESTATIONS OF ANATOMIC COMPRESSION OR INVASION BY NEOPLASMS OF THE MEDIASTINUM

- Vena caval obstruction
- Pericardial tamponade
- Congestive heart failure
- Dysrhythmias
- Pulmonary artery stenosis
- Pulmonary vein obstruction
- Tracheal/bronchial compression
- Esophageal compression
- Vocal cord paralysis
- Horner syndrome
- Phrenic nerve paralysis
- Chylothorax
- Chylopericardium
- Spinal cord compressive syndrome
- Pancoast syndrome
- Postobstructive pneumonitis

From Sabiston DC Jr, Spencer FC. *Surgery of the chest*, 6th ed. Philadelphia: WB Saunders, 1995:584.

Diagnosis

Mediastinal masses commonly present on routine chest radiographs obtained for other purposes. History and physical examination are occasionally useful in diagnosis, especially in patients with one of the rarer symptoms (e.g. hoarseness and Horner syndrome). The age of the patient can also narrow diagnostic possibilities. However, the chest radiograph remains the most important lead to diagnosis, followed by CT of the chest; the latter has revolutionized the diagnosis and evaluation of mediastinal masses and should be part of the routine workup of a mediastinal mass.

Noninvasive Diagnostic Procedures

Computed Tomography

As noted above, chest CT should be routine for all suspected or confirmed mediastinal masses (Figures 16–2–16–4). Although CT is poor with respect to distinguishing between cystic and solid structures, it provides excellent imaging of the mediastinum. Indeed, the diagnosis of certain lesions – such as aortic aneurysms, mediastinal lipomatosis, and pericardial fat

pads – is so straightforward with CT that further search or biopsy is not necessary. CT scanning is the most common technique used to obtain fine-needle aspiration (FNA) biopsies and to provide information about invasion. Additionally, if biopsy or resection is indicated, CT can assist in the selection of the surgical approach (left chest, right chest, mediastinoscopy, or median sternotomy).

Magnetic Resonance Imaging

Magnetic resonance imaging is superior to CT imaging in three specific circumstances: when preoperative determination of a tumor's invasion of vascular or neural structures is crucial, when coronal or radial body sections are necessary, and when contrast material cannot be given intravenously because of renal disease or known allergy to contrast (Table 16–1). Gadolinium can be used to provide additional vascular contrast with MRI but is generally unnecessary because the high inherent contrast between mediastinal masses and cardiovascular structures generally suffices to define those masses. For lesions below the aortic arch, electrocardiographic gating can improve image quality. The ability to perform T1- and T2-weighted images allows discrimination of mediastinal masses from mediastinal fat on T1-weighted images and from the heart and chest wall on T2-weighted images. The use of the combination of these sequences can usually clearly delineate mediastinal masses from surrounding soft tissues. Finally, all neoplasms have higher T1 and T2 values than inflammatory lesions, with bronchogenic carcinoma generating the greatest T1 and T2 values. The difference between T1 and T2 values for bronchogenic carcinoma and chronic inflammatory processes has been shown to be significant.

For lesions close to the thoracic inlet, MRI is probably better than CT at identifying invasion of the brachial plexus and vertebral foramina. Similarly, MRI can clarify lesions at the inferior aspect of the mediastinum that invade the diaphragm. It is the method of choice for evaluation of neurogenic lesions, vascular anomalies, and anomalies of the aortic arch. However, MRI also has some disadvantages: longer times for acquisition of data, greater expense, and unavailability at some institutions. Also, patients are less likely to tolerate MRI because of claustrophobia and difficulties inherent in lying still for longer periods.

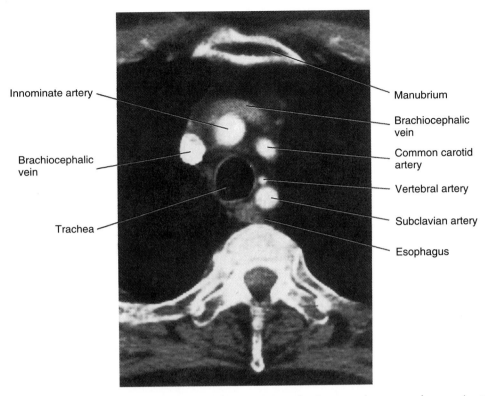

Figure 16-2. Normal upper mediastinal anatomy in an adult male. Computed tomography scan is at the level of the manubrium. Contrast medium has been injected. (From Moss AA, Gamsu G, Genant HK. *Computed tomography of the body*, 2nd ed. Philadelphia: WB Saunders, 1992:44.)

Ultrasonography

Ultrasonography is used in some situations to determine the nature of the mediastinal mass, particularly whether cystic or solid; it may also be used to direct FNA biopsies (Table 16–2). Although the value of ultrasound in differentiating cystic and solid masses is recognized, the use of ultrasound has probably been supplanted in most institutions by CT, MRI, and radionuclide scintigraphy. It is particularly useful in evaluating masses in children because lying still is not as critical. Additionally, endoscopic ultrasound is increasingly useful in evaluating lesions of the esophagus and various periesophageal structures.

Radionuclides

Several radionuclide agents are useful in evaluating mediastinal masses. Thyroid scintigraphy with iodine-131 or iodine-123 may be helpful in patients with obscure substernal anterosuperior compartment lesions. Technetium use in the mediastinum is complicated because the salivary glands secrete technetium, which is swallowed, so the entire esophagus is invariably positive. However, technetium can help to identify areas of gastric mucosa in the esophagus if scanning is performed immediately after several glasses of liquid are swallowed to clear the esophagus.

^{131}I-metaiodobenzylguanine can help to identify pheochromocytomas or functioning paragangliomas anywhere in the body, including the mediastinum. Subsequent CT or MRI scanning is necessary to delineate the anatomy of 'hot spots' identified in this way. Selenomethionine scans often can localize parathyroid adenomas and thymic cysts. Finally, gallium scanning has been used to distinguish benign from malignant anterior mediastinal masses, especially to differentiate lymphomas from benign lesions. Institutional expertise in these techniques is at least as important as the choice of diagnostic technique.

Biochemical Markers

All patients with anterior mediastinal masses, particularly young men, should have determinations of levels of alpha-fetoprotein, beta-human chronic gonadotropin (β-hCG),

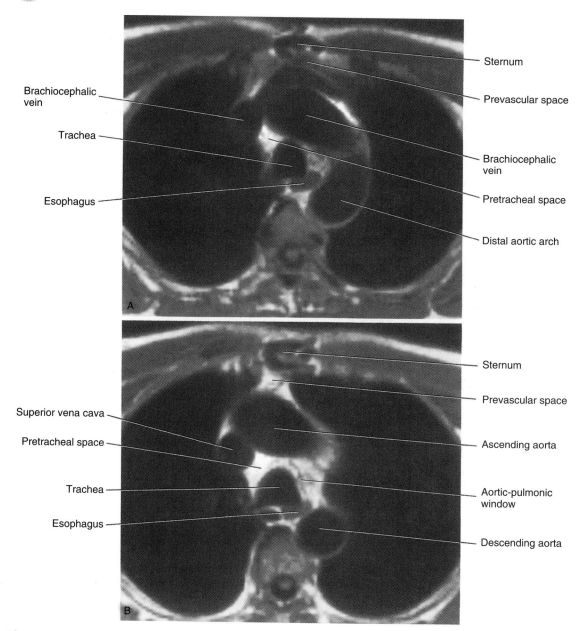

Figure 16–3. Normal mediastinal anatomy in an adult male demonstrated on a spin-echo cardiac-gated image. **A** is at the level of the lower aortic arch; **B** is at the level of the aortic-pulmonic window. (From Moss AA, Gamsu G, Genant HK. *Computed tomography of the body*, 2nd ed. Philadelphia: WB Saunders, 1992:47.)

and carcinoembryonic antigen. Serum levels of alpha-fetoprotein, β-hCG, or both increase in the presence of nonseminomatous malignant germ-cell tumors or some teratomas and carcinomas.

Pheochromocytomas are accompanied by increases in serum catecholamines and in several urinary metabolites – e.g. catecholamines, vanillylmandelic acid, and homovanillic acid. These markers are more valuable in following patients after treatment – i.e. to detect recurrence – than in screening. The levels of these

substances should be determined in patients who present with flushing, tachycardia, or headache for which there is no other explanation. Some paravertebral masses – such as paragangliomas, ganglioneuromas, and some neuroblastomas – can also elaborate norepinephrine and epinephrine.

Invasive Biopsy Procedures

The decision to biopsy mediastinal masses is not straightforward. Biopsy before resection is

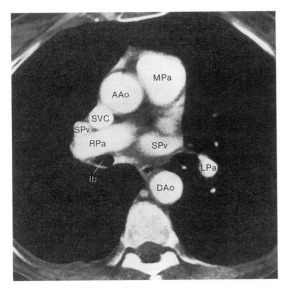

Figure 16–4. Normal mid-mediastinal anatomy. The descending left pulmonary artery (LPa) is posterolateral to the basal bronchus, and the right pulmonary artery (RPa) is in front of the intermediate bronchus (Ib). The superior vena cava (SVC) and right superior pulmonary vein (SPv) are in front of the right pulmonary artery. The main pulmonary artery (MPa) is to the left of the ascending aorta (AAo). (From Moss AA, Gamsu G, Genant HK. *Computed tomography of the body*, 2nd ed. Philadelphia: WB Saunders, 1992:48.)

not necessary in some cases and potentially harmful in others. The likelihood of a positive biopsy depends on several factors: (1) local symptoms; (2) the location and extent of the lesion; (3) tumor markers; and (4) gallium uptake by the lesion.

Locally asymptomatic lesions should not undergo biopsy before removal if they do not extend beyond the anterior compartment, show no increase in levels of tumor markers, and do not take up gallium. In particular, biopsy of a clinically suspected well encapsulated thymoma usually is not necessary and may be associated with spread of tumor cells within the pleural space. For patients with invasive thymoma and symptoms such as severe chest pain, dyspnea, cough, dysphagia, pleural effusion, and superior vena caval obstruction, incisional or FNA biopsy should be performed. The important point here is to distinguish epithelial neoplasms from lymphoma, where resection would not be carried out.

Bulky adenopathy should always undergo biopsy, since surgical intervention is seldom the primary means for treating these lesions. Lesions in the superior mediastinum can be easily accessed by mediastinoscopy while anterior mediastinal lesions usually require a parasternal mediastinotomy. Lesions in the middle mediastinum (visceral), just deep to the sternum, can be sampled by way of subxyphoid mediastinoscopy, whereas other middle-mediastinal lesions require FNA or thoracoscopic techniques. Lesions in the posterior mediastinum require either FNA or a thoracoscopic approach.

Tissue usually should be obtained in patients with mediastinal masses in whom levels of alpha-fetoprotein or β-hCG are increased though the presence of these markers make the diagnosis of germ-cell tumor. These neoplasms are treated primarily with systemic chemotherapy with resection reserved for residual disease. Occasionally, chemotherapeutic treatment for oncologic emergencies may be initiated on the basis of increased levels, *per se*, of tumor

TABLE 16–1 • *Computed Tomography (CT) and Magnetic Resonance Imaging (MRI) in the Evaluation of Mediastinal Masses*		
CT Superior	**MRI Superior**	**CT and MRI Equal**
Spatial resolution	Multiplanar imaging capability and no contrast needed	Detection of pure fluid collections
Detection of bony destruction	Identification of complex fluid collection	Detection of chest wall invasion
Detection of calcification	Soft tissue differentiation	Evaluation of vascular obstruction (contrast CT)
Detection of lung nodules	Tumor vs fibrosis	
Evaluation of lung parenchyma	Tumor vs obstructive pneumonitis	
Single study of screening for lung, liver, adrenals	Evaluation of: Brachial plexus Neural foramina Diaphragm Bone marrow	
	Mediastinal tissue invasion	

From Moore EH. Radiologic evaluation of mediastinal masses. *Chest Surg Clin North Am* 1992;2:1.

Tumors	Ultrastructure
Carcinoid	Dense core granules, fewer tonofilaments and desmosomes
Lymphoma	Absence of junctional attachments and epithelial features
Thymoma	Well-formed desmosomes, bundles of tonofilaments
Germ-cell	Prominent nucleoli, even chromatin, scant desmosomes, rare tonofilaments
Neuroblastoma	Neurosecretory granules, synaptic endings

TABLE 16–2 • *Ultrastructural Characteristics of Mediastinal Tumors*

From Sabiston DC Jr, Spencer FC. *Surgery of the chest*, 6th ed. Philadelphia: WB Saunders, 1995:588.

markers. In contrast, increased concentrations of catecholamines in serum or urine contraindicate biopsy, since disturbance of a pheochromocytoma or pharmacologically active paraganglioma before preparation with alpha- and beta-blockade is dangerous.

Gallium uptake is useful in differentiating lymphomas from thymoma but is rarely used for diagnostic purposes. Gallium is avidly taken up by lymphomas and other inflammatory processes, whereas it is usually taken up by bronchogenic carcinomas, rarely taken up by thymomas, and unpredictably taken up by carcinoids and germ-cell tumors.

Method of Biopsy

Fine-needle aspiration is diagnostic in approximately 75% of mediastinal masses, although it lacks the precision to stage mediastinal and pulmonary malignancies. It is important to emphasize that the primary benefit of FNA of patients is to prevent needless surgical intervention. Accordingly, in a candidate for surgery, a diagnosis other than lymphoma, small-cell carcinoma, or stage IIIB non-small-cell bronchogenic carcinoma will not obviate surgery, since all other diagnoses of solid tumor require surgical staging or resection. FNA usually is adequate for diagnosis of lymphoma since material must be obtained for phenotypic markers and flow cytometry to adequately characterize these malignancies. In cases where lymphoma is suspected, FNA should be avoided.

Although a core biopsy may suffice for the diagnosis of a specific lymphoma, most often more invasive and definitive approaches such as cervical mediastinoscopy, anterior or parasternal mediastinoscopy, and videothoracoscopy are necessary. Needle biopsy of a well encapsulated mass is superfluous. In summary, FNA is inconsistently useful for diagnosis of diseases of the mediastinum, and its use must be carefully assessed. However, complications of FNA are rare.

Surgical approaches to obtain tissue from mediastinal lesions include cervical mediastinoscopy, extended cervical mediastinoscopy, anterior mediastinotomy (Chamberlain procedure), subxyphoid mediastinoscopy, and videothoracoscopy. The diagnosis of lymphoma usually requires a large tissue sample to identify the subtype, especially for non-Hodgkin's lymphomas. Also, lesions at different sites vary with respect to accessibility. Thus, cervical mediastinoscopy, performed through a small incision in the suprasternal notch, can sample masses in the superior mediastinum, i.e. lymph nodes in the subcarinal and paratracheal location (levels 1, 2, 3, 4, 7, and 10 in the American Thoracic Society staging system). Anterior mediastinotomy (parasternal) performed through a small incision usually in the second intercostals space on either side can sample lymph nodes in the para-aortic position (levels 5 and 6 on the left) or anterior mediastinal masses. These procedures can be performed in the outpatient setting, have a very low complication rate, and do not delay chemotherapy or radiotherapy. A portion of the specimen should be sent fresh for formal evaluation of T- and B-cell subpopulations and a sample should be sent for bacterial and fungal culture.

The use of mediastinoscopy to sample large masses that compromise the airway or elicit clinical signs of superior vena caval obstruction is not contraindicated. Anesthetic management and control of the airway is critically important (Figure 16–5). Mediastinoscopy poses no greater risk of bleeding for patients with superior vena caval syndrome than for others undergoing mediastinoscopy.

Subxyphoid mediastinoscopy, performed through an incision below the xiphoid process, is an unusual procedure. It is used to obtain biopsies of tissues located inferiorly in the mediastinum. Videothoracoscopic approaches to either the left or right side of the mediastinum are straightforward and obtain adequate tissue samples with minimal morbidity.

However, thoracoscopic biopsies are not currently being done routinely as outpatient procedures, although the potential for this exists.

Lesions Masquerading as Mediastinal Tumors

A variety of lesions may mimic mediastinal masses radiographically or clinically (Table 16–3).

Substernal Goiter

Substernal goiters usually present as anterosuperior mediastinal masses, even though ectopic thyroid tissue can also be found in retrotracheal and retroesophageal locations. Essentially, all substernal thyroids descend into the mediastinum from the neck; primary mediastinal thyroids are vanishingly rare. Two thirds of patients with a substernal goiter complain of a neck mass. Most are otherwise asymptomatic. Some 25% complain of dyspnea or dysphagia. The occurrence of symptoms does not herald malignancy. CT and MRI scans are the most useful studies in the diagnosis and evaluation of these lesions (Figure 16–6). Modern radioactive iodine-131 scans can delineate the substernal goiter, although there is some debate about the incidence of false negative scans.

Most substernal goiters can be resected through cervical incisions. The lesion usually

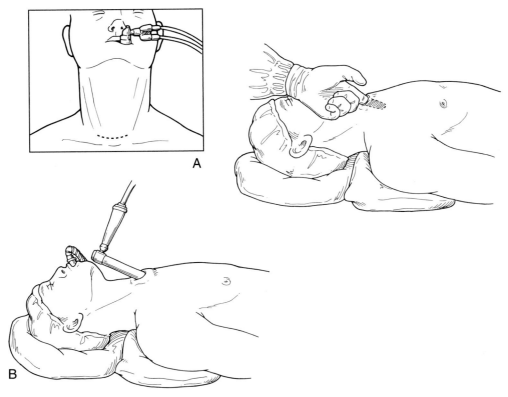

Figure 16–5. Cervical mediastinoscopy. **A**, The endotracheal tube is positioned at the left corner of the mouth, with the anesthesia equipment to the patient's left side. The shoulders are elevated on an inflatable pillow, the top of the head is aligned with the top of the operating table, and the occiput rests on a ring cushion. The incision is positioned one fingerbreadth superior to the clavicular heads. Following transverse division of the subcutaneous fat and platysma, the balance of the dissection is carried out vertically in the midline plane. The strap muscles are separated. The thyroid isthmus is retracted superiorly and the dissection is carried down to the anterior surface of the trachea at the level of the second or third tracheal ring. Once the pretracheal plane is reached, and the last areolar tissue has been dissected from the anterior surface of the trachea, the index finger is inserted into the mediastinum, staying on the anterior surface of the trachea. **B**, The mediastinoscope is inserted and advanced along the pretracheal plane. Dissection of the pretracheal and paratracheal spaces is facilitated with the use of an insulated sucker, which can also be used to cauterize bleeding points following nodal biopsy. A long length of gauze packing should always be available as should a sternal saw or Lubschke knife for the rare occasion when emergency sternotomy might be necessary for control of bleeding.

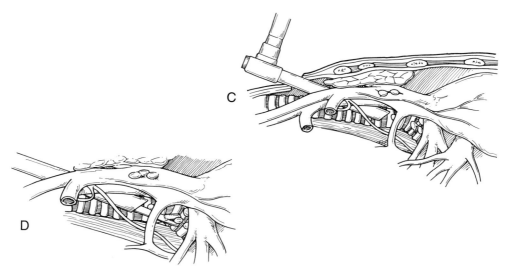

Figure 16–5. Continued. **C,** The lateral 'cut out' view shows the mediastinoscope passing down the right side of the trachea. Dissection with a sucker tip aids in unroofing the nodes. **D,** Each time the mediastinoscope is inserted, care must be taken to ensure its insertion immediately adjacent to the trachea. Biopsies are routinely taken from right peritracheal, bronchial, and subcarinal lymph node areas. Dissection along the left peritracheal and tracheobronchial angle regions must be done with extreme care to avoid injury to the adjacent left recurrent laryngeal nerve. Prior to biopsying the lymph node, it should be mobilized as much as possible to ensure that it is the lymph node and not a major vessel. Particular care must be taken to avoid mistaking the azygos vein for a right tracheobronchial angle lymph node. Even when the operator is quite experienced, a long aspirating needle should be placed in the lymph node and suction applied to the attached syringe, to confirm that the structure to be biopsied is not a vessel, or a flattened lymph node closely applied to the surface of a major vessel. (Redrawn from Urschel HC Jr, Cooper JD. *Atlas of thoracic surgery*. New York: Churchill Livingstone, 1995:61, 63.)

does not extend beyond the uppermost portion of the anterosuperior compartment and ligation of the vascular supply in the neck allows delivery of the mediastinal goiter to the neck.

The reported incidence of malignancy has ranged from 2% to 20%. These data are particularly pertinent to the decision to recommend surgery for asymptomatic substernal goiters. Weighing in the balance the frequency of malignancy (about 2–20%), the potential danger of acute airway obstruction, and the relative safety of the surgical procedure, surgical excision seems reasonable even in asymptomatic patients. This balance in favor of surgery can obviously be tilted against it by the presence of medical complications.

TABLE 16–3 • *Common False Tumors of the Mediastinum*

Previsceral Compartment (Anterior)	Visceral Compartment	Paravertebral Sulci (Posterior)
Aneurysm of ascending aorta, innominate artery or subclavian artery	Aneurysm of the heart or aortic arch	Diaphragmatic hernias
Abnormal dilatation of superior vena cava or azygos vein	Pericarditis	Aneurysm of descending aorta
Sternal or chondrosternal tumors	Enlarged lymph nodes	Tumor of the esophagus
Lymphangiomas	Mediastinitis	Megaesophagus
	Aneurysm of pulmonary artery	Extralobar sequestration
		Pott's abscess
		Meningocele
		Extramedullary hematopoiesis

From Pearson FG, Cooper JD, Deslauriers J. *Thoracic surgery*, 2nd ed. New York: Churchill Livingstone, 2002:1658.

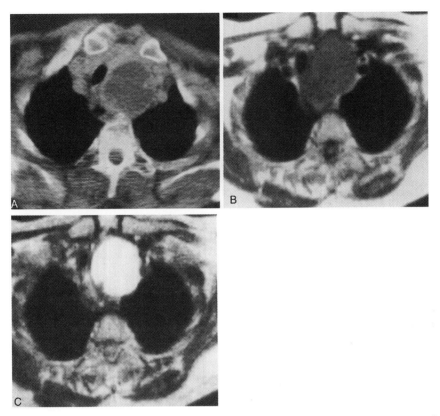

Figure 16–6. Mediastinal extension of a goiter. **A,** Computed tomography (CT) scan shows an inhomogeneous mass with a lower-density center in the upper mediastinum, displacing the trachea and esophagus from left to right. **B,** T1-weighted magnetic resonance image shows the mass as inhomogeneous. The great vessels displaced toward the left are better seen than on CT scan. **C,** On T2 weighting, the mass shows a marked increase in signal intensity, greater than that of fat, owing to a colloid cyst within the goiter. (From Moss AA, Gamsu G, Genant HK. *Computed tomography of the body*, 2nd ed. Philadelphia: WB Saunders, 1992:96.)

Cystic Hygromas

Mediastinal lymphangiomas typically extend from cervical cystic hygromas along the phrenic nerve into the chest. Cystic hygromas may be evident at birth or may not be discovered until later in life. Symptoms are caused by infection, hemorrhage, or continued growth. Resection is accomplished by combined cervicomediastinal approaches. Some of these lesions gradually regress spontaneously without surgical intervention. Sclerosis (e.g. injection of tetracycline) is possible but is generally not effective.

Lesions Originating from the Thoracic Skeleton

Most skeletal lesions in the mediastinum are bony tumors that project from the thoracic spine. Chordomas of the spine are ectopic embryonic remnants of primitive notochords that may be manifest in the paravertebral sulcus. CT scanning usually shows destruction of vertebral bodies in association with soft tissue mass. These tumors are malignant and require extensive excision and reconstruction of the spinal cord. As a rule, 5-year survival is poor.

Other lesions associated with the thoracic skeleton are paravertebral abscesses caused by staphylococcal hematogenous infections of paraspinal muscles, similar to retroperitoneal abscesses. The treatment of these is the same as for all infectious lesions – i.e. drainage and appropriate antibiotic treatment.

An anterior meningocele may occur in the paravertebral sulcus. These are generally asymptomatic masses discovered incidentally on CT scan. They may be confused with primary neurogenic tumors. Patients with anterior meningoceles often have peripheral neurofibromatosis, skeletal abnormalities, or both. Myelography or MRI is crucial in the diagnosis of these lesions. If the diagnosis is made preoperatively, no treatment is needed unless symptoms become manifest.

Extramedullary Hematopoiesis

Hematopoietic tissue can present in the mediastinum, typically in the posterior mediastinum. This process of extramedullary hematopoiesis develops as a compensatory mechanism in patients with abnormal bone marrow function. It may be manifest in several organs, such as the adrenals, liver, lymph nodes, and lungs. Large masses of extramedullary hematopoiesis are designated as erythroblastoma and myelolipoma (Figure 16–7). Consideration of this diagnosis is appropriate in patients with blood dyscrasias, especially thalassemia, who present with mediastinal masses. The tissue is pathologically characteristic, so FNA is often diagnostic. Resection is not indicated if the diagnosis is made preoperatively.

Vascular Lesions

Vascular lesions in the mediastinum may be either arterial or venous lesions and either pulmonary or systemic (Table 16–4). Validation of lesions suspected of being vascular requires either angiography or MRI scanning to avoid dangerous and potentially fatal biopsy. Appropriate therapy depends on the diagnosis.

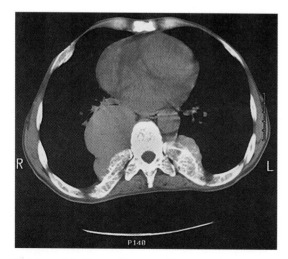

Figure 16–7. A 40-year-old man with beta-thalassemia and extramedullary hemopoiesis. A computed tomography scan shows lobulated right and left paravertebral paraosseous masses. The posterior ribs are markedly expanded and osteopenic. These are typical signs of extramedullary hemopoiesis. (From Pearson FG, Cooper JD, Deslauriers J: Thoracic Surgery, 2nd ed. New York, Churchill Livingstone, 2002, p 1597.)

Esophageal Lesions

Several benign esophageal lesions such as diverticula, duplications, large leiomyomas, hiatal hernias, and achalasia may present as mediastinal masses. Esophageal carcinoma with extramural spread, bulky adenopathy, or contained perforation can manifest as bulky visceral or posterior mediastinal masses. Chest CT scan with oral contrast can differentiate most of these lesions. Formal contrast studies and esophagoscopy are reserved for puzzling circumstances.

Pulmonary Lesions

Pulmonary lesions may manifest primarily as mediastinal masses, particularly as mediastinal adenopathy. Small-cell lung cancer often presents as bulky adenopathy with either a small or endobronchial primary lesion. Extralobar sequestration may also present on the chest radiograph as a paramediastinal mass in a patient with recurrent pneumonia.

Subdiaphragmatic Lesions

Subdiaphragmatic lesions may present as mediastinal masses. The gastrointestinal tract (typically the stomach) may herniate through the esophageal hiatus posteriorly (to form a hiatal hernia) or through the foramen of Morgagni anteriorly. Pancreatic pseudocysts rarely present as mediastinal masses; they occur in patients with characteristic histories of previous pancreatitis or known abdominal pancreatic pseudocysts (Figure 16–8). These lesions should be drained by laparotomy rather than thoracotomy.

Anterior Mediastinal Neoplasms

Lesions of the Thymus

Thymoma

Thymomas appear benign histologically even when they are invasive. They derive from either cortical or medullary epithelial cells. They are the most common of the thymic malignancies. Five histologic grades have been described, based on lymphocytic infiltration: lymphocytic, lymphoepithelial (mixed), epithelial, spindle cell, and unclassified. Thus, a lymphocytic thymoma consists of 65–80% lymphocytes. Mixed thymomas are tumors with 50% lymphocytes

TABLE 16–4 • *Cardiovascular Abnormalities that may Appear as a Mediastinal Mass*

Mediastinal Location	Systemic Venous System	Pulmonary Arterial System	Pulmonary Venous System	Systemic Arterial System
Anterior				Aortic stenosis (poststenotic dilatation) Ascending aortic aneurysm
Middle	Superior vena caval aneurysm Partial anomalous pulmonary venous return to the superior vena cava Azygos vein enlargement	Pulmonary valve stenosis Idiopathic dilatation of pulmonary trunk Congenital absence of the pulmonary valve Pulmonary embolism Pulmonary arterial hypertension Anomalous left pulmonary artery	Pulmonary venous varix Pulmonary venous confluence	Aortic stenosis Right aortic arch Transverse arch aortic aneurysm Aneurysm/fistula of the coronary artery
Posterior				Coarctation and pseudocoarctation Descending aortic aneurysm Tortuous innominate artery
Superior	Aneurysms of the innominate veins Persistent left superior vena cava Hemiazygos vein enlargement	Aneurysm of the ductus	Partial anomalous pulmonary venous return to the innominate vein Total anomalous pulmonary venous return (supracardiac)	Cervical aortic arch Coarctation of the aorta Transverse arch aortic aneurysm

From Sabiston DC Jr, Spencer FC. *Surgery of the chest*, 6th ed. Philadelphia: WB Saunders, 1995:586.

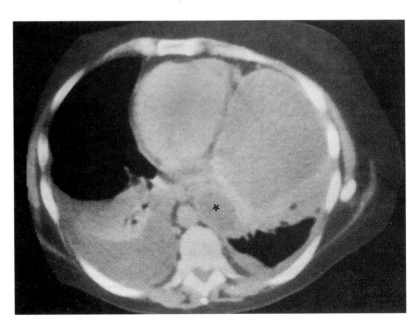

Figure 16–8. Mediastinal extension of pancreatic pseudocyst in a 41-year-old patient with pancreatitis. Computed tomography shows a thick-walled cyst (asterisk) to the left of the descending aorta that has entered the posterior mediastinum through the aortic hiatus. Bilateral pleural effusions are present. Air in the left pleural space is from a previous thoracentesis. (From Moss AA, Gamsu G, Genant HK. *Computed tomography of the body*, 2nd ed. Philadelphia: WB Saunders, 1992:88.)

and 50% epithelial cells. In epithelial thymomas, 65–80% of the cells are epithelial cells. Spindle cell tumors have a characteristic appearance, and unclassified tumors are typically too undifferentiated to classify. The number of mitotic figures in these tumors is very low, so cytologic preparations always appear benign.

A second classification depends on the relative predominance of thymic medullary or thymic cortical cells. Medullary tumors are less aggressive, with rare recurrences, while cortical thymomas (and the most aggressive subtype, thymic carcinoma) tend to recur and metastasize. Differentiation between lymphomas and thymomas can be difficult without substantial tissue and often cannot be made with needle biopsy.

Tumor stage at the time of treatment indicates prognosis better than tumor grade. Stage I lesions (encapsulated) are generally considered benign. Tumor–node–metastasis (TNM) staging has not been widely adopted. A peculiar characteristic of the benign histologic appearance of many of these lesions is that invasion of adjacent structures, and thus the stage of the tumor, can usually be more easily determined by the surgeon at the time of operation than by the pathologist at the time of microscopy. Thymomas most commonly are differentiated as being either 'encapsulated' or 'invasive' opposed to 'benign' or 'malignant.'

Thymoma is the most common primary neoplasm of the mediastinum, comprising approximately 15% of all thymic lesions. These tumors occur with equal frequency in men and women 40–60 years of age. Some 75% present in the anterior mediastinum; more than 90% are visible on the chest radiograph (Figure 16–9).

The mainstay of therapy, even for extensive lesions, is surgical resection. Most surgeons, even those experienced in thoracoscopy, recommend median sternotomy for the procedure. Most recurrences are local, either in the pleural space or in the mediastinum. Distant recurrences, when they do develop, are most often in bone. Recurrences are potentially curable, requiring several therapeutic methods, including repeated surgical exploration.

All patients in whom an invasive thymoma has been resected should receive postoperative radiotherapy, which is strongly recommended for all but stage I patients. Surgery alone yields a recurrence rate of approximately 30%, whereas radiation and surgery together yield a recurrence rate of approximately 5%. Whether noninvasive encapsulated thymomas respond to irradiation is unsettled. Dosage is usually 3500–5000 rad over 3–6 weeks. A dosage of more than 5000 rad does not increase the response rate but does increase the frequency of complications. Patients with thymomas, even when the disease is unresectable, recurrent, or metastatic, often respond to treatment with cisplatin, doxorubicin, and cyclophosphamide.

Paraneoplastic Syndromes

Myasthenia gravis is the most common thymoma-associated systemic syndrome. Patients with myasthenia gravis present with muscle weakness that intensifies with repetitive activity. The pathophysiology of myasthenia gravis entails the autoimmune-mediated binding of antibodies to the acetylcholine receptor, followed by their lysis by complement-mediated factors (Figure 16–10). Striking clinical improvement may occur after thymectomy without any change in measurable immune parameters, including the absence of change in the serum levels of autoantibodies.

Myasthenia gravis is present in approximately one third of patients with thymomas. This disorder may either precede or follow the development of thymoma by many years. Any type of thymic tumor may occur in patients with myasthenia gravis.

Among patients with myasthenia gravis without thymomas, remission can be expected in up to one half: in about 20%, remissions are completely drug-free; in up to 30%, remission is maintained by drugs – i.e. a combined remission rate of 50%. Improvement can be expected in one third to one half of patients; no change is evident in 10%, and a rare patient gets worse after surgery. Patients with myasthenia gravis and thymoma may fare more poorly after resection than do those without a thymoma: their symptomatic improvement after surgery may be less, although recent data suggests no difference in ultimate remission rates. Combined cervical and mediastinal incisions have been recommended to accomplish a maximal thymectomy, although a transcervical approach has been shown to produce equivalent results (Figure 16–11). Postoperative radiotherapy decreases the recurrence rate after resection in patients with invasive disease.

Pure red-cell aplasia occurs in 5% of patients with thymomas. It is a rare disorder that results in a severe normochromic normocytic anemia. Erythroid precursors in the bone marrow are decreased or absent, so reticulocytosis is markedly decreased. Between 33% and 50%

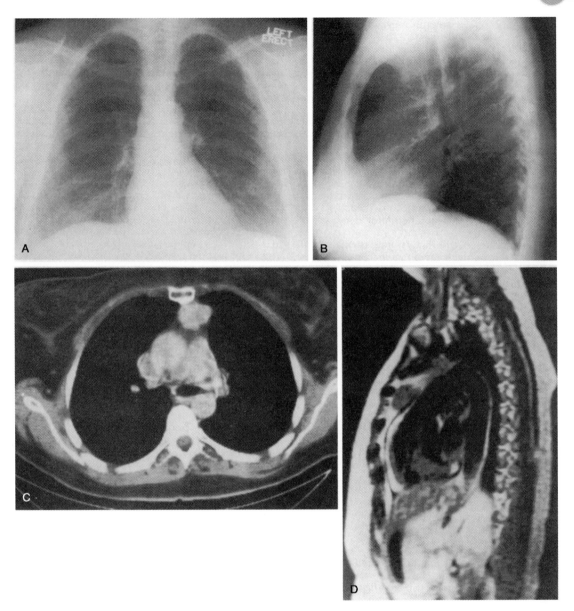

Figure 16–9. A, B, Chest films of a benign thymoma in a patient with myasthenia gravis. The tumor is poorly visualized; the only abnormality is the irregularity of the anterior cardiac border. **C,** Computed tomography image of the tumor. The tumor is clearly visualized in the anterior mediastinum. **D,** Magnetic resonance imaging of the mediastinum indicates a separation between the tumor and the pericardium. (From Sabiston DC Jr, Spencer FC. *Surgery of the chest*, 6th ed. Philadelphia: WB Saunders, 1996:594.)

of patients with red-cell aplasia have thymomas. Thymectomy produces remissions in approximately 40% of patients. It is more likely to be effective in patients with thymoma or thymic enlargement (remissions in up to 50% of patients) than in patients without thymomas.

Hypogammaglobulinemia occurs in 5–10% of patients with thymomas. It is more common in patients with both thymoma and rheumatoid arthritis, ulcerative colitis, many cytopenias, and some extrathymic cancers. Thymectomy has not proved beneficial.

Extrathymic cancers develop in up to 20% of patients who survive thymoma, most commonly as lymphomas, bronchogenic carcinomas, and thyroid cancers. The management of these patients should be determined by the extrathymic malignancy and not by the previous thymoma.

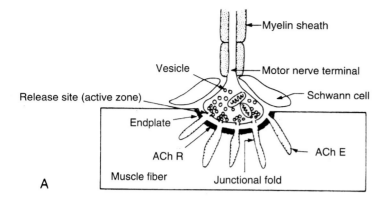

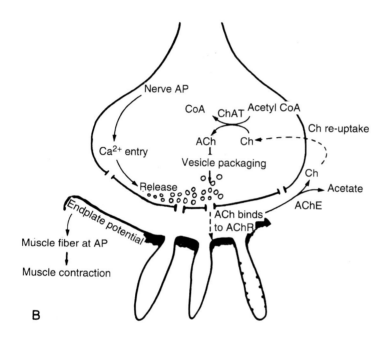

Figure 16–10. A, Schematic representation of the neuromuscular junction. **B,** Magnification showing details of the mechanisms of acetylcholine release, degradation, and binding to receptors, leading to muscle contraction. (From Pascuzzi RM. Introduction to the neuromuscular junction and neuromuscular transmission. *Semin Neurol* 1990;10:1.)

Thymic Carcinoma

These are epithelial neoplasms of thymic origin with considerably more cytologic and architectural features of malignancy than are manifested by thymomas. Several subtypes exist, with significant differences in outcomes after surgical resection. Patients with low-grade lesions (squamous cell carcinoma, mucoepidermal carcinoma, and basaloid carcinoma) have a higher survival rate. However, treatment of high-grade lesions (lymphoepithelioid lesions, small-cell or neuroendocrine lesions, clear-cell and sarcomatoid carcinomas, and anaplastic tumors) yield only a 15% long-term survival. All high-grade lesions should be considered for resection, followed by postoperative chemotherapy, since the more malignant group of tumors may respond to cisplatin-based regimens. These malignancies often

are positive for Epstein–Barr virus (EBV) or demonstrate EBV-associated nuclear antigens in carcinoma cells. However, not all thymic carcinomas demonstrate a linkage to EBV.

Thymic Carcinoid

These are distinctly uncommon neuroendocrine cell neoplasms that may present with a paraneoplastic syndrome. Patients in whom the tumors have a small-cell appearance on histology need postoperative chemotherapy; those in whom the histology is carcinoid require resection alone.

Thymolipomas

These are tumors of fatty tissue within the thymus gland. They are benign tumors that

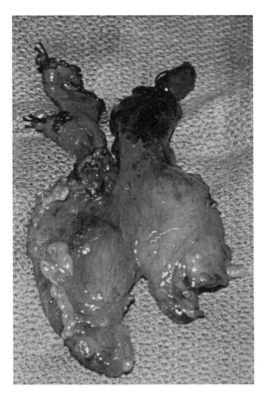

Figure 16–11. Photograph of a thymectomy specimen that was removed by transcervical thymectomy. (From Pearson FG, Cooper JD, Deslauriers J. *Thoracic surgery*, 2nd ed. New York: Churchill Livingstone, 2002:1632.)

masquerade as cardiomegaly (Figure 16–12). If the diagnosis is made preoperatively, they are best followed with scans and do not require resection. However, concern about possible malignancy usually necessitates resection.

Thymic Hyperplasia

True hyperplasia is a large bulky benign tumor that most commonly presents in young boys with massive thymic enlargement. This true hyperplasia occurs in children after treatment of malignancies and recovery from other systemic disease states. It is a common form of presentation in patients who develop bulky thymus glands after treatment for Hodgkin's lymphoma (rebound hyperplasia).

Tumors of Lymph Nodes

Together, lymphomas and metastatic cancer constitute the most common mediastinal masses. The anterior mediastinum not only is the most common site of primary mediastinal lymphomas but also can be invaded by cervical or visceral disease. Inflammatory causes of mediastinal adenopathy may imitate hilar adenopathy and lymph node disease (Table 16–5).

Lymphoma

Lymphomas constitute 10–15% of mediastinal masses in adults. They make up 20% of anterosuperior mediastinal masses and 20% of middle mediastinal masses, ranking second in frequency in both compartments. Lymphomas are rare in the posterior mediastinum. The numerous classifications proposed for lymphoma are generally no better for determining prognosis or managing patients than is simple classification into either Hodgkin's or non-Hodgkin's lymphoma.

Fully 20–30% of patients with lymphoma are asymptomatic, even with bulky malignant disease. Of the symptomatic patients, 60–70% have symptoms of local invasion and 30–35% have systemic symptoms, including fever, weight loss, and pruritus (so-called B type symptoms). Local symptoms include chest heaviness, discomfort, and cough. Tracheal or bronchial compression can cause associated wheezing or stridor. Dysphagia is an unusual complaint. Superior vena cava syndrome is a rare presentation.

Diagnosis requires significant tissue samples. FNA biopsies are not adequate in most circumstances, although the yield improves with radiologic (ultrasound or CT) techniques that target-specific areas of the mediastinal mass. The yield is relatively low, but so is the complication rate. Therefore, an attempt is not unreasonable, especially in patients for whom general anesthesia is problematic. The most efficacious way of obtaining tissue from a mass in the anterior mediastinum is via a parasternal mediastinotomy either with or without excision of the second costal cartilage.

Mediastinal Hodgkin's Disease

The age distribution of patients with mediastinal Hodgkin's disease is bimodal – 20–30 years of age or more than 50 years of age. Among young adults, men and women are affected equally, although mediastinal lymphoma is more common in older men than in older women. The nodular sclerosing subtype of Hodgkin's disease accounts for almost 90% of patients who present with mediastinal invasion. Of these, half have only mediastinal disease and the other half have mediastinal

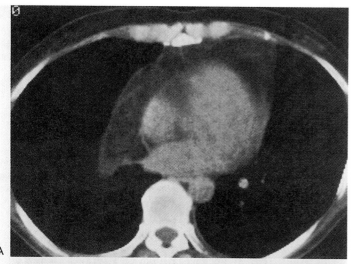

A

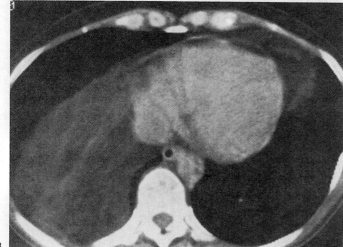

B

Figure 16–12. Mediastinal thymolipoma. Computed tomography scans through the lower thorax show a low-density mass in the anterior mediastinum, in front of the heart and on the right extending to the posterior chest wall. Strands of fibrous tissue course through the mass. At thoracotomy, a 10 kg thymolipoma was removed. (From Moss AA, Gamsu G, Genant HK. *Computed tomography of the body*, 2nd ed. Philadelphia: WB Saunders, 1992:86.)

disease with associated neck disease. Systemic symptoms of night sweats, fever, malaise, and weight loss are common. Mild local symptoms such as pain and cough are not uncommon. Severe local symptoms, such as superior vena cava syndrome, are very uncommon.

Chest radiographs reveal superior mediastinal masses that typically arise in the anterior compartment. CT of the chest discloses a predictable pattern of contiguous spread. The disease typically begins in the anterior mediastinal/paratracheal area and spreads to other mediastinal lymph node groups and subsequently to the hila and into the lungs (Figure 16–13). This consistent progression of Hodgkin's disease of the mediastinum correlates with the staging of the disease.

Non-Hodgkin's Lymphoma

Whereas about 75% of patients with Hodgkin's disease present with mediastinal disease, only

TABLE 16–5 • *Adenopathy in Sarcoid and Lymphoma*			
	Unilateral Hilar	**Paratracheal**	**Prevascular (anterior mediastinum)**
Sarcoid	Rare	Common	Uncommon
Lymphoma	Common	Common	Common

From Meholic A, Ketai L, Lofgren R. *Fundamentals of chest radiology.* Philadelphia: WB Saunders, 1996:216.

Consequently, they may contain elements of skin, bone, cartilage, intestinal and respiratory epithelium, and neurovascular tissue. About 80% of these lesions are benign. A dermoid cyst (benign cystic teratoma) is a variant that contains sebaceous material within a lining of squamous epithelium.

The lesions occur most often in adolescents or adults; the incidence is equal in males and females. About one third of the patients are asymptomatic, but symptoms tend to develop if the cysts become infected and erode into the pericardial space, the pleural space, or a bronchus (Figure 16–17). Occasionally, episodes of hypoglycemia occur in patients with benign mediastinal teratomas and are relieved by resection of the tumor. Approximately one-third of these lesions demonstrate areas of calcification.

Malignant Germ-Cell Tumors

The origin of malignant germ-cell tumors is unclear. The several different types behave differently and require different therapies.

Malignant mediastinal teratomas typically include elements of mature (benign) teratoma, immature teratoma, choriocarcinoma, yolk sac carcinoma, embryonal carcinoma, and seminoma in various proportions. These tumors produce either alpha-fetoprotein or β-hCG, the presence of either of which is diagnostic for malignant as opposed to benign tumor.

The embryologic origins of **mediastinal seminomas** are unclear. One theory holds that they derive from somatic cells of the branchial cleft. The other holds that they derive from extragonadal or embryonic yolk sac germ cells arrested near the developing thymus in the course of their migration along the urogenital ridge to the gonad.

Pure seminomas constitute 50% of all germ-cell tumors of the mediastinum. They occur principally in men 20–40 years of age; fewer than 5% occur in women. Mediastinal seminomas are the most common of the malignant germ-cell tumors of the mediastinum. They often present with intrathoracic metastases that preclude excision (Figure 16–18). A CT scan or ultrasound of the testicles is necessary to rule out a primary lesion that originates in the testicles. Serum levels of alpha-fetoprotein and β-hCG rarely increase in patients with mediastinal seminomas; if their levels are increased, nonseminomatous elements likely are present.

Seminomas are exquisitely radiosensitive. Radiotherapy is appropriate primary therapy for early-stage lesions, as is surgical resection. Criteria for resectability are that the patient is asymptomatic and the mass is confined to the anterior mediastinum, without evidence of either regional or distant metastatic disease. Only complete resections contribute to cure or palliation. Even after complete resection, radiation therapy (4500–5000 rad) improves outcome. Chemotherapy benefits those patients whose lesions appear histologically to be particularly malignant and therefore suggest a high risk of failure. A *cis*-platinum based regimen usually is employed. Chemotherapy given to patients with disseminated disease can yield 5-year disease-free survivals of 60–90%. Extensive disease and prior radiotherapy presage poorer prognosis.

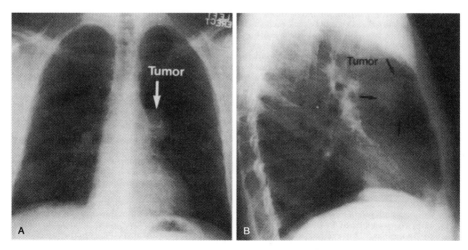

Figure 16–17. Chest films of a teratoma of the anterior mediastinum. (From Sabiston DC Jr, Spencer FC. *Surgery of the chest*, 6th ed. Philadelphia: WB Saunders, 1996:597.)

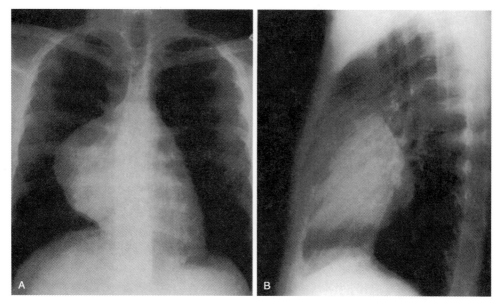

Figure 16–18. Chest films of a seminoma in an asymptomatic 17-year-old man. (From Sabiston DC Jr, Spencer FC. *Surgery of the chest*, 6th ed. Philadelphia: WB Saunders, 1996:598.)

Nonseminomatous tumors are less common than seminomatous malignant germ-cell tumors but occur in the anterior mediastinum. Nonseminomatous tumors usually are quite bulky at presentation and present with symptoms of compression or invasion of local thoracic structures. Patients usually have systemic symptoms of weight loss, fatigue, and fever. In 85–95%, there is at least one site of distant metastasis. Serum hCG or alpha-fetoprotein levels higher than 500 mg/mL are diagnostic of nonseminomatous malignant, germ-cell tumors. Nonseminomatous malignant germ-cell tumors include pure and mixed embryonal carcinomas, teratocarcinomas, choriocarcinomas, and endodermal sinus (or yolk sac) tumors.

The typical patient is a young male (median age of 35 years). In all patients with these tumors, hCG or alpha-fetoprotein levels in serum are increased. Nonseminomatous tumors usually demonstrate a heterogeneous density on CT scan, whereas seminomas tend to have a homogeneous density (Figure 16–19). These tumors are relatively more frequent in patients with Klinefelter syndrome.

Embryonal carcinomas occur in both adults and children and are clinically similar to seminomas. Choriocarcinomas typically present in young adult men, half of whom have gynecomastia as a result of the production of β-hCG by the tumor. This β-hCG is a specific tumor marker in these patients and helps in following the course and recurrence of the disease.

Endodermal sinus (yolk sac) tumors occur in both adults and children. They occur infrequently in the mediastinum and more commonly in sacrococcygeal teratomas and in the gonads. They produce alpha-fetoprotein no matter where they are located; the blood level of this protein helps in following therapy.

Teratocarcinomas are mixed-cell lesions. They are similar to embryonal and endodermal sinus tumors in that they occur in adults and children and may present with distant metastases.

Management of these tumors does not involve surgery initially, since the lesions are generally bulky and unresectable at presentation. Treatment with chemotherapy and radiotherapy is the mainstay. More aggressive regimens, particularly the addition of cisplatin, improve the results of treatment of extragonadal nonseminomatous tumors. In such responders who are left with a residual mass, resection is appropriate. Testicular tumors are more chemosensitive than all extragonadal tumors, and retroperitoneal tumors are more sensitive than mediastinal tumors. The chemotherapy regimens include bleomycin, cisplatin, vinblastine, and etoposide. These regimens can yield complete response rates of 40–60% and 30–50% long-term survivors.

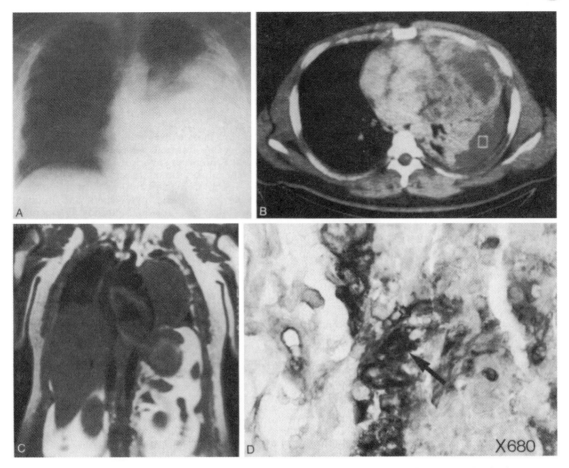

Figure 16–19. A, Chest film of a 28-year-old man with a malignant germ-cell tumor who had respiratory distress. **B,** Computed tomography scan shows a large left anterior mass with lobar collapse and a large pleural effusion. **C,** Coronal magnetic resonance imaging delineates pulmonary artery encasement. **D,** Raised serum titer and positive staining for alpha-fetoprotein (dark-stained areas within the cytoplasm) established the diagnosis of a nonseminoma (×680). (Courtesy of D. Thomas B. Clark, Duke University Medical Center, Durham, NC.)

Any residual mass following chemotherapy should be resected if two conditions are met: the patient has had a good response to the chemotherapy and levels of tumor markers in serum fall to normal. Residual tumor must be removed to assess whether it is a benign teratoma or necrotic tumor mass that can degenerate and redevelop malignancy. If the tumor markers do not fall but the tumor shrinks, surgery is of no benefit.

A few mediastinal germ-cell tumors are composed of a single cell type. Testicular biopsy or testicular CT is necessary in patients with such mediastinal germ-cell tumors to rule out a primary testicular neoplasm. Testicular biopsy is indicated if a mass is palpated, if high-resolution ultrasound is abnormal, and if CT demonstrates involvement of pelvic or retroperitoneal lymph nodes.

Middle Mediastinal Masses

Bronchogenic Cysts

Mediastinal cysts constitute 20% of all mediastinal masses, and bronchogenic cysts make up 60% of all mediastinal cysts. Symptoms are present in two thirds of patients, usually from compression of adjacent structures. If the diagnosis of a bronchogenic cyst is made preoperatively and patients are asymptomatic, observation is an appropriate course. If there is any question of malignancy – based on radiographic appearance, positive cytology, or evidence of enlargement or recurrence – the lesion should be resected (Figure 16–20). The presence of symptoms – especially pain, cough, or hemoptysis – suggests the advisability of resection. The presence of an air–fluid level indicates connection with the bronchopulmonary tree (rare) and the likelihood of recurrent infection, and indicates that resection is in order. Symptoms tend to develop with time, and resection at an asymptomatic stage may be best in healthy subjects. Video-assisted techniques offer the opportunity to resect these benign lesions with low morbidity. Depending on location, many of these may be resected through the mediastinoscope.

Esophageal Cysts

Esophageal cysts are periesophageal lesions that possess some form of gastroesophageal epithelial lining, but rarely is there communication with the esophagus. Diagnosis is possible with esophageal ultrasound, chest CT scan, or contrast studies of the upper gastrointestinal tract (Figure 16–21). Resection is the therapy of choice, whether by thoracoscopic or open technique.

Neuroenteric Cysts

Neuroenteric cysts make up 5–10% of foregut lesions and are associated with vertebral anomalies. They possess not only endodermal but also ectodermal or neurogenic elements. They are usually connected by a stalk to the meninges and spinal cord. They present in infants before 1 year of age and are uncommon in adults. A CT scan showing a cystic mediastinal

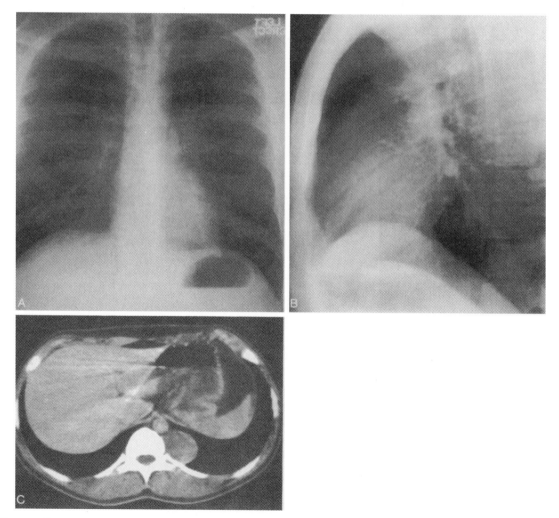

Figure 16–20. A, B, Chest films of a bronchogenic cyst in an asymptomatic 21-year-old man. **C,** Computed tomography image shows the paraspinal sulcus location of the cystic mass. (From Sabiston DC Jr, Spencer FC. *Surgery of the chest*, 6th ed. Philadelphia: WB Saunders, 1996:608.)

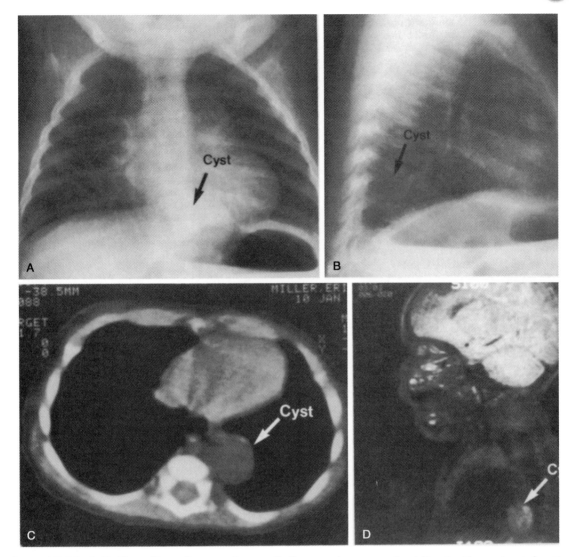

Figure 16–21. A, **B**, Chest films of an enteric cyst. **C**, Computed tomography delineates the anatomic location but does not further differentiate the mass from a neurogenic tumor. **D**, Magnetic resonance imaging shows the cystic nature of the mass and its relationship to the esophagus. (From Davis RD Jr, Sabiston DC Jr. Primary mediastinal cysts and neoplasms. In: Sabiston DC Jr, ed. *Essentials of surgery*. Philadelphia: WB Saunders, 1987)

lesion associated with a vertebral abnormality such as congenital scoliosis, hemivertebrae, and spina bifida should prompt consideration of neuroenteric cysts.

Posterior Mediastinal Masses

Neurogenic Tumors

The most common masses in both children and adults used to be neurogenic tumors. In recent decades, although these tumors continue to be the most common malignancy in children, in adults they have become less common than either thymomas or lymphomas. They now represent approximately 15% of all mediastinal masses in adults. Furthermore, in adults, the malignancy rate of neurogenic tumors is less than 10% (and probably only 1–2%). In children, fully 50% of these lesions are malignant.

Neurogenic tumors develop from the embryonic neural crest cells around the spinal ganglia and from either sympathetic or parasympathetic components (Table 16–6). Almost all these lesions form in the paravertebral sulci in association with intercostal nerves. Lesions can also develop from vagus and phrenic nerves. Most of the lesions are asymptomatic, although some patients manifest symptoms of

TABLE 16–6 • *Classification of Neurogenic Tumors of the Mediastinum*		
Tumor Origin	**Benign**	**Malignant**
Nerve sheath	Neurilemmoma Neurofibroma Melanotic schwannoma Granular cell tumor	Neurofibrosarcoma
Ganglion cell	Ganglioneuroma	Ganglioneuroblastoma Neuroblastoma
Paraganglionic	Chemodectoma Pheochromocytoma	Malignant chemodectoma Malignant pheochromocytoma

From Pearson FG, Cooper JD, Deslauriers J. *Thoracic surgery*, 2nd ed. New York: Churchill Livingstone, 2002:1732.

spinal cord compression or have cough, dyspnea, chest wall pain, and hoarseness. Horner's syndrome is an unusual presentation.

Most patients with neurogenic tumors are asymptomatic, so the initial diagnosis is usually made on chest radiographs obtained for other reasons. A rare patient may present with a pheochromocytoma or a chemically active neuroblastoma or neuroganglia. In all symptomatic patients, serum catecholamine levels and 24-hour urine levels of homovanillic acid and vanillylmandelic acid should be determined.

An MRI scan is necessary to rule out intraspinal extension through the neural foramen along the nerve roots (so-called dumbbell tumors). These patients may rarely present with symptoms of spinal cord compression. About 10% of patients with mediastinal neurogenic tumors have extension through a vertebral foramen. Although the vast majority of these lesions are benign, approximately 1 to 2% are malignant. The CT scan typically shows a smoothly rounded homogeneous density abutting the vertebral column (Figure 16–22). Nerve sheath tumors account for 65% of all mediastinal neurogenic tumors.

Tumors of Nerve Sheath Origin

Benign lesions are classified as either neurilemoma (schwannoma) or neurofibromas. Neurilemomas are more common than neurofibromas. Some 25–40% of patients with nerve sheath tumors have multiple neurofibromatosis (von Recklinghausen's disease).

Malignant tumors (neurogenic sarcomas or malignant schwannomas) are unusual. The incidence of malignancy is greater in tumors in patients with von Recklinghausen's disease (10–20%).

Neurilemomas are well encapsulated, firm, and grayish tan. Melanotic schwannomas are grossly pigmented, and many of them extend into the vertebral canal. In general, the prognosis with any malignant tumor of nerve sheath origin is poor. Neurogenic sarcomas occur at the extremes of age – in the first and second decades of life and in the sixth and seventh decades. The primary method of treatment is resection, by either thoracotomy or video-assisted resection. MRI scanning is necessary to identify any intraspinal extension. If intraspinal extension is present, it should be resected at the same time with neurosurgical assistance. Postoperative radiation is always given.

Endocrine Tumors

Many primary mediastinal lesions produce hormones or antibodies that cause systemic symptoms that may characterize a specific syndrome (Table 16–7).

Mediastinal Pheochromocytoma

These tumors usually cause no symptoms. Occasionally, however, they do present with varying degrees of hypertension, diabetes, and hypermetabolism. The tumors produce epinephrine, norepinephrine, or both. Vanillylmandelic acid and homovanillic acid are the chief urinary excretion products but epinephrine and norepinephrine may also be secreted in the urine. Normal values of vanillylmandelic acid in the urine are 2–9 mg/24 h. Normal levels of epinephrine in the urine should be less than 50 mg/24 h; normal norepinephrine levels in urine should be less than 150 μg/24 h.

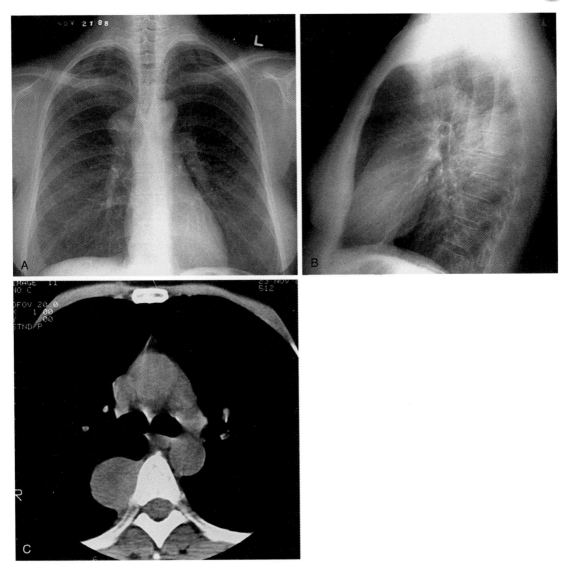

Figure 16–22. A 52-year-old asymptomatic woman with a right posterior, paravertebral, oval, well defined mass on posteroanterior (**A**) and lateral (**B**) chest radiographs. **C**, Computed tomography scan showing the typical location of the neurofibroma. (From Pearson FG, Cooper JD, Deslauriers J. *Thoracic surgery*, 2nd ed. New York: Churchill Livingstone, 2002:1593.)

TABLE 16–7 • *Systemic Syndromes Caused by Mediastinal Neoplasm Hormone Production*	
Syndrome	**Tumor**
Hypertension	Pheochromocytoma, chemodectoma, ganglioneuroma, neuroblastoma
Hypoglycemia	Mesothelioma, teratoma, fibrosarcoma, neurosarcoma
Diarrhea	Ganglioneuroma, neuroblastoma, neurofibroma
Hypercalcemia	Parathyroid adenoma/carcinoma, Hodgkin's disease
Thyrotoxicosis	Thyroid adenoma/carcinoma
Gynecomastia	Nonseminomatous germ-cell tumors
Precocious puberty	Nonseminomatous germ-cell tumors

From Sabiston DC Jr, Spencer FC. *Surgery of the chest*, 6th ed. Philadelphia: WB Saunders, 1995:585.

Large masses may be visible on the chest radiograph but in most patients CT scans are necessary to visualize the tumors. On MRI, a nonhomogeneous mass with a flow void will be visualized. ^{131}I-metaiodobenzylguanidine scintigraphy is particularly useful in mediastinal lesions: it can be used to localize lesions not seen on other scans.

The tumors may produce functioning peptides that can cause Cushing syndrome, secretory diarrheas, and polycythemia vera. In the thorax, these lesion probably derive from neuroendocrine cells and typically develop in the paravertebral sulci. Surgical excision is the treatment of choice. However, the patient should first undergo alpha-blockade with phenoxybenzamine for 1 week and then beta-blockade with metoprolol or propranolol. Typically, the intravascular volume of these patients is contracted and will normalize during the period of alpha-blockade. For emergency surgery, simultaneous alpha- and beta-blockade and fluid restoration are necessary.

Parathyroid Adenomas

Normal parathyroid glands occur in abnormal positions in 20% of the population – in the lower part of the neck, in the thymic capsule, or in the anterior mediastinum. Approximately 20% of parathyroid adenomas localize to the mediastinum: 80% in the anterior mediastinum and 20% in the visceral compartment (Figure 16–23). It is unusual to be able to identify these lesions either by chest radiography or by CT scan. Usually, a search in the mediastinum begins only after a negative neck exploration for hyperparathyroidism. After a negative exploration of the neck, further search using MRI, technetium scanning, thallium scanning, single photon emission computed tomography (SPECT) scanning, and venous sampling for parathyroid hormone can help to localize the lesion (Figure 16–24). Transcervical thymectomy may also be carried out at the time of the initial exploration if the adenoma is unable to be located in the neck.

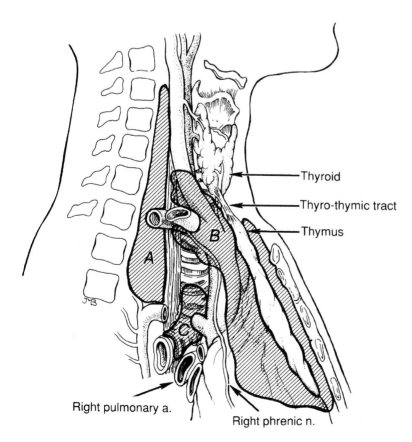

Thyroid

Thyro-thymic tract

Thymus

Right pulmonary a.

Right phrenic n.

Figure 16–23. The three regions in which mediastinal ectopic parathyroid glands are found. **A**, Retroesophageal and paraesophageal region, which spans both the neck and the upper mediastinum down to the level of the carina (ectopic upper parathyroid IV). **B**, Anterior mediastinum, including thymus and posteriorly the pericardium, the aortic arch, and the great vessels of the upper mediastinum (ectopic lower parathyroid III). **C**, Mid-mediastinal compartment in front of carina and mainstem bronchi. Note the close proximity anteriorly of the right pulmonary artery. This area extends out of view along the left main bronchus underneath the aortic arch into the aortopulmonary window. (From Pearson FG, Cooper JD, Deslauriers J. *Thoracic surgery*, 2nd ed. New York: Churchill Livingstone, 2002:1762.)

Other Mediastinal Tumors

Mesenchymal Tumors

These tumors constitute approximately 2% of all tumors that occur in the mediastinum. More than half of these mesenchymal lesions are malignant, however, and they run the entire gamut of soft tissue tumors. Their management resembles that of soft tissue tumors in the rest of the body; resection is indicated if possible.

Fatty Tumors

Some fatty tumors, if they can be reliably identified before surgery, do not require resection. Lipomatosis is overgrowth of mature fat seen as a widening of the mediastinum. It results from

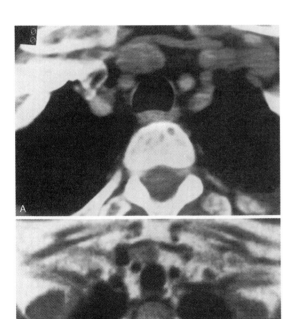

Figure 16–24. Superior mediastinal parathyroid adenoma in a patient with recurrent hyperparathyroidism following neck exploration. **A,** Computed tomography scan demonstrates a 2 cm mass immediately in front of the trachea. **B,** T1-weighted magnetic resonance at the same level demonstrates the mass, which is low in signal intensity and can be readily distinguished from mediastinal fat. (From Moss AA, Gamsu G, Genant HK. *Computed tomography of the body*, 2nd ed. Philadelphia: WB Saunders, 1992:97.)

endogenous obesity, steroids, or Cushing's disease and should not be resected. Lipomas can form in the mediastinum and do not require resection unless they appear to be growing rapidly. Large lipomas can cause respiratory embarrassment and may require resection for symptomatic reasons, although this is extremely rare.

Lipoblastomatosis is an unusual benign lesion seen principally in children. It is associated with fatty overgrowth in the mediastinum and compression of structures. Resection is the treatment of choice. Liposarcomas of the mediastinum are extremely rare. On CT scanning, the density of these masses is midway between that of fat and water. The lesions are large and ill defined. They cause local symptoms, including superior vena caval obstruction and tracheobronchial compression and should be resected.

Superior Vena Cava Syndrome

In the first part of the 20th century, the most common causes of the superior vena cava (SVC) syndrome were benign mediastinal diseases, specifically syphilitic aneurysms. Currently, malignant tumors, such as lymphoma, bronchopulmonary cancers, thymic malignancies, and germ-cell tumors of the mediastinum, account for more than 90% of SVC obstructions. Lung cancer is most common, especially small-cell cancer, although lymphoma is also common. Other malignancies are rare. Some 5–10% of cases of SVC obstruction are due to benign causes. Most result from invasive monitoring techniques, such as the placement of central venous lines, Swan–Ganz catheters, and interventional techniques, such as the placement of pacemakers and central venous catheters for chemotherapy that result in thrombosis of the superior vena cava.

Congestion of venous outflow from the head, neck, and upper extremities results in swelling of the face, neck, arms, and upper chest. Patients may have headaches, dizziness, tinnitus, and a bursting sensation. In addition, the face may appear cyanotic even although capillary refill is normal. Venous hypertension in SVC syndrome may lead to serious consequences (e.g. jugular venous and cerebrovascular thrombosis). At times, this syndrome may require urgent treatment, though this is unusual.

Chest radiography may show mediastinal widening but is nonspecific. CT scanning, using intravenous contrast, can document SVC obstruction but must show opacification of the SVC above the mass and nonopacification below to establish the diagnosis. Thrombosis, compression, and invasion of the SVC are common causes. If the CT scan is nondiagnostic, venography using arm veins may demonstrate caval obstruction, especially for the SVC syndrome that is secondary to chronic fibrosing mediastinitis or indwelling intravenous catheters or pacemaker leads. Radioactive iodine scans may be useful for SVC obstruction secondary to goiter.

In order to obtain tissue for diagnosis, FNA may be diagnostic. Experienced surgeons can perform mediastinoscopy safely in this group of patients. Intraoperative complications, including bleeding, are rare, but the airway management may be complicated. Patients with the SVC syndrome, or any large anterior mediastinal mass, often must be intubated and extubated while awake so that airway obstruction can be prevented during the surgical procedure.

If the underlying disease is malignant, it is important to obtain tissue from the mediastinal neoplasm causing the SVC syndrome in order to direct therapy. Because the SVC syndrome may cause cerebral venous thrombosis, it is an oncologic emergency. Even with respiratory symptoms, tissue should be obtained before treatment is instituted. The treatment of choice is radiation therapy: 3000–4000 rad for 4 days.

Additional medical measures include salt restriction, diuretic treatment, steroid administration, and anticoagulation. Although radiotherapy is the mainstay of treatment, patients with small-cell carcinoma, lymphoma, and undifferentiated carcinoma should be treated with systemic chemotherapy. Intravascular stenting with expandable venous stents has been successful in some patients and is appropriate therapy for poor-risk patients who do not respond to radiotherapy. Surgical resection may be part of a multidisciplinary plan for certain low-risk patients (Table 16–8).

For benign causes of SVC syndrome, treatment must be tailored to the specific origin. Substernal goiters should be resected. Aneurysmal disease causing SVC syndrome requires cardiopulmonary bypass and repair. Anticoagulation and antibiotic administration are the best initial treatments of idiopathic thrombophlebitis or septic thrombophlebitis and iatrogenic thrombosis of the SVC. Failure of these approaches calls for the use of fibrinolytic agents such as urokinase and streptokinase.

The treatment of SVC syndrome in patients with chronic fibrosing mediastinitis is controversial. Replacement of the SVC with vein or ringed polytetrafluoroethylene (PTFE) grafts is possible, but the technique is reserved for those with severe symptoms recalcitrant to medical treatment. The best approach in this case is median sternotomy. Unless the benign process continues to progress, however, most symptoms will resolve without surgery as collaterals develop.

TABLE 16–8 • *Indications and Contraindications for Superior Vena Cava Resections*

Indications	Contraindications
Neoplasms	
Non-small-cell lung tumors	SVC syndromes related to unresectable tumors
Anterior mediastinal tumors	
Primary SVC tumors	
Vascular	
Primary saccular aneurysms	Obstructed SVC with a rich collateral vein circulation
Primary malformations	
Trauma	
Iatrogenic, blunt, or penetrating SVC, superior vena cava	Abnormal walls of the proximal veins

From Pearson FG, Cooper JD, Deslauriers J. *Thoracic surgery*, 2nd ed. New York: Churchill Livingstone, 2002:1775.

Key Readings

Hainsworth JD, Greco FA. Germ cell neoplasms and other malignancies of the mediastinum. *Cancer Treat Res* 2001;105: 303–325.

Marchevsky, A. The mediastinum. *Pathology* 1996;3: 339–348.

Strollo DC, Rosado-de-Christenson ML, Jett JR. Primary mediastinal tumors: part II. Tumors of the middle and posterior mediastinum. *Chest* 1997;112: 1344–1357.

Selected Readings

Aisenberg AC. Primary large cell lymphoma of the mediastinum. *Semin Oncol* 1999;26: 251–258.

Graeber GM, Tamim W. Current status of the diagnosis and treatment of thymoma. *Semin Thorac Cardiovasc Surg* 2000;12: 268–277.

Iyoda A, Yusa T, Hiroshima K, *et al.* Castleman's disease in the posterior mediastinum: report of a case. *Surg Today* 2000;30: 473–476.

Murray JG, Breatnach E. Imaging of the mediastinum and hila. *Curr Opin Radiol* 1992;4: 44–52.

Reeder LB. Neurogenic tumors of the mediastinum. *Semin Thorac Cardiovasc Surg* 2000;12: 261–267.

Ronson RS, Duarte I, Miller JI. Embryology and surgical anatomy of the mediastinum with clinical implications. *Surg Clin North Am* 2000;80: 157–169, x–xi.

Suster S, Moran CA. Neuroendocrine neoplasms of the mediastinum. *Am J Clin Pathol* 2001;115: S17–A27.

Wood DE. Mediastinal germ cell tumors. *Semin Thorac Cardiovasc Surg* 2000;12: 278–289.

Wright CD, Mathisen DJ. Mediastinal tumors: diagnosis and treatment. *World J Surg* 2001;25: 204–209.

Yoneda KY, Louie S, and Shelton DK. Mediastinal tumors. *Curr Opin Pulm Med* 2001;7: 226–233.

Index